The Evolution of the Immune System
Conservation and Diversification

The Evolution of the Immune System

Conservation and Diversification

Davide Malagoli

Department of Life Sciences
Biology Building, University of Modena
and Reggio Emilia, Modena, Italy

AMSTERDAM • BOSTON • HEIDELBERG • LONDON
NEW YORK • OXFORD • PARIS • SAN DIEGO
SAN FRANCISCO • SINGAPORE • SYDNEY • TOKYO

Academic Press is an imprint of Elsevier

Academic Press is an imprint of Elsevier
125 London Wall, London EC2Y 5AS, United Kingdom
525 B Street, Suite 1800, San Diego, CA 92101-4495, United States
50 Hampshire Street, 5th Floor, Cambridge, MA 02139, United States
The Boulevard, Langford Lane, Kidlington, Oxford OX5 1GB, UK

British Library Cataloguing-in-Publication Data
A catalogue record for this book is available from the British Library

Library of Congress Cataloging-in-Publication Data
A catalog record for this book is available from the Library of Congress

ISBN: 978-0-12-801975-7

For information on all Academic Press publications
visit our website at https://www.elsevier.com/

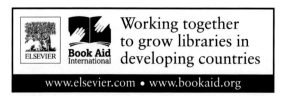

Working together
to grow libraries in
developing countries

www.elsevier.com • www.bookaid.org

Typeset by Thomson Digital

Dedication

**To my teachers, my students,
and all the people who taught me something.**

Contents

3.   Lymphocyte Populations in Jawless Vertebrates: Insights
     Into the Origin and Evolution of Adaptive Immunity

Yoichi Sutoh, Masanori Kasahara

4.   The Evolution of Lymphocytes in Ectothermic
     Gnathostomata

Giuseppe Scapigliati, Francesco Buonocore

7.   Antiviral Immunity: Origin and Evolution in Vertebrates
Jun Zou, Rosario Castro, Carolina Tafalla

8.   Lectins as Innate Immune Recognition Factors: Structural, Functional, and Evolutionary Aspects
Gerardo R. Vasta

**14. The Evolution of Major Histocompatibility Complex
in Teleosts**
Masaru Nonaka, Mayumi I. Nonaka

Contributors

Numbers in Parentheses indicate the pages on which the author's contributions begin.

Alice Accorsi (1), Stowers Institute for Medical Research, Kansas City; Howard Hughes Medical Institute, Stowers Institute for Medical Research, Kansas City, MO, United States

Sophie A.O. Armitage (241), Institute for Evolution and Biodiversity, University of Münster, Münster, Germany

Loriano Ballarin (29), Department of Biology, University of Padova, Padova, Italy

Megan A. Barela Hudgell (295), Department of Biological Sciences, The George Washington University, WA, United States

Steve Bird (87), Molecular Genetics, Department of Biological Sciences, University of Waikato, Hamilton, New Zealand

Daniela Brites (241), Swiss Tropical and Public Health Institute, Basel, Switzerland

Francesco Buonocore (69), Department for Innovative Biology, Agro-Industry and Forestry, University of Tuscia, Viterbo, Italy

Rosario Castro (173), Animal Health Research Center (CISA-INIA), Carretera de Algete a El Casar, Valdeolmos (Madrid), Spain

Francesca Cima (29), Department of Biology, University of Padova, Padova, Italy

Russell F. Doolittle (275), Departments of Chemistry & Biochemistry and Molecular Biology, University of California, San Diego, La Jolla, CA, United States

Nicola Franchi (29), Department of Biology, University of Padova, Padova, Italy

Preethi Golconda (295), Department of Biological Sciences, The George Washington University, WA, United States

Masanori Kasahara (51), Department of Pathology, Hokkaido University Graduate School of Medicine, Sapporo, Japan

Davide Malagoli (1), Department of Life Sciences, Biology Building, University of Modena and Reggio Emilia, Modena, Italy

Cheng Man Lun (295), Department of Biological Sciences, The George Washington University, WA, United States

Miki Nakao (151), Department of Bioscience and Biotechnology, Faculty of Agriculture, Kyushu University, Hakozaki, Fukuoka, Japan

Masaru Nonaka (331), Department of Biological Sciences, Graduate School of Science, The University of Tokyo, Tokyo, Japan

Mayumi I. Nonaka (331), Department of Biological Sciences, Graduate School of Science, The University of Tokyo, Tokyo, Japan

Matan Oren (295), Department of Biological Sciences, The George Washington University, WA, United States

Enzo Ottaviani (225), Department of Life Sciences, University of Modena and Reggio Emilia, Modena, Italy

Giuseppe Scapigliati (69), Department for Innovative Biology, Agro-Industry and Forestry, University of Tuscia, Viterbo, Italy

Christopher J Secombes (87), Scottish Fish Immunology Research Centre, University of Aberdeen, Zoology Building, Tillydrone Avenue, Aberdeen, United Kingdom

L. Courtney Smith (295), Department of Biological Sciences, The George Washington University, WA, United States

Valerie J. Smith (1), Scottish Oceans Institute, School of Biology, University of St Andrews, St Andrews, Fife, United Kingdom

Tomonori Somamoto (151), Department of Bioscience and Biotechnology, Faculty of Agriculture, Kyushu University, Hakozaki, Fukuoka, Japan

Yoichi Sutoh (51), Emory Vaccine Center and Department of Pathology and Laboratory Medicine, Emory University, Atlanta, GA, United States

Carolina Tafalla (173), Animal Health Research Center (CISA-INIA), Carretera de Algete a El Casar, Valdeolmos (Madrid), Spain

Jos P.M. van Putten (311), Department of Infectious Diseases and Immunology, Utrecht University, Utrecht, The Netherlands

Gerardo R. Vasta (205), Department of Microbiology and Immunology, University of Maryland School of Medicine, UMB, and Institute of Marine and Environmental Technology, Columbus Center, Baltimore, MD, United States

Carlos G.P. Voogdt (311), Department of Infectious Diseases and Immunology, Utrecht University, Utrecht, The Netherlands

Tiehui Wang (87), Scottish Fish Immunology Research Centre, University of Aberdeen, Zoology Building, Tillydrone Avenue, Aberdeen, United Kingdom

Jun Zou (173), Scottish Fish Immunology Research Centre, University of Aberdeen, Zoology Building, Aberdeen, United Kingdom

Preface

Lord, we know what we are, but know not what we may be.

Shakespeare

"Evolution" is a fascinating term that may be used in several different contexts. In everyday life, evolution refers to what is in progress, and will change in a short time. In natural history and comparative anatomy, the word "evolution" still means change, but on a much longer period. Changes are continuous, and there is no need to be a paleontologist or a biologist to know that during geological eras several organisms got extinct, and new different species replaced them, profiting of the free ecological niches.

"Immunity," is a well-known concept as well. The struggle to survive does not consist only of the ability to escape the predator and to catch the prey. It also requires contrasting potential pathogens, and limiting the expansion of microorganisms that have beneficial effects only as long as they are kept within the proper boundaries. Again, to be a scientist or a Doctor of Medicine is not necessary to understand that a good health implies a good functioning of the immune system, working 24/7 to prevent the pathogen widespread into the organism.

However, if the theory of evolution and the indispensable role of the immune system are obvious concepts for everyone, the evolution of the immune system is a less obvious topic. Scientists have no clues of the immune system of the extinct organisms because it does not leave traces in fossils. And since the largest part of immunologists is represented by individuals with a medical education, it is frequently ignored that apparently simple organisms, such as flies, snails, and sea urchins present an incredible ability to discriminate between numerous microorganisms and to elicit an efficacious immune response, without using antibodies.

This book will help the reader to gain a modern and open view of the evolution of the immune systems in multicellular organisms. Since the immune system is not leaving hints of its functioning in fossil records, it is fundamentally a comparative analysis of information from as much present-day models as possible. In these respects, the book gives the reader a complete overview of the most studied models and of the hot topics in comparative immunology. I would like to remark at this point that the outline of the book is conceived to allow a comparative analysis of different immune components, as it focuses on the several aspects shared by the immune systems of all the metazoans, highlighting conserved components and remarking the important features that diversified along evolutionary lineages.

The book consists of three sections:

Section 1 is entitled The Players of Cell-Based Immunity in Metazoans and it contains an up-to-date description of the cells involved in the immune response in the principle nonmammalian models. Chapter: Hematopoiesis and Hemocytes in Pancrustacean and Molluscan Models highlights the similarities and the differences of the hemocytes described in Molluscs and Pancrustacea, and it gives a detailed description of the hematopoiesis and of the maturational niches observed in these vast, highly populated and extremely divergent taxa. Closer to humans, the Chordate phylum is considered in detail, starting from the sister-group of vertebrates (the Tunicates, chapter: Origin and Functions of Tunicate Hemocytes) and moving to lampreys (chapter: Lymphocyte Populations in Jawless Vertebrates: Insights Into the Origin and Evolution of Adaptive Immunity) and bony fish (chapter: The Evolution of Lymphocytes in Ectothermic Gnathostomata). In these chapters, the evolution of one of the most interesting cell type, that is, the lymphocyte, is described, and the functional convergence of the lymphocyte-like system of lampreys is also presented, in order to give the reader the opportunity to get in touch with the stunning evolutionary plasticity of the immune system.

Section 2 focuses on The Evolution of Immune-Related Soluble Factors. The section kicks off with a detailed and complete analysis of the cytokines observed in vertebrates to date (chapter: Vertebrate Cytokines and Their Evolution). Molecular details are provided, helping the reader in identifying which are the molecular components more conserved during vertebrate diversification. Chapter: Vertebrate Cytokines and Their Evolution also resumes the knowledge about potential homologs of vertebrate cytokines observed in nonvertebrate models. With a similar approach and detail, other basic and fundamental components of humoral immune response are described in chapters: The Evolution of Complement System Functions and Pathways in Vertebrates (the complement system) and Antiviral Immunity: Origin and Evolution in Vertebrates (antiviral molecules). Lectins, and more precisely galectins and F-type lectins, are the amazing protagonists of chapter: Lectins as Innate Immune Recognition Factors: Structural, Functional, and Evolutionary Aspects. Here, the numerous roles played by these molecules are presented, and the structural details are described to highlight the number of interactions that these molecules can entertain. The second section ends with the description of the origin and the evolution of the neuro-immune cross-talk, encompassing more than 30 years of studies in this field (chapter: Origin and Evolution of the Neuro-Immune Cross-Talk in Immunity).

Section 3 introduces the reader to The Evolution of Diversity in Immune System. Here, some of the most fascinating discoveries of the last decade are presented. Chapter: The Immune-Related Roles and the Evolutionary History of Dscam in Arthropods is centered on Dscam, a molecule representing an extreme example of somatic diversification in Pancrustacea. Respecting in full the layout of the book, the chapter: The Immune-Related Roles and the Evolutionary History of Dscam in Arthropods reviews the involvement of Dscam in pancrustacean immunity. Dscam evolutionary history is also presented, together with potential developments for future research. Similarly, chapter: Structural and Functional Diversity of Fibrinogen-Related Domains describes the diversity developed by fibrinogen-related domains during the evolution of metazoans. Still on the topic of highly variable molecules, chapter: Genomic Instability and Shared Mechanisms for Gene Diversification in Two Distant Immune Gene Families: The Plant *NBS-LRR* Genes and the Echinoid *185/333* Genes presents the 185/333 protein family in sea urchins and highlights the mechanisms for gene diversification that 185/333 genes share with the evolutionary remote NBS-LRR genes of higher plants. The evolution of Toll-like receptors is reviewed in chapter: The Evolution of the Toll-Like Receptor System, and the selective microbial pressures that drive Toll-like receptors adaptation is described in detail. The book ends up with a focus on the major histocompatibility complex (MHC) of teleosts. This group of bony fish is the most diverse among vertebrates, and its MHC presents several unique features that are presented in the final chapter: The Evolution of Major Histocompatibility Complex in Teleosts.

This Book provides a new and original perspective about the evolution of the immune system, and it will help scientists from different educational paths and at different stages of their career to appreciate the conserved traits and the original innovations of immune systems.

Davide Malagoli
Department of Life Sciences,
University of Modena and Reggio Emilia,
Italy

Chapter 1

Hematopoiesis and Hemocytes in Pancrustacean and Molluscan Models

Valerie J. Smith*, Alice Accorsi**,†, Davide Malagoli‡
*Scottish Oceans Institute, School of Biology, University of St Andrews, St Andrews, Fife, United Kingdom; **Stowers Institute for Medical Research, Kansas City, MO, United States; †Howard Hughes Medical Institute, Stowers Institute for Medical Research, Kansas City, MO, United States; ‡Department of Life Sciences, Biology Building, University of Modena and Reggio Emilia, Modena, Italy

1 INTRODUCTION

All animals are at risk of damage from microorganisms, parasites, toxins, abrasive particles, or other threats that may kill or bring about somatic cell or tissue injury with longer-term detriment to health. The immune system is the key player in implementing surveillance and response to counter such threats, and the efficacy of its recognition and reactivity abilities is independent of the taxonomic or phylogenetic status of the species. This holds true for both long- and short-lived species, and both vertebrates and invertebrates.

Invertebrate immune systems are often divided into cellular and humoral components.[1] Cellular components include the circulating blood cells, called hemocytes, as the dominant representatives. The renewal of hemocytes is usually referred to as hematopoiesis or hemopoiesis.[2] The existing literature on invertebrate hematopoiesis is greatly exceeded by that on hemocyte morphology and functions. Notwithstanding, comparative studies on hematopoiesis are crucial for the understanding of the molecular basis of hemocyte proliferation, differentiation, and maturation, especially in models of economic relevance. For mammals and most other vertebrates, which have both innate and adaptive immune responses, the immune cells are derived from either a progenitor of a myeloid or a lymphoid lineage, both originating mainly from the bone marrow, but differentiating and maturing in secondary sites around the body.[3–5] In protostome and deuterostome invertebrates, by contrast, the circulating blood cells that participate in host defense may come from a variety of tissues or organs and there is no clear distinction of myeloid or lymphoid cell lineages equivalent to that of vertebrates. In protostomes, to which the Pancrustacea and Mollusca belong, the available evidence points to them originating in one or more dedicated parts of the connective tissues; for example, in the lymph gland in insects,[6] in the cephalothorax in decapods,[7,8] in the connective tissue at the base of the gills in bivalves,[9,10] in the pericardial walls in gastropods,[11] or in the white gland in cephalopods.[12,13] The anatomies of the various species and their adaptations to different environments make almost impossible a homogenous description of hematopoiesis and hemocyte lineages in invertebrates. As a general concept, however, hemocytes are cells of mesodermal origin, arising from the coelom and referred to as hemocytes in pancrustaceans and mollusks because the coelom is reduced in these animals to the circulatory fluids contained within a cavity enclosing the heart and main body organs, known as the hemocoel.[2] In this chapter, the hematopoietic organs and the different hemocytes present in relevant pancrustacean and molluscan models are described.

2 HEMATOPOIESIS IN PANCRUSTACEAN MODELS

Pancrustacea is a recently identified invertebrate clade that includes the two largest, most studied and representative groups of arthropods, namely, all hexapods and crustaceans.[14–17] This clade comprises a monophyletic group that contains millions of species, all highly diverse in their development, anatomy, and physiology. They are united, however, through molecular data derived from comparisons of nuclear rRNA genes, mitochondrial rRNA genes, and certain protein-coding genes.[14] Members of the clade are believed to have diversified from a common ancestor in the Silurian, 420–430 million years ago.[18]

Here, we consider certain key model species that are scientifically and/or economically important, and thus well-studied. In both insects and crustaceans, the hemocytes are present in the hemocoel during both larval and adult life stages throughout life. Holometabolous insects (as represented by *Drosophila melanogaster*) undergo a complete metamorphosis in the transition from larval to adult stage and they usually present a discontinuous hematopoiesis, limited to embryonic and larval life stages.[19,20] This may be because in these insects the adult and final stage is principally devoted to reproduction,[21] and it is relatively a short part of the lifespan.[20] Conversely, decapods, the best-known crustacean clade, are generally iteroparous (ie, have multiple reproduction cycles) and grow after sexual maturity. Thus, hematopoiesis in these animals tends to be continuous.[22]

2.1 Insect Hematopoiesis

Fruit flies, especially *D. melanogaster,* are widely used models for understanding development and immunity, and, with respect to hematopoiesis, have been employed to study the process from early- stage embryos onwards. In this animal, hematopoiesis occurs in successive waves of cell proliferation.[19] The first wave, where immature hemocytes (prohemocytes) form a loose mass of cells, occurs in the head mesoderm during early embryonic development.[19,23] These embryonic prohemocytes then migrate in a regulated way,[24,25] along the dorsal blood vessel and the ventral neural chord, to permeate the entire embryo.[19,23,26] In this phase, embryonic hemocytes acquire phagocytic capability.[19,24] Embryonic hemocytes maintain their activity in larvae and persist even after metamorphosis into adult flies.[19,26] In *Drosophila* larvae, immature hemocytes migrate to the hemolymph and populate specific niches.[27] These niches are segmentally divided hematopoietic-microenvironments, in which the hemocytes may proliferate de novo during larval stages.[27] Experimental manipulation of larvae promotes the dispersal of the hemocytes from the hematopoietic niches to the circulation, but they rapidly return to their home niche.[28] The peripheral nervous system plays a fundamental role in regulating this hemocyte homing and the proliferation in the hematopoietic niches, indicating that the functional connection between immune and nervous systems may be crucial for hematopoiesis in the *Drosophila* larvae.[28] In this insect, the main hematopoietic organ is the lymph gland that begins its formation during late embryogenesis. The lymph gland is hematopoietically active only in larvae.[19] It arises from the cardiogenic mesoderm of the embryo, a feature reminiscent of hematopoiesis in mammals, where circulating cells derive from the hemangioblasts.[29] The lymph gland accounts for most of the larval hematopoiesis in *Drosophila*, and it remains in close contact with the dorsal blood vessel, a circulatory organ with heart-like activity.[29] Despite the lymph gland hosting hemocyte proliferation and differentiation, in the absence of immune challenges, the hemocytes are retained by the lymph gland and released immediately after pupation.[19] The larval lymph gland has a lobular organization, and the anterior (primary) pair of lobes are the most important for the development of hemocytes, with the primary lobe having cortical zone containing maturing hemocytes.[23] The inner layer, defined as the medullary lobe, contains immature hemocytes, usually described as prohemocytes.[23] The primary lobe also includes the posterior signaling center (PSC), with specialized and unique hemocytes, which are not immediately recognizable either as the maturing hemocytes or as immature prohemocytes.[23] The PSC exerts control over the proliferation and differentiation of the prohemocytes, and it also controls hemocyte maturation in the primary lobe. At the end of the larval period, the lymph gland reaches its maximum size, and after pupation it dissociates and releases all the hemocytes, irrespective of their level of maturation.[19] The mediators and signaling pathways that regulate the release of hemocytes from the lymph gland are unknown at present.[6] Transmission electron microscopy observations, plus analysis using hemocyte markers, indicate that the release of hemocytes from the lymph gland after pupation may occur as a consequence of localized degeneration of the gland basement membranes and through augmented hemocyte motility.[30] This means that adult fruit flies, which can live for approximately 4 weeks, are able to survive after metamorphosis without a hematopoietic organ.[28,30] Adults therefore rely on protection from the larval hemocytes that persist in the circulation and produce immune humoral factors, such as prophenoloxidase (proPO) activating components and antimicrobial peptides (AMPs).[1]

The genetic tools available for *D. melanogaster* have allowed the detection of specific markers on maturing cells and of molecular mediators responsible for driving the hemocyte maturation.[31] Recently, the *Drosophila* fibroblast growth factor receptor (FGFR), Heartless, has been shown to play a role in the maturation of larval hemocytes.[31] Two FGF-8-like ligands, Thisbe and Pyramus,[32,33] activate, through Heartless, a signaling pathway essential for hemocyte maturation and lymph gland development. However, several aspects of hemocyte maturation in the lymph gland remain to be elucidated, but it is worth noting that in *Drosophila,* the extracellular matrix is involved in the process.[31] Trol, a *perlecan* homolog, is a heparan sulfate-containing proteoglycan that negatively regulates the availability of Thisbe and Pyramus. Acting on ligand availability, Trol intervenes in Heartless signaling within the lymph gland and regulating hemocyte maturation and lymph gland lobe differentiation.[31]

There is less detailed information about hematopoiesis for other insect species, although in the silkworm, *Bombyx mori,* and the hornworm, *Manduca sexta* (Lepidoptera), embryonic hematopoiesis also involves the head mesoderm, as in *Drosophila,* and, in larvae, it takes place in the thoracic mesoderm-derived organ, the lymph gland, or the hematopoietic producing organ (HPO), positioned on imaginal disks of the wings.[34] In *B. mori*, the lymph gland dissociates during metamorphosis.[6,34,35] A further similarity to *D. melanogaster* is the presence of compact islets of prohemocytes surrounded by loose islets of differentiated hemocytes in *B. mori* larval HPO. The compact and loose islets of *B. mori* HPO structurally resemble the medullary and cortical zones of the *Drosophila* lymph gland, respectively.[35] The PSC of *Drosophila* does not have an equivalent counterpart in the silkworm lymph gland, but it has been proposed that a specific group of hemocytes present in the silkworm HPO, the reticular cells, may play a role in controlling the hemocyte proliferation and differentiation.[36] Studies on insects undergoing incomplete metamorphosis are much less frequent and provide less detailed data.[6] The hematopoietic organs and the reticular cells have been investigated also in some orthopteran insect models, such as locusts and grasshoppers. The importance of reticular cells in the hematopoietic tissues of these insects is implied by the term, reticulo-hematopoietic organ.[37,38] Whereas holometabolous insects such as *D. melanogaster* and *B. mori* possess distinct embryonic and larval sites for hematopoiesis and any adult hematopoietic organs, the hemimetabolan insects *Locusta migratoria* and *Euprepocnemis shirakii* have a functional lymph gland at adult stage that is tightly associated with the dorsal blood vessels.[6] As in *D. melanogaster*, the lymph glands of *L. migratoria* and *E. shirakii* comprise two layers containing hemocytes at different degrees of maturation.[6,38–40] Very recently, it has been observed that the hematopoietic tissue may not be the main source of new hemocytes in adult *L. migratoria*.[41] A drop in the number of circulating hemocytes occurs immediately after injection of β-1,3-glucan (fungal membrane component) into the locusts. Hemocyte replenishment seemingly followed the mitotic activity of the circulating hemocytes rather than that of the hematopoietic tissue.[41]

2.2 Crustacean Hematopoiesis

Among crustaceans, the hematopoiesis has been studied in detail only in decapods, principally, shrimp and crayfish. In these invertebrates, it takes place in a dedicated tissue located on the dorsolateral surface of the foregut, in the cephalothorax.[7,8] In penaeid shrimp it is large and composed of lobules, full of small, undifferentiated, proliferative, immature cells (again, termed prohemocytes).[42] The lobules may also extend into the bases of the pereiopods (walking legs)[43] or along the ophthalmic and antennal arteries in the vicinity of the pericardial region.[42,44–46] In other species, particularly crab, the tissue is small and diffuse,[47] making it less conspicuous than the hematopoietic tissue in shrimp or crayfish.

The exact processes by which the hemocytes develop within the hematopoietic organ is not fully understood, but in the shrimp, *Penaeus monodon*, the smaller agranulated cells tend to occur at the periphery of the lobules, while the larger, more granulated cells are present in the center.[42] This pattern of distribution is believed to reflect a gradient of maturation, with mature cells released from lobule center into the hemocoel.[42] Previous authors, working on other decapod species, hold a different view, and have considered that maturation takes place in the circulation, as low numbers of dividing cells, resembling prohemocytes, may be present in the hemolymph.[48–50] However, it is possible that under certain conditions—for example, following nonself challenge or injury-induced blood loss—hematopoiesis might be upregulated to repopulate the hemolymph, with new defense cells thus driving partially matured prohemocytes into the circulation prematurely. Certainly, the number of mitotic cells in the circulation rises approximately two- to fivefold (from <1%) after such treatments.[51–54] Increased levels of mitosis have also been reported to occur within the hematopoietic tissue by immune stimulation.[53]

Whatever the stimulus, a variety of signaling events directly or indirectly induces cell division within the hematopoietic tissue itself. Work on crayfish, *Pacifastacus leniusculus*, has shown that prokineticin-like cytokines, named astakines, and transglutaminases (TGases) play important roles in the process.[55,56] Astakines cause upregulation of hematopoiesis, transiently increasing the total hemocyte count in a dose-dependent manner[55] while concomitantly suppressing TGase activity.[56] Similar events are likely to occur in other decapod species, as a gene encoding an astakine homolog has been found in *P. monodon*.[55–57] Moreover, a further study on *P. monodon* has shown that astakine levels are influenced not only by TGase, but also by a crustin AMP.[58] Depletion of these two proteins results in elevated levels of astakine and increased hemocyte proliferation, despite astakine mRNA levels remaining unaffected.[58] Other factors reported to be involved in hematopoiesis are thymosins.[59] Well-known to be associated with tissue repair and cell migration through interaction with ATP-synthase in vertebrates, two β-thymosins have been found to participate in a complex way to regulate hematopoietic stem cell proliferation and differentiation in *P. leniusculus*, and to induce expression of Astakine-1.[59] Both β-thymosin-1 and β-thymosin-2 stimulate migration of cells in vitro, but β-thymosin-2 does so in combination with Astakine-1.[59] β-Thymosin-1 also causes a transitory increase in the number of circulatory semigranular cells, whereas both thymosins induce the expression of Astakine-1.[59] Interestingly, the two thymosin isoforms suppress production of reactive oxygen species (ROS) by the respiratory burst by enhancing superoxide production,[59] so it is interesting to speculate whether these findings are indicative of some kind of selection process within the hematopoietic tissue, with ROS used as a means of deleting superfluous or deleterious hemocytes.

3 MOLLUSCAN HEMATOPOIESIS

With more than 100,000 living species, the Mollusca is the second largest phylum of metazoans after the Arthropoda. The group contains species with wide variation in body plans, physiology, and anatomical specialization. They may be present in freshwater, the sea, or terrestrial environments[60] and show diversity in reproductive strategies and life histories. However, the immune systems of this group have received rather less research attention than that given to arthropods, with most directed at economically important bivalves and gastropods, and, to a lesser extent, cephalopods. These taxa are sometimes grouped together, along with scaphopods, in the monophyletic subphylum Conchifera.[60] To the best of our knowledge, almost nothing is known about the hemocytes or their production and maturation in members of the lesser-known groups of Solenogastres, Caudofoveata, Polyplacophora, or scaphopod. Research on the immune systems of Conchifera dates back to the early 1970s and has been done on a wide range of species. Unfortunately, there is no commonly adopted model (such as *D. melanogaster*) that has received intensive research underpinned by full genome-sequence data. However, recent sequencing of the genomes from the oyster, *Crassostrea gigas*,[61] and the owl limpet, *Lottia gigantea*,[62] together with the developing of transcriptome databases, for example, for the mussel, *Mytilus galloprovincialis*,[63] and for the apple snail, *Pomacea canaliculata*,[64] should prompt new studies that will enable integration of morphological, physiological, and molecular findings.

3.1 Bivalves

As with pancrustaceans, bivalves and gastropods have open circulatory systems and possess populations of circulating hemocytes involved in host defense. Although there is a respectable body of literature on the morphology and functionality of these immune cells (see Section 5.3), hematopoiesis is very poorly characterized. It has been generally thought that hemocytes originate from the connective tissue and/or mantle,[9,65,66] and although some may mature before entering the circulation,[67–70] evidence is accumulating that mitosis may also occur after hemocyte release to the hemolymph, as demonstrated by the clam, *Tapes philippinarum*.[71] These clam cells are positive for the stem cell marker, CD34.[71] Also in oysters, a family of transcription factors *Cg-tal,* homologous to

Tal1/SCL, has been reported to be expressed during ontogeny of *C. gigas.*[72,73] This family of transcription factors is known to be involved in the hematopoietic process of vertebrates.[74] Challenge of oysters with *Vibrio* spp. has further been reported to induce the production of new hemocytes, and to upregulate the expression of certain genes, such as *Cg-runx1* and *Cg-BMP7,* which encode proteins involved in hemocyte proliferation.[75] Another recent study has provided some indication that at least some prohemocytes emerge from the basement of the gill epithelium in oysters,[10] which bears out the early proposition by Cuenot that bivalve hemocytes originate in the gills.[76] It is also noteworthy that molecular analyses of developing *C. gigas* juveniles have indicated that hematopoiesis-related factors are expressed in the hemocytes rather than in the connective tissue, suggestive that, as in pancrustacean models, the hematopoietic cells could derive from the vessel and/or artery endothelial cells.[72] In the scallop, *Chlamys farreri,* several molecules associated with the proliferation and differentiation of prohemocytes have been identified and characterized from the circulating hemocytes. These include Cf-Ets,[77] Cf-Runt, and Cf-CBFβ.[78] *Cf-runt* is similar to the mammalian *runt* gene, so it is possible that the encoded protein is necessary for hematopoiesis, and the recruitment of new hemocytes to the circulation after immune challenge.[78] Runt is a conserved family of transcription factors that has also been identified in crayfish.[53] A similar transcription factor, named *lozenge,* is present also in *D. melanogaster,* and is believed to control crystal cell commitment during embryogenesis.[6] These molecular studies are providing evidence that progenitors of fully differentiated hemocytes can occur in the circulation of bivalves, where presumably they continue to mature; but much remains unknown. This evidence also supports the hypothesis that in bivalves the proliferation of circulating hemocytes may occur as a consequence of an immune challenge, as already observed in insect larvae and crustaceans.[6,79] In the near future, information from genome sequencing of *C. gigas* or other bivalves should enable clarification of the contradictory views and permit a better understanding of the relationship between the different hemocyte lineages.

3.2 Gastropods

Hematopoiesis occurs in gastropods in specific and well-defined tissues positioned close to the reno-pericardial zone.[80,81] There is no evidence of proliferation in the circulating hemolymph. In the freshwater snail, *Biomphalaria glabrata,* the hematopoietic tissue, described as the amoebocyte-producing organ (APO), constitutes a cluster of cells between the pericardium and the posterior mantle epithelia.[82] The hematopoietic cells are contained in the stroma, composed of small fibroblasts and smooth muscle cells surrounded by blood sinuses.[82] Immune challenge with the trematode parasite, *Schistosoma mansoni,* induces mitotic activity in this tissue,[83] and transplantation of the hematopoietic tissue from a *S. mansoni*-resistant strain to a susceptible strain confers resistance to *S. mansoni* in the new host that otherwise would succumb to the parasite.[84] In the freshwater gastropod,

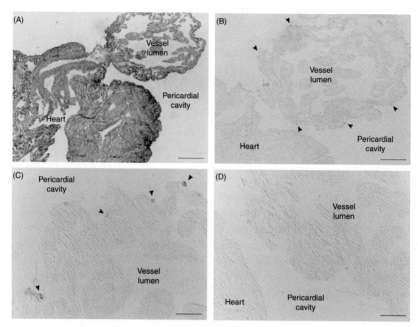

FIGURE 1.1 **Hematopoietic tissue in the gastropod, *P. canaliculata*.** The heart is localized in the pericardial cavity, where it is connected with both afferent and efferent cardiac vessels. (A) heart and ctenidial/pulmonary vein as revealed by Azan–Mallory stain; (B) immunohistochemical staining with the mitotic marker, phospho-Ser10 histone H3, shows positive cells *(arrowheads)* around the vein on the side facing the pericardial cavity; (C) higher magnification of (B) showing proliferative cells *(arrowheads)*, giving rise to new hemocytes; (D) negative control. Bars: (A) = 120 μm; (B) = 100 μm; (C, D) = 40 μm.

Planorbarius corneus, the hematopoietic tissue is located between the mantle cavity and the pericardium, with mature hemocytes transported to the circulation via the blood sinuses.[85] In *P. canaliculata*, new hemocytes seem to originate close to the heart, as a highly conserved mitotic marker, phospho-Ser10 histone H3, has revealed that positive cells are localized in the fluid that fills the pericardial cavity.[86] Mitotic figures have been noted as adhering to the external epithelium of the ctenidial/pulmonary vein that faces the pericardial cavity[86] (Fig. 1.1). In other gastropods the hematopoietic tissue is less defined, but in the lymnaeids and the land slug, *Incilaria fruhstorferi,* the formation of new hemocytes seems to happen either in the connective tissues or the vascular system, but, as yet, the process has not been fully described or characterized.[87,88]

3.3 Cephalopods

Unlike all other mollusks, cephalopods have a closed circulatory system with high systemic blood-pressure and a high rate of delivered oxygen.[89] The circulating hemocytes (once called leucocytes) are produced in the white body,[90] which is localized in the orbital pits of the cranial cartilages, behind the eyes and close to the optic ganglia.[91] This organ has been described for three cephalopod species, namely *Octopus vulgaris*, *Octopus briareus*, and the squid, *Sepia officinalis*. It usually takes the form of internal strings of precursors of hemocytes, surrounded by external connective tissue.[12,92] These hemocyte precursors are generated by proliferating cells known as leucoblasts or hemocytoblasts, and are thought to migrate from the strings into the vascular sinuses for differentiation and maturation.[12,92] Light and electron microscopy studies suggest that hemoblasts proliferate, transform, and mature in the white body.[92] During maturation, the young cells enlarge and modify their nuclear organization and cytoplasmic organelles before entering the circulatory system as mature hemocytes.[12] In *O. vulgaris*, proliferative activity in the white body has been demonstrated both in vitro[93] and in vivo.[90] The majority of young cells resident in the white body are either proliferating or maturing cells that show immunocompetence, but their phagocytic capacity is lower than that of the circulatory hemocytes.[90]

4   HEMATOPOIESIS IN PANCRUSTACEAN AND MOLLUSCAN MODELS: FINAL CONSIDERATIONS

From the accounts above, it is clear that there are differences in the location and structure of the hematopoietic tissues and in the hematopoietic process between members of the pancrustaceans and the mollusks. In general, hematopoiesis in pancrustaceans occurs in tissues/organs associated with the main blood vessels, which in embryos are little more than cellular masses. In larvae through to adults, it takes place in more defined tissues, often in the pericardial region of the hemocoel, which has, in older papers, been described as the so-called "lymphoid organ."[44] In these tissues there are layers of hemocytes at different stages of maturation that are released into the open circulatory system upon maturation. The release of hemocytes is not continuous, but dependent on either developmental or immunological cues. By contrast, in mollusks, the hematopoietic tissues tend to be more varied, with new hemocytes produced continuously throughout the animal's lifespan, albeit with some upregulation following non-self stimulation. The best studied molluscan groups are bivalves and gastropods, and, in the latter, the APO or its equivalent occur in the pericardial region, a position comparable to that of the decapod hematopoietic tissue.

5   HEMOCYTES IN PANCRUSTACEAN AND MOLLUSCAN MODELS

The finding of conserved elements between pancrustacean and molluscan model species is significantly harder when it comes to the description of hemocyte types. Insect, crustacean, and molluscan hemocyte types and morphologies have been reviewed several times,[2,6,68,69,94–97] but differences in the naming and classification of the various hemocyte types are so numerous as to make it almost impossible to present a generalized and widely accepted system. Here, a general morphological description, considering the main functions of the cells, will be presented with some consideration given to their likely lineages.

5.1 Hemocytes and Their Lineages in Insects

In 1981, Rowley and Ratcliffe[2] tried to rationalize the nomenclature of insect hemocyte types and identified six main types, although not all occur in every species. The hemocyte types they defined are: prohemocytes, plasmatocytes, granular cells, cystocytes, spherule cells, and oenocytoids[2] (Table 1.1).

D. melanogaster is generally regarded as having just three hemocyte types in both its larval and adult stages. According to Williams[98] these are, in order of decreasing abundance: plasmatocytes, crystal cells, and lamellocytes (Fig. 1.2). This seems to be a derived condition because other dipterans, such as Calliphora vomitoria, also possess oenocytoids.[99] In addition to these cells, some authors have reported the presence of small and round cells, considered to be immature hemocytes, and so are called prohemocytes.[97,100] However, the presence of pro-hemocytes in the circulation of adult Drosophila spp. is at odds with the view of other authors, in that hemocyte proliferation and differentiation occur only during embryo and larval development.[1,6] Plasmatocytes are the dominant cell type in Drosophila spp., but they may transform into lamellocytes upon parasitoid infection.[101] Drosophila plasmatocytes are agranular and have considerable phagocytic capacity, whereas the lamellocytes, which remain agranular, are larger and nonphagocytic. Instead they adhere and contribute to encapsulation of parasites that may gain entry to the larval body[1,6,100–102] (Fig. 1.2). By contrast, crystal cells, which contain granules of the proPO activating system, do not display significant morphological changes after immune challenge[98] and show no phagocytic activity.[1,6,100] It is not clear if crystal cells can be considered to be derived from a different cell lineage from plasmatocytes.[6,100–102]

In D. melanogaster embryos, the hemocytes that move along fixed routes and invade the developing larva are mainly plasmatocytes (approximately 95%), along with a few crystal cells.[96] Usually lamellocytes are absent in embryos.[19] As described in Section 2.1, in the absence of an immune challenge the circulating hemocytes observed in late embryos are evident in the hemolymph of D. melanogaster larvae, along with a few lamellocytes.[103] Immature cells occupy the medullary zone of the primary lobes of the lymph gland in Drosophila, while maturing plasmatocytes occupy the cortical zone together with a minority of crystal cells, as revealed by the expression of a number of specific cell markers.[19] At present, there is no evidence supporting the existence of two separate hemocyte lineages in the lymph gland of Drosophila[6,102,103] (Fig. 1.3A). It should be noted that larval hematopoiesis occurs also in specific niches along the larval body, producing plasmatocytes only.[28] Data obtained on D. melanogaster hemocytes and their development are of great value for understanding hematopoiesis in fruit flies, but unfortunately the findings do not necessarily apply to other flies, even of the same genus.[97]

TABLE 1.1 Morphological and Functional Features of the Six Main Circulating Hemocyte Types Identified Among Insect Orders Following the Classification by Rowley and Ratcliffe (1981)[2]

	Prohemocyte	Plasmatocyte	Granular Cell	Cystocyte	Spherule Cell	Oenocytoid
Size	6–13 μm	10–15 μm	8–20 μm	8–15 μm	8–16 μm	12–30 μm
Shape	Round to oval, high N/C ratio	Round to spindle shaped	Round to oval	Round, high N/C ratio	Oval to spindle shaped	Round to oval
Inclusions in the cytoplasm	A few granule-like inclusions	None/moderate/large number of granules	Many granules with variable structure	Many granules with variable structure	Large and spherular inclusions	Homogeneous cytoplasm
Percentage	Less than 5%	30–60%	30–60%	30–60%	Less than 5%	1–2%
Reaction in vitro	Highly stable, formation of small protoplasmic extensions	Stable, formation of protoplasmic extensions and ameboid movement	Unstable, degranulation with formation of vacuoles	Unstable, quick degeneration, degranulation, increase of nucleus refractivity, formation of "islet of coagulation"	Highly stable, formation of rare protoplasmic extensions	Highly stable, no formation of protoplasmic extensions
Function in vivo	Mitotic division, direct differentiation to plasmatocytes	Phagocytosis, encapsulation, basement membrane formation, wound repair, nodule formation, metamorphosis	Phagocytosis, nodule formation, encapsulation, melanin formation, hemolymph coagulation, wound repair, hormone transport	Coagulation, encapsulation, nodule formation, and phagocytosis	Uncertain. In B. mori they are involved in silk production	Uncertain. They may be involved in melanization process and reactions to parasites

(Continued)

TABLE 1.1 Morphological and Functional Features of the Six Main Circulating Hemocyte Types Identified Among Insect Orders Following the Classification by Rowley and Ratcliffe (1981)[2] (cont.)

	Prohemocyte	Plasmatocyte	Granular Cell	Cystocyte	Spherule Cell	Oenocytoid
Orders in which the hemocyte type has been described	Blattoidea Coleoptera Collembola Diptera Hemiptera Hymenoptera Lepidoptera	Blattoidea Coleoptera Collembola Diptera Hemiptera Hymenoptera Lepidoptera Orthoptera	Blattoidea Coleoptera Collembola Diptera Hemiptera Hymenoptera Lepidoptera Orthoptera Phasmatodea	Blattoidea Coleoptera Hemiptera Orthoptera Phasmatodea	Coleoptera Collembola Diptera Hemiptera Lepidoptera Orthoptera	Coleoptera Diptera Hemiptera Hymenoptera Lepidoptera Orthoptera
Synonyms	Proleukocyte Proleukocytoid	Amoebocyte Leukocyte Macronucleocyte Macrophage Phagocyte	Granular leukocyte	Coagulocyte Explosive corpuscle	Adipohemocyte Coarsely granular cell Eruptive cell Eleocyte Spherulocyte	Crystal cells in dipterans may be a special type of oenocytoid Oenocytes

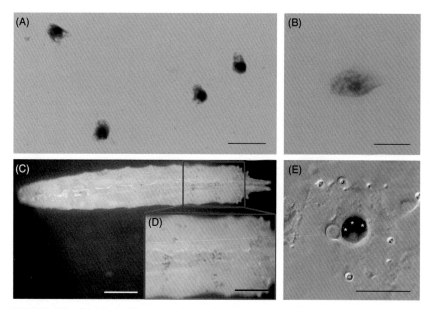

FIGURE 1.2 Circulating hemocytes in the hemolymph of larva of the dipteran, *D. melanogaster*. Three different types of hemocytes are shown, namely: (A) plasmatocytes, the most abundant in the hemolymph; (B) lamellocytes, which are larger and more flattened than the plasmatocytes; (C) crystal cells, which are highly unstable in vitro, and show cytoplasmic melanin synthesis; (D) two-fold magnification of the red square in (C); (E) crystal cells collected and observed after heat treatment (30 min at 60°C). The crystalline inclusions in the crystal cells are indicated with white asterisks. Bars: (A, B, E) = 20 μm; (C) = 500 μm; (D) = 250 μm.

Lepidoptera is the most studied insect group after the Diptera, and the information on their hemocytes is extensive.[97,104] In lepidopteran larvae, the most common cell type is the granulocyte, or granular hemocyte. These cells have high phagocytic ability,[104] and so are functionally similar to plasmatocytes in *Drosophila*, but, unlike fruit fly plasmatocytes, lepidopteran granulocytes contain numerous cytoplasmic granules. Another difference between *Drosophila* and lepidopterans is that plasmatocytes in lepidopterans are agranular and seem to be functionally comparable to *Drosophila* lamellocytes, as their main function is encapsulation of parasitoids or pathogens too big for being phagocytosed.[104] However, lepidopteran plasmatocytes are also able to engulf large particles in vitro, indicating that they might display some phagocytic activity also in vivo.[96] A third type of hemocyte observed in lepidopteran larvae is the oenocytoid, a cell functionally equivalent to *Drosophila* crystal cells, as it contains granules of proPO.[104,105] A fourth, and so far uncharacterized, hemocyte type present in lepidopterans is the spherulocyte (Table 1.1). Its function is thought to be associated with transport of cuticular components,[106] but this has yet to be fully confirmed.[104] Finally, mention needs to be made of reticular cells (or reticulocytes), whose role in insect hemocyte development has yet to be

(A)   (B)   (C)

D. melanogaster   *B. mori*   *P. monodon*

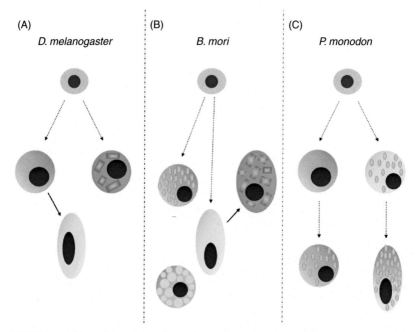

FIGURE 1.3   Schematic representation of the hemocytes described in Pancrustacea on the basis of their functions. (A) *D. melanogaster*; (B) *B. mori*; (C) *P. monodon*. *Gray cells* represent undifferentiated precursors that give rise to mature hemocytes (in some cases through intermediary cell stages). Cell lineages in Pancrustacea have not been clearly determined as of yet, and the most widely accepted scenarios are represented by *dashed arrows*. *Red* indicates cells endowed with phagocytic activity. These may have either an agranular (hyaline), a granular, or a semigranular cytoplasm. *Yellow* indicates cells involved in encapsulation of large pathogens, and these, again, may or may not contain cytoplasmic granules. *Green* indicates cells with crystal-like inclusions, some of which may promote the production of ROS or activate the proPO cascade. Solid arrows indicate that there may be interconversion between hemocyte types, as on *Drosophila* spp. or *B. mori*. Blue indicates spherule cells, typically present in some insect species, but whose function(s) have yet to be elucidated. In *P. monodon,* the semigranular and phagocytic cells are thought to develop from hyaline cells, with a second lineage in which nonphagocytic granular cells mature through a sequence of intermediary semigranular cell stages. In decapods, proPO activity is confined to semigranular and granular cells only.

clarified (Table 1.1). Reticulocytes are found in several insect species, including lepidopteran or hemimetabolan insects, such as *L. migratoria*.[6] Reticulocytes are not circulatory hemocytes and are found only in the lymph gland.[107] Grigorian and Hartenstein[6] have suggested that they may represent immature hemocytes able to mature into the other hemocyte types. Mandal et al.[108] however, consider that reticulocytes may play a regulatory role in hemocyte proliferation and differentiation in hematopoietic organs, similar to the PSC cells in the *D. melanogaster* lymph gland.

Although the existence of separate hemocyte lineages in the *D. melanogaster* lymph gland has not been established,[102,103] (Fig. 1.3A), lepidopteran circulatory hemocytes have been proposed recently to develop from two separate cell lineages.[35] By injecting prohemocytes obtained from a GFP-expressing *B. mori* lymph gland into wild-type larvae, three different fluorescently labelled cell types (granulocytes, plasmatocytes, and oenocytoids) can be observed at the end of the experiments.[35] In vitro experiments demonstrate that, in the silkworm, mature plasmatocytes can develop into oenocytoids, which is not the case for mature granulocytes. These findings point to the existence of two hemocyte lineages in *B. mori*: the first one differentiating into granulocytes, and a second one differentiating into plasmatocytes and the plasmatocyte-derived oenocytoid[35] (Fig. 1.3B). That both plasmatocytes and granulocytes in lepidopterans can divide in circulation has been shown by bromodeoxyuridine (BrdU) incorporation experiments[109] and by the use of monoclonal antibodies.[110] However, the results supporting the existence of two hemocyte lineages in silkworms are in disagreement with the observations of Beaulaton,[111] who reported that hemocytes in *B. mori* larvae are all derived from the plasmatocytes.

The classification of hemocyte lineages in insects is further complicated by the transformation of one hemocyte type into another one (Fig. 1.3). The interconversion between cell types in insects has been reported several times,[6] and further studies, focused on specific cell markers, are necessary to elucidate distinction of cell types and lineages. It has also been suggested that the nomenclature of the insect needs to be updated in order to avoid misunderstandings or misleading synonyms, for example, plasmatocytes in *Drosophila* are hemocytes with different morphology and functions than plasmatocytes in other insects[96,97] (Table 1.1). This revision of hemocyte nomenclature would seem wise, but at present most authors adhere to the original names.[6,97] On the basis of the descriptions presented in this chapter, larvae of flies and butterflies possess three main functional families of circulating hemocytes: one has high phagocytic activity, the second is able to encapsulate large pathogens, and the third is involved in ROS production and activation of the proPO cascade (Fig. 1.3). These three hemocyte groups are usually all present in the hemolymph and cooperate in the insect immune response, although their proportion may change in relation to the immune challenge considered.[97,101] It remains to be established if three functional groups in other insects also stem from separated hemocyte lineages, or if they all derive from the same precursor through differentiated processes of maturation. The possible interconversion between cell types suggests that they may derive from the same embryonic/larval stem cell, though by different and species-specific pathways.[19,96,97]

5.2 Hemocytes and Their Lineages in Crustaceans

Nearly all studies on crustacean immunity have been on decapods, particularly shrimp, crab, and lobster. Across these groups, a common pattern emerges of at least three main cell types, distinguishable morphologically by their degree of granulation (Fig. 1.3C). They can also be physically separated by density gradient centrifugation[112] and distinguished by monoclonal antibody markers,[46,113–116] flow cytometry,[117] or activated cell sorting.[118] The three main hemocyte types are termed hyaline cells, semigranular cells, and granular cells,[7,8] with, in some species, a small population of prohemocytes also present.[54] The prohemocytes are relatively rare (about 2% or fewer of the total number of hemocytes in the circulation), but are distinguishable by their small size, spherical shape, and large nuclear to cytoplasm ratio.[54] Subdivisions of large and small granular cells have also been noted occasionally in the literature[7] but it is unclear if these represent truly distinct functional categories. In shrimp, the dominant cells are the semigranular and granular cells, with the hyaline cells relatively uncommon in the circulation.[8,114] A similar situation occurs in crayfish[112] and lobster,[119] and in all these decapods the semigranular cells are generally accepted as being those most responsible for phagocytosis.[119–121] However, in crab the hyaline cells are dominant, and are the ones that are chiefly responsible for phagocytosis.[121,122] Across all decapods studied, the granular hemocytes appear to have no phagocytic capability, but, together with the semigranular cells and hyaline cells (if present), they contribute to encapsulation reactions.[8,123] The granular cells, and to a lesser extent the semigranular cells, are also the main repositories of important immune proteins, such as antimicrobial proteins[8,124] or factors involved in activation of proPO.[8,112] It is interesting to note that, at least in crab, only the hyaline cells and the semigranular cells exhibit the phenomenon of ETosis, where ET stands for extracellular traps.[125] This is a relatively recently discovered cell-death pathway that aids entrapment and clearance of infective agents from the blood. The process was first reported for mammalian neutrophils, but is now known to be an ancient process[125,126] that entails the expulsion of decondensed chromatin from the nucleus to the extracellular environment in a controlled and regulated way.[125,127] The released nuclear material forms a mesh that becomes studded with antimicrobial proteins derived from the granules of the disrupted cell,[125,127] which entraps bacteria or other microorganisms, preventing their spread around the body. More importantly, the entrapped microbes are brought into close contact with the antimicrobial proteins on the chromatin fibers and are killed.[127] In crab, neither the granular cells nor the prohemocytes show the response,[125] offering further evidence that two cell lineages exist in decapods. Whilst bivalve hemocytes are also able to undergo this cell death process,[125] it is unclear whether cytosolic or nuclear proteins released from ETotic cells stimulate hematopoiesis to replace lost cells.

In keeping with their immature status, crustacean prohemocytes in general tend to show a lack of immune reactivity, as they also appear to be incapable of phagocytosis or a respiratory burst, and do not seem to contain antibacterial proteins (Smith, VJ, unpublished observations). The prohemocytes are, however, able to undergo cell division in the circulation in vivo.[54] Indeed, very low numbers of mitotic cells have been noted in the circulation of shrimp and other decapods,[51–53,128] but it is still unclear whether these are prohemocytes, or a rare, previously unrecognized type of mature hemocyte.

The lineages to which the various hemocyte types belong remain uncertain; van de Braak et al.[42] consider that two lines of cells are produced independently from the hematopoietic stem cells in *P. monodon*. One line is proposed to develop into the granular cells through a sequence of intermediary semigranular cell stages, with the final maturation step taking place in the connective tissue.[42] The other cell lineage is postulated to develop from hyaline cells into a separate semigranular cell type[42] (Fig. 1.3C). Based on histological and ultrastructural analysis of the hematopoietic tissue in Chinese shrimp, *Fenneropenaeus chinensis,* Zhang et al.[46] concur with the notion that hemocytes originate from two separate lineages within the hematopoietic tissue. The finding that similarly sized prohemocytes, enriched in the hemolymph from crab, *Hyas arenaeus*[54] and *Carcinus maenas* (Smith, VJ, unpublished observations), may be either granulated or agranular, lends some further credence to this idea.

5.3 Hemocytes and Their Lineages in Mollusks

Molluscan hemocytes have been described mainly in bivalves, with a few studies made on gastropods and cephalopods. However, the absence of available molecular databases means that classification of the cells remains based mainly on morphological, cytochemical, and functional characteristics, without the possibility to define separate cell lineages. Key features that define the cells include the presence or absence of cytoplasmic granules; acidic, basic, or neutral staining of the granules; phagocytic activity.

5.3.1 Bivalves

Bivalves generally possess three discernable hemocyte morphologies: hyaline cells (sometimes also described as hyalinocytes or agranulocytes), which lack conspicuous cytoplasmic granules; granular cells (also described as granulocytes)[9,129,130]; and small agranular cells, possibly prohemocytes (also known as hemoblast-like cells).[69,70,131,132] In the oysters, *Crassostrea virginica* and *Crassostrea rhizophorae*, and immediately in the mussel, *Perna viridis,* prohemocytes may comprise 3–10% of the total circulating cell number.[69,70,131,132] In other species, these are either absent, or so rarely seen that they have been overlooked by researchers.[67] The proportion of hyaline and granular cells varies from species to species, but wide fluctuations in hemocyte subpopulations may occur in response to different bacterial challenges.[133–135] For example, in *C. virginica* and *C. rhizophorae*, the hyaline cells have been reported to comprise 70–80% of the hemogram,[70,131] with high values also reported for the clam, *Chamelea gallina*, the brown mussel, *Perna perna*, and the scallop, *Argopecten irradians*.[67,69] The remaining proportion of the hemocyte pool is made up of granular cells irrespective of size or staining properties of the granules.[67,69,70,131] In other bivalve species, such as in the blue mussel, *Mytilus edulis*; the cockle, *Cerastoderma edulis*; and the razor shell, *Ensis siliqua*, the proportion of hyaline cells is much lower (6–16%), with basophilic and acidophilic granular cells dominant.[134] *C. edulis* is unusual in also possessing large, vacuolated, spherical agranular cells.[134] Other bivalves with a high population of granular hemocytes include *M. galloprovincialis, Cerastoderma glaucum, P. viridis,* and the clams, *Ruditapes decussatus* and *T. philippinarum.*[67,69,136]

In some species phagocytic activity is usually carried out by the dominant cell type, whether it be the hyaline cells, as in oysters,[67,69,70,131] or the granular cells, as in blue mussel and other bivalves.[68,69,133,134] Thus, phagocytosis may not be executed by exclusively either hyaline or granulated hemocytes in bivalves, but it is species-specific. Rather, phagocytic activity seems to be associated more with the presence in the hemocytes of AMPs,[137] lysozyme, esterases, and/or an ability to undergo the respiratory burst.[68,69] Concerning *P. viridis, M. edulis,* and the giant clam, *Tridacna crocea,* authors[69] have further reported that hyaline hemocytes have no phagocytic ability, but they play a central role in coagulation, and could contribute to limiting blood loss and healing wounds.

With regard to the relationship of the different hemocyte types to each other in bivalves, much remains unclear. Few studies have identified cell-specific markers, although monoclonal antibodies have been developed to distinguish the various hemocyte populations of *M. edulis.*[138,139] Ottaviani et al.[140] and, subsequently, Rebelo and coworkers[70] suggest that bivalves possess only one cell lineage, with the different morphologies representing various maturational stages and/or degranulation events. However, other researchers[9,129] support the hypothesis that granulocytes and hyalinocytes are two separate cell lineages with different immunological roles. The general absence of cell-specific molecular markers confounds testing these conflicting views. Notwithstanding, Dyrynda et al.[139] were able to trace hemocytic changes during ontogenic development of *M. edulis,* using a panel of monoclonal antibodies. Interestingly, the antibodies raised against hemocytes from mature adult mussels also show reactivity with cells from both the trochophore and veliger larvae of *M. edulis,* indicating that epitopes on adult mussel hemocytes are also present at much earlier stages in the life.[139] As of yet, it is still unknown whether *M. edulis* hyaline cells are immature hemocytes (perhaps equivalent to prohemocytes), or if they are fully and terminally differentiated cells. Further studies on the hematopoietic tissue, and prohemocytes capitalizing on new genome sequence data,[61,63] should reveal more about the origin and development of hemocyte stem cells, thus shedding light on how hemocytes in this hugely economically important group of mollusks mature and relate to each other.

5.3.2 Gastropods

Gastropods possess three types of hemocytes: agranular or hyaline cells (sometimes termed amoebocytes), granular hemocytes, and small spherical cells with big nuclei that may represent immature cells (ie, prohemocytes)[80,81] (Fig. 1.4). However, variations occur in functionality of different morphological types. For example, in the freshwater snails, *B. glabrata, Biomphalaria straminea,*

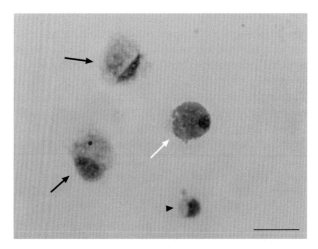

FIGURE 1.4 Circulating hemocytes in the hemolymph of the gastropod *P. canaliculata*, showing three morphologically distinct hemocyte types. The small round hemocytes with high nucleus/cytoplasm ratio are prohemocytes *(arrowhead)*. Mature hemocytes are larger, and the cytoplasm may be either agranular *(black arrows)* or granular *(white arrow)*. In *P. canaliculata,* the agranular large hemocytes are the most abundant in the hemolymph. Bar = 10 μm.

and abalone, *Haliotis tuberculata,* the hyaline cells are the most abundant in the hemolymph.[132,141] In *Biomphalaria* spp. the different roles of the hyalinocytes and granulocytes during the immune response are not completely clear. They both show acid phosphatase and peroxidase activities,[142] but the main phagocytic activity seems to be played by the fixed phagocytes with a developed lysosomal apparatus in connective tissues in several organs.[142] In abalones *H. tuberculata* and *Haliotis discus discus,* granulocytes are almost absent and the hyaline cells exhibit adhesion, aggregation, and phagocytic activities.[132,143] In the pond snail, *Lymnaea stagnalis,* both hyaline cells and granular cells are present,[80] and phagocytosis mainly involves the granular cells.[144,145] Recently, light and electron microscopic studies, together with flow cytometry, has shown that the apple snail, *P. canaliculata,* possesses three distinct populations of hemocytes, namely, the small cells resembling the prohemocytes, the agranular cells, and the granular cells[146] (Fig. 1.4). All, except the prohemocyte-like cells, are capable of phagocytosis.[146] Lack of specific cell markers for these cells is the principal reason for the limited number of studies correlating the immune functions with hemocyte subpopulations, and limits our understanding of the lineages of gastropod hemocytes.

5.3.3 Cephalopods

The classification of hemocyte types in cephalopods is uncertain. Early studies considered that these invertebrates possess only one type of mature hemocyte,[13] but a more recent study has identified two populations in octopus,

O. vulgaris.[147] The dominant population is the large granulocyte, with a U-shaped nucleus and basophilic granules in the cytoplasm, whereas the remainder are hemocytes with a round nucleus, occupying almost the entire cell and few granules in the cytoplasm.[147] Immune reactivity, such as phagocytosis and ROS and nitric oxide production, are more evident in the large granulocytes than in the smaller circulating cells.[90,147] The morphology of the small agranular cell type, coupled with its apparent lack of immune reactivity, indicates that it might be immature cells, equivalent perhaps to the prohemocytes in other pancrustacean and molluscan species, rather than a terminally differentiated and fully functional defense cell.[147] The two hemocyte morphologies described in *O. vulgaris* are not evident in all the octopus species. In the octopus, *Eledone cirrhosa,* only granulocytes with phagocytic, bactericidal, and ROS production ability are present.[148,149] Indeed, a study on *S. officinalis* has reported the existence of only one cell type that has phagocytic capacity.[150] It has a variable number of eosinophilic granules, and some vesicles containing acid phosphatase, lysozyme, and proPO.[150] As reported for bivalves,[129,140] it remains to be established if in cephalopods the large granulocytes and the small agranulocytes derive from separate and postmitotic lineages.

With regard to functionality, early studies reported that cephalopod hemocytes in the circulation show relatively low levels of phagocytosis, at least compared to other molluscan species, and have been considered, by at least some authors, to have less of a role in inflammation than in wound healing.[13,92] Certainly it has been known for some time that cephalopod hemocytes migrate to wounds and assume a fused shape, forming a barrier that protects the damaged area from infection.[92] However, transcriptomic and proteomic research has established that circulating hemocytes in cephalopods do express a number of immune-related genes and proteins.[90,147,151–154] Unfortunately, despite their economic importance, the immune system of cephalopods has received considerably less research interest than other mollusks.

6 CONCLUDING REMARKS

Although the main taxa discussed in this chapter are widely separated in evolutionary terms, and, as a consequence, have great diversity in form and life history, some trends are apparent. All possess hematopoietic tissue of mesodermal origin that is in close contact with the hemal cavity. These tissues generally comprise layers of undifferentiated, developing, and fully or semimature cells, although, sometimes, maturing cells may be present in the circulation, probably through internal or external stimuli. As yet, our understanding of the specific signals and pathways involved in the initiation and regulation of hematopoiesis remains poor. Notwithstanding, increasing availability of genomic, transcriptomic, and proteomic data should enable us to unlock these processes. Of particular importance is to understand if and how the generation, timing, and release of new hemocytes may be influenced by different types of stimuli. Does the phenotypic character of the emergent cells (eg, in terms of their repertoire of cell surface pattern-recognition receptors) vary among different types of pathogen-associated molecular patterns, in order to respond more efficiently to continued threats from invasive microorganisms?

Likewise, there is a dearth of information about the factors that determine what type of cell the stem and prohemocytes mature into. Certainly, members of the pancrustaceans and mollusks share a number of commonalities in the morphology and functionality of their mature hemocytes, although very little is known about the cell lineages, how they age, and the longevity of the different cell types in the hemocoel. An even more intriguing question is the pluripotency of their stem cells. To what degree can such cells generated in the hematopoietic tissue transform into other cells, for instance, neural cells? Such a scenario is not as implausible as once would have been thought, following the discovery that adult-born neurons in crayfish, *P. leniusculus,* can be derived from hemocytes.[155] Invertebrate blood cells and immune systems continue to surprise us.

ACKNOWLEDGMENTS

Part of this work was funded by Grant A.006@FONDRESNOM@02BI-MALAGBIO (Department of Life Sciences, University of Modena and Reggio Emilia, Modena, Italy) and Fondazione di Vignola (Vignola, MO, Italy) grant to DM. Thanks goes to Dr Elisabeth Dyrynda (Heriot Watt University, Edinburgh, Scotland) for helpful discussions on the manuscript.

REFERENCES

1. Lemaitre B, Hoffmann J. The host defense of *Drosophila melanogaster*. *Annu Rev Immunol* 2007;**25**:697–743.
2. Rowley AF, Ratcliffe NA. Insects. In: Ratcliffe NA, Rowley AF, editors. *Invertebrate blood cells*, vol. 2. London and New York: Academic Press; 1981. p. 421–88.
3. Tavian M, Péault B. Embryonic development of the human hematopoietic system. *Int J Dev Biol* 2005;**49**:243–50.
4. Martinez-Agosto JA, Mikkola HKA, Hartenstein V, Banerjee U. The hematopoietic stem cell and its niche: a comparative view. *Genes Dev* 2007;**21**:3044–60.
5. Dorshkind K. Not a split decision for human hematopoiesis. *Nat Immunol* 2010;**11**:569–70.
6. Grigorian M, Hartenstein V. Hematopoiesis and hematopoietic organs in arthropods. *Dev Genes Evol* 2013;**223**:103–15.
7. Bauchau AG. Crustaceans. In: Ratcliffe NA, Rowley AF, editors. *Invertebrate blood cells*, vol. 2. London and New York: Academic Press; 1981. p. 385–420.
8. Smith VJ, Roulston C, Dyrynda EA. The shrimp immune system. In: Alday-Sanz A, editor. *The shrimp book*. Nottingham: Nottingham University Press; 2010. p. 89–148.
9. Cheng TC. Bivalves. In: Ratcliffe NA, Rowley AF, editors. *Invertebrate blood cells*. London and New York: Academic Press; 1981. p. 233–300.
10. Jemaà M, Morin N, Cavelier P, Cau J, Strub JM, Delsert C. Adult somatic progenitor cells and haematopoiesis in oysters. *J Exp Biol* 2014;**217**:3067–77.

11. Sullivan JT. Hematopoiesis in three species of gastropod following infection with *Echinostoma paraensi*. *Trans Am Microsc Soc* 1988;**107**:355–61.

12. Cowden RR. Some cytological and cytochemical observations on the leucopoietic organs, the "white bodies", of *Octopus vulgaris*. *J Invertebr Pathol* 1972;**19**:113–9.

13. Cowden RR, Curtis SK. Cephalopods. In: Ratcliffe NA, Rowley AF, editors. *Invertebrate blood cells*, vol. 1. London and New York: Academic Press; 1981. p. 301–23.

14. Shultz JW, Regier JC. Phylogenetic analysis of arthropods using two nuclear protein-encoding genes supports a crustacean + hexapod clade. *Proc Biol Sci* 2000;**267**:1011–9.

15. Giribet G, Edgecombe GD. Reevaluating the arthropod tree of life. *Annu Rev Entomol* 2012;**57**:167–86.

16. Sasaki G, Ishiwata K, Machida R, Miyata T, Su ZH. Molecular phylogenetic analyses support the monophyly of hexapoda and suggest the paraphyly of entognatha. *BMC Evol Biol* 2013;**13**:236.

17. Rehm P, Meusemann K, Borner J, Misof B, Burmester T. Phylogenetic position of myriapoda revealed by 454 transcriptome sequencing. *Mol Phylogenet Evol* 2014;**77**:25–33.

18. Grimaldi DA. 400 million years on six legs: on the origin and early evolution of hexapoda. *Arthropod Struct Dev* 2010;**39**:191–203.

19. Wood W, Jacinto A. *Drosophila melanogaster* embryonic haemocytes: masters of multitasking. *Nat Rev Mol Cell Biol* 2007;**8**:542–51.

20. De Loof A. Longevity and aging in insects: is reproduction costly; cheap; beneficial or irrelevant? A critical evaluation of the "trade-off" concept. *J Insect Physiol* 2011;**57**:1–11.

21. Kubrak OI, Kučerová L, Theopold U, Nässel DR. The sleeping beauty: how reproductive diapause affects hormone signaling, metabolism, immune response and somatic maintenance in *Drosophila melanogaster*. *PLoS One* 2014;**9**:e113051.

22. Berrill M. The life cycle of the green crab *Carcinus maenas* at the northern end of its range. *J Crustacean Biol* 1982;**2**:31–9.

23. Jung SH, Evans CJ, Uemura C, Banerjee U. The *Drosophila* lymph gland as a developmental model of hematopoiesis. *Development* 2005;**132**:2521–33.

24. Tepass U, Fessler LI, Aziz A, Hartenstein V. Embryonic origin of hemocytes and their relationship to cell death in *Drosophila*. *Development* 1994;**120**:1829–37.

25. Brückner K, Kockel L, Duchek P, Luque CM, Rorth P, Perrimon N. The PDGF/VEGF receptor controls blood cell survival in *Drosophila*. *Dev Cell* 2004;**7**:73–84.

26. Holz A, Bossinger B, Strasser T, Janning W, Klapper R. The two origins of hemocytes in *Drosophila*. *Development* 2003;**130**:4955–62.

27. Makhijani K, Alexander B, Tanaka T, Rulifson E, Brückner K. The peripheral nervous system supports blood cell homing and survival in the *Drosophila* larva. *Development* 2011;**138**:5379–91.

28. Makhijani K, Brückner K. Of blood cells and the nervous system: hematopoiesis in the *Drosophila* larva. *Fly (Austin)* 2012;**6**:254–60.

29. Mandal L, Banerjee U, Hartenstein V. Evidence for a fruit fly hemangioblast and similarities between lymph-gland hematopoiesis in fruit fly and mammal aorta-gonadal-mesonephros mesoderm. *Nat Genet* 2004;**36**:1019–23.

30. Grigorian M, Mandal L, Hartenstein V. Hematopoiesis at the onset of metamorphosis: terminal differentiation and dissociation of the *Drosophila* lymph gland. *Dev Genes Evol* 2011;**221**:121–31.

31. Dragojlovic-Munther M, Martinez-Agosto JA. Extracellular matrix-modulated Heartless signaling in *Drosophila* blood progenitors regulates their differentiation via a Ras/ETS/FOG pathway and target of rapamycin function. *Dev Biol* 2013;**384**:313–30.

32. Gryzik T, Müller HA. FGF8-like1 and FGF8-like2 encode putative ligands of the FGF receptor Htl and are required for mesoderm migration in the *Drosophila* gastrula. *Curr Biol* 2004;**14**:659–67.

33. Stathopoulos A, Tarn B, Ronshaugen M, Frasch M, Levine M. Pyramus and Thisbe: FGF genes that pattern the mesoderm of *Drosophila* embryos. *Genes Dev* 2004;**18**:687–99.
34. Nardi JB, Pilas B, Ujhelyi E, Garsha K, Kanost MR. Hematopoietic organs of *Manduca sexta* and hemocyte lineages. *Dev Genes Evol* 2003;**213**:477–91.
35. Nakahara Y, Kanamori Y, Kiuchi M, Kamimura M. Two hemocyte lineages exist in silkworm larval hematopoietic organ. *PLoS One* 2010;**5**:e11816.
36. Joo K, Mun J, Lee K, Yu C, Kang S, Seo Y, et al. Three-dimensional reconstruction of hematopoietic organ of *Bombyx mori* larva. *Entomol Res* 2004;**34**:291–8.
37. Zachary D, Hoffmann JA, Porte A. Role of the reticulo-hemopoietic tissue of *Locusta migratoria* in the process of immunization against *Bacillus thuringensis*. *Arch Zool Exp Gen* 1981;**122**:55–63.
38. Lim JY, Lee BH, Kang SW, Wago H, Han SS. Association of reticular cells with CD34+/Sca-1+ apoptotic cells in the hemopoietic organ of grasshopper, *Euprepocnemis shirakii*. *J Insect Physiol* 2004;**50**:657–65.
39. Hoffmann JA. The hemopoietic organs of the two orthopterans *Locusta migratoria* and *Gryllus bimaculatus*. *Z Zellforsch Mikrosk Anat* 1970;**106**:451–72.
40. Francois J. Hemocytes et organe hematopoietique de *Thermobia domestica* (packard) (Thysanura: Lepismatidae). *Int J Insect Morphold Embryol* 1975;**4**:477–94.
41. Duressa TF, Vanlaer R, Huybrechts R. Locust cellular defense against infections: sites of pathogen clearance and hemocyte proliferation. *Dev Comp Immunol* 2015;**48**:244–53.
42. van de Braak CBT, Botterblom MHA, Liu W, Taverne N, van der Knapp WPW, Rombout JHWM. The role of the haematopoietic tissue in haemocyte production and maturation in the black tiger shrimp (*Penaeus monodon*). *Fish Shellfish Immunol* 2002;**12**:253–72.
43. Bell T, Lightner DV. *A handbook of normal penaeid shrimp histology*. Kansas: World Aquaculture Society, Allan Press; 1988 p. 114.
44. Martin GG, Hose JE, Kim JJ. Structure of hematopoietic nodules in the ridgeback prawn, *Sicyonia ingentis*: light and electron microscopic observations. *J Morphol* 1987;**192**:193–204.
45. Hose JE, Martin GG, Tiu S, McKrell N. Patterns of hemocyte production and release throughout the molt cycle in the penaeid shrimp *Sicyonia ingentis*. *Biol Bull* 1992;**183**:185–99.
46. Zhang ZF, Shao M, Kang KH. Classification of haematopoietic cells and haemocytes in Chinese prawn, *Fenneropenaeus chinensis*. *Fish Shellfish Immunol* 2006;**21**:159–69.
47. Johnson P. *Histology of the blue crab,* Callinectes sapidus. New York: Praeger Press; 1980 p. 440.
48. Ghiretti-Magaldi A, Milanese C, Tognon G. Hemopoiesis in crustacea decapoda: origin and evolution of hemocytes and cyanocytes of *Carcinus maenas*. *Cell Differ Dev* 1977;**6**:167–86.
49. Martin GG, Hose JE, Choi M, Provost R, Omori G, McKrell N, et al. Organization of hematopoietic tissue in the intermoult lobster *Homarus americanus*. *J Morphol* 1993;**216**:65–78.
50. Chaga O, Lignell M, Söderhäll K. The haemopoietic cells of the feshwater crayfish, *Pacifastacus leniusculus*. *Anim Biol* 1995;**4**:59–70.
51. Sequeira T, Tavares D, Arala-Chaves M. Evidence for circulating hemocyte proliferation in the shrimp *Penaeus japonicus*. *Dev Comp Immunol* 1996;**20**:97–104.
52. Hammond JA, Smith VJ. Lipopolysaccharide induces DNA synthesis in a sub-population of haemocytes from the swimming crab, *Liocarcinus depurator*. *Dev Comp Biol* 2002;**26**:227–36.
53. Söderhäll I, Bangyeekhun E, Mayo S, Söderhäll K. Hemocyte production and maturation in an invertebrate animal; proliferation and gene expression in hematopoietic stem cells of *Pacifastacus leniusculus*. *Dev Comp Immunol* 2003;**27**:661–72.
54. Roulston C, Smith VJ. Isolation and *in vitro* characterisation of prohaemocytes from the spider crab, *Hyas araneus* (L.). *Dev Comp Immunol* 2011;**35**:537–54.
55. Söderhäll I, Kim YA, Jiravanichpaisal P, Lee SY, Söderhäll K. An ancient role for a prokineticin domain in invertebrate hematopoiesis. *J Immunol* 2005;**174**:6153–60.

56. Lin X, Söderhäll K, Söderhäll I. Transglutaminase activity in the haemopoietic tissue of a crustacean, *Pacifastacus leniusculus*, importance in hemocyte homeostasis. *BMC Immunol* 2008;**9**:58.
57. Hsiao CY, Song YL. A long form of shrimp astakine transcript: molecular cloning, characterization and functional elucidation in promoting hematopoiesis. *Fish Shellfish Immunol* 2010;**28**:77–86.
58. Chang YT, Lin CY, Tsai CY, Siva VS, Chu CY, Tsai HJ, et al. The new face of the old molecules: crustin Pm4 and transglutaminase type I serving as RNPs down-regulate astakine-mediated hematopoiesis. *PLoS One* 2013;**8**:e72793.
59. Saelee N, Noonin C, Nupan B, Junkunlo K, Phongdara A, Lin X, et al. β-Thymosins and hemocyte homeostasis in a crustacean. *PLoS One* 2013;**8**:e60974.
60. Ponder WF, Lindberg DR. *Phylogeny and evolution of the Mollusca*. Berkeley: University of California Press; 2008.
61. Zhang G, Fang X, Guo X, Li L, Luo R, Xu F, et al. The oyster genome reveals stress adaptation and complexity of shell formation. *Nature* 2012;**490**:49–54.
62. Simakov O, Marletaz F, Cho SJ, Edsinger-Gonzales E, Havlak P, Hellsten U, et al. Insights into bilaterian evolution from three spiralian genomes. *Nature* 2013;**493**:526–31.
63. Gerdol M, Venier P. An updated molecular basis for mussel immunity. *Fish Shellfish Immunol* 2015;**46**:17–38.
64. Accorsi A, Ottaviani E, Ross E, Gotting K, Sánchez Alvarado A. Regeneration of adult sensory tentacle and eyes in *Pomacea canaliculata*. *Inv Surv J* 2015;**12**:90.
65. Mix MC. A general model for leucocyte cell renewal in bivalve mollusks. *Mar Fish Rev* 1976;**38**:37–41.
66. Elston R. Functional morphology of the coelomocytes of the larval oysters (*Crassostrea virginica* and *Crassostrea gigas*). *J Mar Biol Assoc UK* 1980;**60**:947–57.
67. Matozzo V, Rova G, Marin MG. Haemocytes of the cockle *Cerastoderma glaucum*: morphological characterisation and involvement in immune responses. *Fish Shellfish Immunol* 2007;**23**:732–46.
68. Donaghy L, Lambert C, Choi KS, Soudant P. Hemocytes of the carpet shell clam (*Ruditapes decussatus*) and the manila clam (*Ruditapes philippinarum*): current knowledge and future prospects. *Aquaculture* 2009;**297**:10–24.
69. Wang Y, Hu M, Chiang MW, Shin PK, Cheung SG. Characterization of subpopulations and immune-related parameters of hemocytes in the green-lipped mussel *Perna viridis*. *Fish Shellfish Immunol* 2012;**32**:381–90.
70. Rebelo Mde F, Figueiredo Ede S, Mariante RM, Nóbrega A, de Barros CM, Allodi S. New insights from the oyster *Crassostrea rhizophorae* on bivalve circulating hemocytes. *PLoS One* 2013;**8**:e57384.
71. Matozzo V, Marin MG, Cima F, Ballarin L. First evidence of cell division in circulating haemocytes from the manila clam *Tapes philippinarum*. *Cell Biol Int* 2008;**32**:865–8.
72. Tirapé A, Bacque C, Brizard R, Vandenbulcke F, Boulo V. Expression of immune-related genes in the oyster *Crassostrea gigas* during ontogenesis. *Dev Comp Immunol* 2007;**31**:859–73.
73. Barreau-Roumiguière C, Montagnani C, Escoubas JM. Characterization of a Tal/SCL-like transcription factor in the pacific oyster *Crassostrea gigas*. *Dev Comp Immunol* 2003;**27**:793–800.
74. Green T. Master regulator unmasked. *Nature* 1996;**383**:575.
75. Zhang T, Qiu L, Sun Z, Wang L, Zhou Z, Liu R, et al. The specifically enhanced cellular immune responses in Pacific oyster (*Crassostrea gigas*) against secondary challenge with *Vibrio splendidus*. *Dev Comp Immunol* 2014;**45**:141–50.
76. Cuénot L. Le sang et les glandes lymphatiques. In: Lacaze-Duthiers H, editor. *Archives de zoologie expérimentale et énérale*. Paris: Académiedes Sciences; 1891 pp. 13–90.

77. Ma H, Wang J, Wang B, Zhao Y, Yang C. Characterization of an ETS transcription factor in the sea scallop *Chlamys farreri*. *Dev Comp Immunol* 2009;**33**:953–8.
78. Yue F, Zhou Z, Wang L, Sun R, Jiang Q, Yi Q, et al. The essential roles of core binding factors CfRunt and CfCBFβ in hemocyte production of scallop *Chlamys farreri*. *Dev Comp Immunol* 2014;**44**:291–302.
79. Bachère E, Gueguen Y, Gonzalez M, de Lorgeril J, Garnier J, Romestand B. Insights into the anti-microbial defense of marine invertebrates: the penaeid shrimps and the oyster *Crassostrea gigas*. *Immunol Rev* 2004;**198**:149–68.
80. Sminia T. Structure and function of blood and connective tissue cells of the fresh water pulmonate *Lymnaea stagnalis* studied by electron microscopy and enzyme histochemistry. *Cell Tissue Res* 1972;**130**:497–526.
81. Sminia T, Gastropods. In: Ratcliffe NA, Rowley AF, editors. *Invertebrate blood cells*, vol. 1. London: Academic Press; 1981. p. 191–232.
82. Jeong KH, Lie KJ, Heyneman D. The ultrastructure of the amebocyte-producing organ in *Biomphalaria glabrata*. *Dev Comp Immunol* 1983;**7**:217–28.
83. Sullivan JT. Mitotic responses to injected extracts of larval and adult *Schistosoma mansoni* in *Biomphalaria glabrata*: effects of dose and colchicine treatment. *J Parasitol* 2007;**93**:213–5.
84. Sullivan JT, Spence JV. Factors affecting adoptive transfer of resistance to *Schistosoma mansoni* in the snail intermediate host, *Biomphalaria glabrata*. *J Parasitol* 1999;**85**:1065–71.
85. Ottaviani E. Histological and immunocytochemical studies on the origin of haemocytes in the freshwater snail *Planorbarius corneus* (L.) (Gastropoda, Pulmonata). *Z mikrosk-anat Forsch* 1988;**102**:649–54.
86. Accorsi A, Ottaviani E, Malagoli D. Effects of repeated hemolymph withdrawals on the hemocyte populations and hematopoiesis in *Pomacea canaliculata*. *Fish Shellfish Immunol* 2014;**38**:56–64.
87. Monteil JF, Matricon-Gondran M. Hemocyte production in trematode-infected *Lymnaea truncatula*. *Parasitol Res* 1991;**77**:491–7.
88. Furuta E, Yamaguchi K, Shimozawa A. Blood cell-producing site in the land slug, *Incilaria fruhstorferi*. *Kaibogaku Zasshi* 1994;**69**:751–64.
89. Wells MJ, Smith PJS. The performance of the octopus circulatory system: a triumph of engineering over design. *Experientia* 1987;**43**:487–99.
90. Novoa B, Tafalla C, Guerra A, Figueras A. Cellular immunological parameters of the octopus *Octopus vulgaris*. *J Shellfish Res* 2002;**21**:243–8.
91. Bolognari A. Morfologia, struttura e funzione del "corpo bianco" dei Cefalopodi. I. morfologia. *Arch Zool Ital* 1949;**34**:79–97.
92. Ford LA. Host defense mechanisms of cephalopods. *Annu Rev Fish Dis* 1992;**2**:25–41.
93. Necco A, Martin R. Behavior and estimation of the mitotic activity of the white body cells in *Octopus vulgaris*, cultured *in vitro*. *Exp Cell Res* 1963;**30**:588–90.
94. Rizki TM. Alterations in the haemocyte population of *Drosophila melanogaster*. *J Morphol* 1957;**100**:437–58.
95. Ratcliffe NA. Cellular defense responses of insects: unresolved problems. In: Beckage NE, Thompson SN, Federici BA, editors. *Parasites and pathogens of insects*, vol. 1. San Diego: Academic Press; 1993. p. 267–304.
96. Lavine MD, Strand MR. Insect hemocytes and their role in immunity. *Insect Biochem Mol Biol* 2002;**32**:1295–309.
97. Ribeiro C, Brehelin M. Insect haemocytes: what type of cell is that? *J Insect Physiol* 2006;**52**:417–29.
98. Williams MJ. *Drosophila* hemopoiesis and cellular immunity. *J Immunol* 2007;**178**:4711–6.

99. Kaaya GP, Ratcliffe NA. Comparative study of hemocytes and associated cells of some medically important dipterans. *J Morphol* 1982;**173**:351–65.

100. Brehélin M. Comparative study of structure and function of blood cells from two *Drosophila* species. *Cell Tissue Res* 1982;**221**:607–15.

101. Nappi AJ, Vass E, Malagoli D, Carton Y. The effects of parasite-derived immune-suppressive factors on the cellular innate immune and autoimmune responses of *Drosophila melanogaster*. *J Parasitol* 2004;**90**:1139–49.

102. Honti V, Csordás G, Márkus R, Kurucz E, Jankovics F, Andó I. Cell lineage tracing reveals the plasticity of the hemocyte lineages and of the hematopoietic compartments in *Drosophila melanogaster*. *Mol Immunol* 2010;**47**:1997–2004.

103. Krzemien J, Oyallon J, Crozatier M, Vincent A. Hematopoietic progenitors and hemocyte lineages in the *Drosophila* lymph gland. *Dev Biol* 2010;**346**:310–9.

104. Strand MR. The insect cellular immune response. *Insect Sci* 2008;**15**:1–14.

105. Ashida M, Ochiai M, Niki T. Immunolocalization of prophenoloxidase among hemocytes of the silkworm, *Bombyx mori*. *Tissue Cell* 1988;**20**:599–610.

106. Sass M, Kiss A, Locke M. Integument and hemocyte peptides. *J Insect Physiol* 1994;**40**:407–21.

107. Hoffmann J, Zachary D, Hoffmann D, Brehelin M, Porte A. Postembryonic development and differentiation: hemopoietic tissues and their functions in some insects. In: Gupta A, editor. *Insect hemocytes*. Cambridge: University Press; 1979. p. 29–66.

108. Mandal L, Martinez-Agosto JA, Evans CJ, Hartenstein V, Banerjee U. A Hedgehog- and Antennapedia-dependent niche maintains *Drosophila* haematopoietic precursors. *Nature* 2007;**446**:320–4.

109. Gardiner EM, Strand MR. Hematopoiesis in larval *Pseudoplusia includes* and *Spodoptera frugiperda*. *Arch Insect Biochem Physiol* 2000;**43**:147–64.

110. Gardiner EMM, Strand MR. Monoclonal antibodies bind distinct classes of hemocytes in the moth *Pseudoplusia includens*. *J Insect Physiol* 1999;**45**:113–26.

111. Beaulaton J. Hemocytes and hemocytopoiesis in silkworms. *Biochimie* 1979;**61**:157–64.

112. Söderhäll K, Smith VJ. Separation of the haemocytes of *Carcinus maenas* and other decapod crustaceans and phenoloxidase distribution. *Dev Comp Immunol* 1983;**7**:229–39.

113. Rodriguez J, Boulo E, Mialhe E, Bachere E. Characterisation of shrimp haemocytes and plasma components by monoclonal antibodies. *J Cell Sci* 1995;**108**:1043–50.

114. van de Braak CBT, Taverne N, Botterblom MHA, van der Knaap WPW, Rombout JHWM. Characterisation of different morphological features of black tiger shrimp (*Penaeus monodon*) haemocytes using monoclonal antibodies. *Fish Shellfish Immunol* 2000;**10**:515–30.

115. Winotaphan P, Sithigorngul P, Muenpol O, Longyant S, Rukpratanporn S, Chaivisuthangkura P, et al. Monoclonal antibodies specific to haemocytes of black tiger prawn *Penaeus monodon*. *Fish Shellfish Immunol* 2005;**18**:189–98.

116. Lin YB, Zhan W, Li Q, Zhang Z, Wei ZZ, Sheng X. Ontogenesis of haemocytes in shrimp (*Fenneropenaeus chinensis*) studied with probes of monoclonal antibody. *Dev Comp Immunol* 2007;**31**:1073–81.

117. Owens L, O'Neill A. Use of a clinical cell flow cytometer for differential counts of prawn *Penaeus monodon* haemocytes. *Dis Aquat Orgs* 1997;**31**:147–53.

118. Yip ECH, Wong JTY. Fluorescence activated cell-sorting of haemocytes in penaeid prawns. *Aquaculture* 2002;**204**:25–31.

119. Stewart JE, Dingle JR, Odense PH. Constituents of the haemolymph of lobster, *Homarus americanus*. *Can J Biochem* 1966;**44**:1447–59.

120. Fontaine CT, Lightner DV. Observations on the phagocytosis and elimination of carmine particles into the abdominal muculature of the white shrimp, *Penaeus setiferus*. *J Invertebr Pathol* 1974;**24**:141–8.

121. Söderhäll K, Smith VJ, Johansson M. Exocytosis and phagocytosis by isolated haemocyte populations of crustaceans: evidence for cell co-operation in the cellular defence reactions. *Cell Tissue Res* 1986;**245**:43–9.

122. Smith VJ, Ratcliffe NA. Host defence reactions of the shore crab *Carcinus maenas* (L.): *in vitro*. *J Mar Biol Assoc UK* 1978;**58**:367–97.

123. Smith VJ, Ratcliffe NA. Cellular defense reactions of the shore crab, *Carcinus maenas* (L.): *in vivo* haemocytic and histopathological responses to injected bacteria. *J Invertebr Pathol* 1980;**35**:65–74.

124. Sperstad SV, Smith VJ, Stensvåg K. Expression of antimicrobial peptides from *Hyas araneus* haemocytes following bacterial challenge *in vitro*. *Dev Comp Immunol* 2010;**34**:618–24.

125. Robb CT, Dyrynda EA, Gray RD, Rossi AG, Smith VJ. Invertebrate extracellular phagocyte traps show that chromatin is an ancient defence weapon. *Nat Commun* 2014;**5**:4627.

126. Poirier AC, Schmitt P, Rosa RD, Vanhove AS, Kieffer-Jaquinod S, Rubio TP, et al. Antimicrobial histones and DNA traps in invertebrate immunity: evidences in *Crassostrea gigas*. *J Biol Chem* 2014;**289**:24821–31.

127. Brinkmann V, Reichard U, Goosmann C, Fauler B, Uhlemann Y, Weiss DS, et al. Neutrophil extracellular traps kill bacteria. *Science* 2004;**33**:1532–5.

128. Battison A, Cawthorn R, Horney B. Classification of *Homarus americanus* hemocytes and the use of differential hemocyte counts in lobsters infected with *Aerococcus viridans* var. *homari* (Gaffkaemia). *J Invertebr Pathol* 2003;**84**:177–97.

129. Hine PM. The inter-relationships of bivalve haemocytes. *Fish Shellfish Immunol* 1999;**9**:367–85.

130. Hartenstein V. Blood cells and blood cell development in the animal kingdom. *Annu Rev Cell Dev Biol* 2006;**22**:677–712.

131. Ashton-Alcox KA, Ford SE. Variability in molluscan hemocytes: a flow cytometric study. *Tissue Cell* 1998;**30**:195–204.

132. Travers MA, Mirella da Silva P, Le Goïc N, Marie D, Donval A, Huchette S, et al. Morphologic, cytometric and functional characterisation of abalone (*Haliotis tuberculata*) haemocytes. *Fish Shellfish Immunol* 2008;**24**:400–11.

133. Pipe RK, Farley SR, Coles JA. The separation and characterisation of haemocytes from the mussel *Mytilus edulis*. *Cell Tissue Res* 1997;**289**:537–45.

134. Wootten EC, Dyrynda EA, Ratcliffe NA. Bivalve immunity: comparisons between the marine mussel (*Mytilus edulis*), the edible cockle (*Cerastoderma edule*) and the razor-shell (*Ensis siliqua*). *Fish Shellfish Immuol* 2003;**15**:195–210.

135. Parisi MG, Li H, Jouvet LBP, Dyrynda EA, Parrinello N, Cammarata M, et al. Differential involvement of mussel hemocyte sub-populations in the clearance of bacteria. *Fish Shellfish Immunol* 2008;**25**:834–40.

136. Cima F, Matozzo V, Marin MG, Ballarin L. Haemocytes of the clam *Tapes philippinarum* (Adams & Reeve, 1850): morphofunctional characterisation. *Fish Shellfish Immunol* 2000;**10**:677–93.

137. Mitta G, Hubert F, Dyrynda EA, Boudry P, Roch P. Mytilin B and MGD2, two antimicrobial peptides of marine mussels: gene structure and expression analysis. *Dev Comp Immunol* 2000;**24**:381–93.

138. Noël D, Pipe RK, Elston R, Bachère E, Mialhe E. Antigenic characterization of hemocyte subpopulations in the mussel *Mytilus edulis* by means of monoclonal-antibodies. *Marine Biol* 1994;**119**:549–56.

139. Dyrynda EA, Pipe RK, Ratcliffe NA. Sub-populations of haemocytes in the adult and developing marine mussel, *Mytilus edulis*, identified by use of monoclonal antibodies. *Cell Tissue Res* 1997;**289**:527–36.

140. Ottaviani E, Franchini A, Barbieri D, Kletsas D. Comparative and morphofunctional studies on *Mytilus galloprovincialis* hemocytes: presence of two aging-related hemocyte stages. *Ital J Zool* 1998;**65**:349–54.

141. Cavalcanti MG, Filho FC, Mendonça AM, Duarte GR, Barbosa CC, De Castro CM, et al. Morphological characterization of hemocytes from *Biomphalaria glabrata* and *Biomphalaria straminea*. *Micron* 2012;**43**:285–91.

142. Matricon-Gondran M, Letocart M. Internal defenses of the snail *Biomphalaria glabrata*. *J Invertebr Pathol* 1999;**74**:235–47.

143. Donaghy L, Hong HK, Lambert C, Park HS, Shim WJ, Choi KS. First characterization of the populations and immune-related activities of hemocytes from two edible gastropod species, the disk abalone, *Haliotis discus discus* and the spiny top shell, *Turbo cornutus*. *Fish Shellfish Immunol* 2010;**28**:87–97.

144. Adema CM, van Deutekom-Mulder EC, van der Knaap WP, Meuleman EA, Sminia T. Generation of oxygen radicals in hemocytes of the snail *Lymnaea stagnalis* in relation to the rate of phagocytosis. *Dev Comp Immunol* 1991;**15**:17–26.

145. Russo J, Lagadic L. Effects of environmental concentrations of atrazine on hemocyte density and phagocytic activity in the pond snail *Lymnaea stagnalis* (*Gastropoda, Pulmonata*). *Environ Pollut* 2004;**127**:303–11.

146. Accorsi A, Bucci L, de Eguileor M, Ottaviani E, Malagoli D. Comparative analysis of circulating hemocytes of the freshwater snail *Pomacea canaliculata*. *Fish Shellfish Immunol* 2013;**34**:1260–8.

147. Castellanos-Martínez S, Prado-Alvarez M, Lobo-da-Cunha A, Azevedo C, Gestal C. Morphologic, cytometric and functional characterization of the common octopus (*Octopus vulgaris*) hemocytes. *Dev Comp Immunol* 2014;**44**:50–8.

148. Malham SK, Runham NW, Secombes CJ. Phagocytosis by haemocytes from the lesser octopus *Eledone cirrhosa*. *Iberus* 1997;**15**:1–11.

149. Malham SK, Lacoste A, Gélébart F, Cueff A, Poulet SA. A first insight stress-induced neuroendocrine and immune changes in the octopus *Eledone cirrhosa*. *Aquat Living Resour* 2002;**15**:187–92.

150. Le Pabic C, Goux D, Guillamin M, Safi G, Lebel JM, Koueta N, et al. Hemocyte morphology and phagocytic activity in the common cuttlefish (*Sepia officinalis*). *Fish Shellfish Immunol* 2014;**40**:362–73.

151. Collins AJ, Schleicher TR, Rader BA, Nyholm SV. Understanding the role of host hemocytes in a squid/vibrio symbiosis using transcriptomics and proteomics. *Front Immunol* 2012;**3**:91.

152. Castellanos-Martínez S, Arteta D, Catarino S, Gestal C. De novo transcriptome sequencing of the *Octopus vulgaris* hemocytes using illumina RNA-Seq technology: response to the infection by the gastrointestinal parasite *Aggregata octopiana*. *PLoS One* 2014;**9**:e107873.

153. Castellanos-Martínez S, Diz AP, Álvarez-Chaver P, Gestal C. Proteomic characterization of the hemolymph of *Octopus vulgaris* infected by the protozoan parasite *Aggregata octopiana*. *J Proteom* 2014;**105**:151–63.

154. Yazzie N, Salazar KA, Castillo MG. Identification, molecular characterization, and gene expression analysis of a CD109 molecule in the Hawaiian bobtail squid *Euprymna scolopes*. *Fish Shellfish Immunol* 2015;**44**:342–55.

155. Benton JL, Kery R, Li J, Noonin C, Söderhäll I, Beltz BS. Cells from the immune system generate adult-born neurons in crayfish. *Dev Cell* 2014;**30**:322–33.

Chapter 2

Origin and Functions of Tunicate Hemocytes

Francesca Cima, Nicola Franchi, Loriano Ballarin
Department of Biology, University of Padova, Padova, Italy

1 INTRODUCTION

Tunicates, or urochordates, are a subphylum of the phylum Chordata, sharing with other members of the phylum: (1) a permanent or temporary notochord, in the form of a dorsal rod; (2) a central nervous system, in the form of a dorsal tube; (3) a pharynx provided with gill slits or pharyngeal pouches, and a ventral gland secreting iodoproteins (endostyle or thyroid); and (4) a muscular tail.

Tunicates are considered the sister group of vertebrates,[1] forming with the latter the clade Olfactoria. Recently, it has been proposed to classify them as a phylum within the superphylum Chordata.[2] They are traditionally subdivided in three classes: (1) Ascidiacea (benthic and sessile), (2) Thaliacea, and (3) Larvacea or Appendicularia (pelagic).

Ascidians have a free-swimming, tadpole-like larva, an adult sac-like body with two siphons that allow water flux, and a large branchial basket, provided with a ventral endostyle that secretes the mucous net required for filtration. They comprise two orders: Enterogona (including the suborders Phlebobranchia and Aplousobranchia) and Pleurogona (with the suborder Stolidobranchia).[3] Thaliaceans include three orders: the colonial Pyrosomida, and the solitary/colonial Doliolida and Salpida. They have a barrel-like adult body, and, with the exception of Doliolida, are devoid of larval stages.[4,5] Larvaceans or appendicularians resemble the ascidian larvae and use the tail to create the water current for filtration; filters are included in the gelatinous house secreted by the animals themselves.[4] Most of the recent authors consider larvaceans as a sister group of the other tunicates, and thaliaceans as a sister group of Enterogona[5–10] (Fig. 2.1).

Ascidians include about 2300 species, and most of the information on tunicate hemocytes comes from studies on this group of organisms. This review will, then, focus mainly on ascidian hemocytes and will discuss their role in immunity. Where possible, information on circulating cells of pelagic tunicates will be added.

The Evolution of the Immune System. http://dx.doi.org/10.1016/B978-0-12-801975-7.00002-5

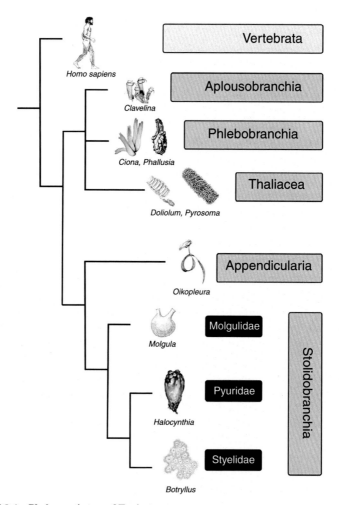

FIGURE 2.1   Phylogenetic tree of Tunicates.

2   ASCIDIAN CIRCULATION

Ascidians have an open circulatory system with a colorless hemolymph that is forced inside blood sinuses and lacunae within the body tissues by the contractions of a tubular hearth. The direction of the peristaltic waves reverses periodically with the consequent reversal of the hemolymph flow.[11,12]

The colorless hemolymph is isotonic with seawater and contains low concentrations of proteins, which are mainly secreted by the hemocytes: they exert important roles in humoral-defense reactions.[12–14]

3 ASCIDIAN HEMOCYTES

Ascidian hemocytes are involved in a variety of functions, such as: (1) storage and transport of nutrients and catabolites, (2) asexual reproduction, (3) tunic synthesis, (4) allorecognition, and (5) defense reactions.[15-17]

3.1 Hematopoietic Tissues

Hematopoietic sites are mainly located in peripharyngeal regions, clearly evident in solitary species as "lymphatic nodules," or clusters of stem cells surrounded by hemocytes at various developmental stages.[12,18,19] In colonial species of the genus *Botryllus*, mitotic figures have been occasionally observed in circulating hemocytes.[20] In the same species, stem cell niches have been identified close to the adult endostyle.[21-23] From this location, they colonize the cell islands, that is, aggregates of hemocytes located along the sides of the endostyle, from which they enter the circulation and contribute to various zooid tissues, germline and hemolymph included.[23]

3.2 Hemocyte Morphology

Many investigators studied the morphology of living and fixed hemocytes and their ultrastructure.[16,17] Various authors have also proposed unifying classification frameworks,[11,12,24] but a certain degree of uncertainty still persists on the terminology and differentiation pathways of ascidian hemocytes. In our opinion, they can be grouped in the following categories: undifferentiated cells, immunocytes (i.e., cells involved in immune defense), and storage cells (Fig. 2.2).

Undifferentiated cells, known as hemoblasts, feature a high nucleus/ cytoplasmic ratio, a well-defined nucleolus, and a basophilic cytoplasm (Fig. 2.2A). The now obsolete term "lymphocyte" has also been used in the literature, both as a synonymous of the term "hemoblast" and to indicate a young hemocyte having entered a differentiation pathway.[18,25,26] In *Botrylloides leachii* and *Botryllus schlosseri*, hemoblasts show positivity to antibodies against mammalian CD-34.[16,23] In *B. schlosseri*, new hemoblasts cyclically enter the circulation to replace the hemocytes that undergo apoptosis at the generation change.[27]

Circulating immunocytes include both phagocytes and cytotoxic cells.

Phagocytes can assume both a spreading and a round morphology. Spreading phagocytes are also known as hyaline amoebocytes: they are multifunctional cells that can actively move toward foreign cells or particles and ingest them. Their cytoplasm contains fine cytoplasmic granules, unresolvable under the light microscope, and shows positivity for lysosomal enzyme activities[15,17,28] (Fig. 2.2B). Upon the ingestion of foreign material, they withdraw their projections, assuming a round morphology (in this phase, they are also called macrophages or macrophage-like cells). Round phagocytes are large cells, with one or more phagosomes (Fig. 2.2C). A detailed study of the properties of round

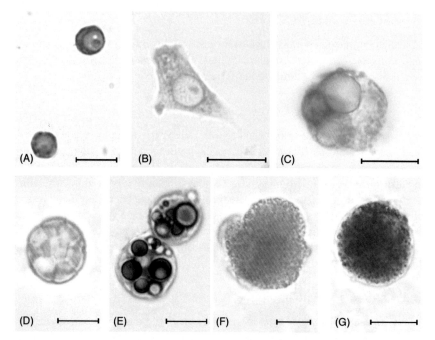

FIGURE 2.2   **Circulating hemocytes of the colonial ascidian *Botryllus schlosseri*.** (A–C, E) fixed hemocytes stained with Giemsa solution; (D, F, G) living hemocytes. (A) hemoblasts; (B) hyaline amoebocytes; (C) macrophage-like cell; (D) living morula cell; (E) fixed morula cells; (F) nephrocyte; (G) blue-pigment cell. Scale bar: 10 μm.

phagocytes in the colonial ascidians *B. leachii* and *B. schlosseri* confirmed the presence of hydrolytic enzymes, as well as of lipids and lipofuscins inside their phagosomes.[15–17] In *B. schlosseri*, the presence of a static and a mobile population of phagocytes have been described, the former homing in ventral islands, on both sides of the endostyle.[29]

   Cytotoxic cells are vacuolated cells containing the enzyme phenoloxidase (PO). They constitute one of the most abundant (sometimes more than 50%) circulating hemocyte-types and are represented, in most cases, by morula cells (MCs), so-called for the berry-like morphology they assume after fixation (Fig. 2.2D–E). In the solitary ascidian *Ciona intestinalis*, PO-containing cells are represented by univacuolar refractile granulocytes, whereas in *Phallusia mammillata*, compartment cells and granular amoebocytes contain the enzyme.[31–33] MCs have a large diameter (10–15 μm) and cytoplasm filled by many vacuoles, uniform in size (around 2 μm in diameter) where the enzyme PO, probably stored as an inactive precursor (proPO), resides.[33] In botryllid ascidians, granular amoebocytes are considered to be the direct precursors of MCs, because they share with the latter similar cytochemical properties and common enzymatic content inside their granules.[15–17]

Storage cells, that is, circulating hemocytes that do not exert immune-related functions, consist of vanadocytes, nephrocytes, pigment cells, and trophocytes.

Vanadocytes, present in Enterogona, can accumulate vanadium (V) up to a concentration of 350 mM (the mean V concentration of seawater is 35 nM) inside their vacuoles, complexed with V-binding proteins. The function of such high V concentration is still unexplained.[34–37]

Nephrocytes, 10–15 μm in diameter, accumulate urate crystals in Brownian motion inside large vacuoles (Fig. 2.2F). They represent a sort of "circulating kidney," as tunicates lack a defined excretory system.[11,12,38,39] Nephrocytes can leave the circulation and contribute to the ascidian pigmentation.[40]

Pigment cells are large hemocytes (up to 40 μm in diameter) containing blue, orange, and/or reddish pigment granules, either in the form of cytoplasmic globules or as crystals in Brownian motion inside a few large vacuoles[11,12,41] (Fig. 2.2G). Their frequency tends to increase with the age of the organism/colony.

Trophocytes represent the most abundant circulating cells of many colonial ascidians. They are large (10–15 μm in diameter), round cells with the cytoplasm filled with many granules, which store nutrients. They sustain bud morphogenesis, especially in species such as *Polyandrocarpa misakiensis*, where buds detach very early from the parental organism.[42–44]

4 IMMUNE ROLE OF TUNICATE HEMOCYTES

4.1 Phagocytosis

Ascidians rely only on innate immunity for their defense, and phagocytes constitute a fraction of approximately 20% of the total immunocytes number.[12,17] The ingestion of foreign materials occurs either in liquid phase (macropinocytosis[45]) or through classical phagocytosis, which is a "zipper-like" process involving integrins.[46] The recognition of nonself molecules by phagocytes requires the presence of surface receptors. Two typical Toll-like receptor (TLR) genes, composed of TIR, transmembrane, and LRR domains, have been identified in the solitary species *C. intestinalis*; they are expressed in both plasma membrane and the endosomes of phagocytes.[47] Also in *B. schlosseri*, preliminary data indicate that TLRs are involved in phagocytosis.[48]

Nonself recognition by phagocytes triggers evolutionary-conserved signal-transduction pathways, such as those mediated by trimeric G-proteins and the protein kinases PKA and PKC.[49,50] In addition, active PI3K, MAPKs, NF-kB, and a transient increase of cytosolic calcium are required.[46,51–53] In addition, genes putatively encoding for MyD88, IRAK, TRAF, NF-kB, and IkB, involved in the signal transduction triggered by activated TIR domains, have been identified in the *Ciona* genome, as well as a gene for CD36, which is a scavenger receptor able to recognize oxidized lipids and surface microbial molecules that are required for phagocytosis of apoptotic cells.[54]

The ingestion of foreign materials is usually associated with the activation of both a membrane oxidase, with the consequent increase in oxygen consumption, and nitric oxide synthase (NOS); this leads to the production of reactive oxygen species (ROS) and reactive nitrogen species (RNS), with microbicidal function.[55,56]

In *B. schlosseri*, as a consequence of nonself recognition, phagocytes produce and release a rhamnose-binding lectin (BsRBL), able to coat the microbial surfaces and act as opsonin.[57] The same lectin, when added to hemocyte cultures, can trigger the phagocyte respiratory burst and exert chemotactic activity toward phagocytes that assume a spreading morphology. Both the transcription of the BsRBL gene and the synthesis of the protein significantly increase during the colonial generation change, when a consistent fraction of circulating hemocytes (~30%) undergoes cell death by apoptosis and is cleared by phagocytes.[58]

In *B. schlosseri*, phagocytosis of apoptotic cells occurs massively during the cyclical generation change[59–61]; the recognition of dying cells is mediated by the exposure of phosphatidylserine and sialic acid, and involves molecules recognized by a polyclonal anti-CD36 antibody.[61,62] The correct clearance of apoptotic cells by phagocytes is required for the completion of the generation change and progression of bud development to adulthood.[63]

Moreover, in *B. schlosseri*, a population of phagocytes is exposed to seawater and adheres to the internal tunic of the oral and atrial siphons. Such sentinel cells are active in immunosurveillance, controlling the entrance to branchial and atrial chambers.[64]

Some tunic cells, probably derived from hemocytes, have phagocytic activity and contribute to protect organisms from pathogens or parasites.[65–68]

4.2 Encapsulation

Circulating phagocytes usually encapsulate any foreign material too large to be ingested by a single cell. The formation of capsule around parasitic crustaceans has been reported in *Ascidiella aspersa*,[69] *Microcosmus savignyi*,[70] and *Styela gibbsii*.[71] In *Molgula manhattensis*, both phagocytes and MCs are recruited in the infectious area during capsule formation.[72] In *C. intestinalis*, the injection of mammalian erythrocytes, BSA, or LPS in the tunic leads to capsule formation following the massive recruitment of hemocytes to the inoculum site.[73–75]

Botryllus scalaris is the only botryllid species reported so far in which capsule formation by circulating phagocytes is involved in allorecognition between contacting, incompatible colonies. In this case, after the fusion of the ampullae and the initial blood-exchange between contacting colonies, circulating phagocytes crowd inside the fused vessels and stimulate the aggregation of hemocytes into large clusters, which are encapsulated by other phagocytes. In this way, the hemocyte-mass plugs the lumen of the fused ampullae and the blood flow is interrupted within a few minutes.[76]

4.3   Cytotoxicity

When hemocytes of *C. intestinalis* and *Styela plicata* are incubated in the presence of mammalian erythrocytes or tumor cells, a rapid cytotoxic reaction can be observed. Cytotoxic reactions require the contact between hemocytes and target cells, are Ca^{2+}-dependent, and are inhibited by sphingomyelin.[77–80] Cytotoxic cells are represented, in both cases, by PO-containing hemocytes[30,80]; their cytotoxicity is related to either the release of active PO in the medium, as in *Styela*[81] and *Ciona*,[82] or to the activity of the enzyme phospholipase A2, modulated by lectins with specificity for galactosides, as in *Ciona*.[83]

In *B. schlosseri*, MC degranulation and the induction of cytotoxicity may be reproduced *in vitro* by exposing hemocytes to the cell-free hemolymph of incompatible colonies[84–86] and can be prevented by PO inhibitors.[87] Cytotoxicity is related to the induction of oxidative stress consequent to the production of ROS by PO, as indicated by the observation that ROS scavengers can suppress the induction of cytotoxicity both in vitro and in vivo, in colony allorecognition, although they have no effect on MC degranulation or PO activity.[87,88] The role of nitric oxide (NO) in the induction of cell death is suggested by the in vitro production of nitrite, when hemocytes are exposed to nonself molecules, and by the decrease of in vitro cytotoxicity in the presence of the NOS inhibitor N^{ω}-nitro-L-arginine methyl ester.[89] The production of NO by hemocytes, after their exposure to either LPS or zymosan, has been reported also in *Phallusia nigra*.[90]

Cytotoxicity is related to the oxidation of polyphenol substrata, likely represented by tunichromes,[91–93] contained inside MCs, by PO, causing the production of ROS and quinones that can damage various kinds of macromolecules.[17,81,88]

4.4   Inflammation

Inflammation in ascidians is characterized by recruitment of circulating cells, extravasation, cell degranulation, and induction of cytotoxicity to the infection area.

S. plicata granulocytes contain histamine, which, when released upon the recognition of nonself, induces an inflammatory reaction by recruiting hemocytes, which, in turn, prompt tunic vessel-contraction and inhibit phagocytosis.[94]

The injection of foreign material (rabbit erythrocytes, BSA, and LPS) into the tunic of *C. intestinalis* leads to an inflammatory reaction because of hemocyte recruitment to the injection area,[75,95,96] hemocyte degranulation, and, eventually, capsule formation[74] and tissue damage.[97] Circulating granulocytes in treated animals increase the transcription of a gene for a member of the CAP-superfamily of proteins.[98]

Tissue transplantation is another cause of inflammation: in solitary species, a higher recruitment of hemocytes has been observed in the case of allografts with respect to autografts; the ultimate rejection of allografts is more rapid in previously challenged animals.[99–101] Graft rejection in *M. manhattensis* involves the recruitment of MCs and induction of cytotoxicity.[19,72] Analogously, in *S. plicata*, MCs are massively recruited in the graft region and contribute to the induction of cytotoxicity.[102]

In colonial ascidians, the induction of inflammation is observable during the nonfusion reaction among genetically incompatible colonies. The phenomenon has been particularly studied in botryllid ascidians. In *Botryllus primigenus* and *B. schlosseri*, it is controlled by a highly polymorphic Fu/HC (fusibility/histocompatibility) allorecognition gene with codominant alleles[103,104]: contacting colonies can fuse into a single chimeric colony, with anastomosis of the tunic and the tunic vasculature, if they share at least one allele at the Fu/HC locus.[105,106] Conversely, a rejection reaction occurs, characterized by the appearance, along the contact border, of a series of cytotoxic foci, called points of rejection (POR), which contain melanin deposits due to PO activity.[85]

In *B. schlosseri*, MCs are the first cells to sense nonself molecules,[107] and, as a consequence of the recognition, they produce and release molecules able to activate phagocytes, stimulate the release of BsRBL, and enhance their recruitment to the site of infection (see further).

The contact among allogeneic colonies leads to partial fusion of the facing tunics with the local disappearance of the limiting cuticles, leakage of humoral factors from one colony to the other, and the selective recruitment of MCs inside the blind endings of the tunic vessels (ampullae) facing the alien colony. Then, MCs migrate into the tunic where they degranulate and release their vacuolar content, in particular, the enzyme PO and its polyphenol substrata and quinones, which are responsible for the induction of cytotoxicity along the contact border.[85,88,89] The involvement of MCs in a nonfusion reaction has been demonstrated also in other botryllid ascidians, such as *Botrylloides simodensis*, *Botrylloides fuscus*, *Botrylloides violaceus*, and *B. leachii*.[106,108–112]

Genes involved in allorecognition and their receptors[113,114] are also expressed by hemocytes, although some uncertainties still persist as to the identity of the allorecognition gene.[113,115]

When incompatible colonies are artificially brought into contact at their cut surfaces, an intense inflammatory reaction is observed in ovoviviparous botryllid ascidians,[106,112,116–118] whereas fusion of tunics and blood vessels always occurs in the case of the viviparous species studied so far, suggesting that the hemocytes of these species have lost their ability for allorecognition. This can be related to the necessity to prevent the immune system from attacking the brooded embryos, which share only one allele at the Fu/HC locus with the mother colony, and might undergo rejection/resorption, as they are exposed to the circulation for more than a week.[119] In partial confirmation of the above statement, the PO activity of the hemolysate of viviparous species is much lower than that of ovoviviparous ones.[120,121]

5 HUMORAL FACTORS PRODUCED BY HEMOCYTES

5.1 Phenoloxidase

Chaga[122] was the first to describe a DOPA-oxidase activity, ascribable to PO, in ascidians. Today, the presence of PO activity in ascidian hemocytes is widely reported in both solitary and colonial species.[123] PO is assumed to be stored as an inactive proenzyme (proPO) inside the vacuoles of PO-containing hemocytes, and, analogous to what is known in arthropods,[124] is activated by plasmatic serine proteases once released outside the cells.

In solitary species, PO is involved in cytotoxic responses triggered by foreign material[81,82,125]; in colonial ascidians, the enzyme contributes to the formation of the POR along the contact border among genetically incompatible colonies.[85,88,89,109,111,120]

Ascidian POs have a molecular weight ranging between 60 and 90 kDa, in agreement with molecular data predicting a molecular weight of 92 and 87 kDa for *Ciona intestinalis* POs.[31,82,126–128] Electrophoretic data indicate that ascidian PO monomers interact to form dimers.[31,82,126]

The analysis of nucleotide and deduced amino-acid sequences of PO from *C. intestinalis,*[128] *B. schlosseri,* and *P. misakiensis*[123] confirmed their high similarity with arthropod hemocyanins.

5.2 Lectins

Hemocytes are generally considered responsible for the synthesis and release of humoral lectins, the presence of which, in the ascidian hemolymph, has been described in various species.[129] Only in a few cases, a definite role in immunity has been ascertained.[58]

In the solitary species *Halocynthia roretzi*, a 120-kDa lectin, produced by MCs, recognizes LPS and other constituents of the microbial walls and also agglutinates bacteria; it can act as opsonin, facilitating the phagocytosis of microbes.[130]

In *B. schlosseri*, BsRBL can agglutinate yeast, mammalian erythrocytes, and some bacterial strain. At high concentration, the lectin can trigger MC degranulation.[58]

The genes for two galectins of 32 and 37 kDa have been identified in *C. intestinalis*.[131] They are overexpressed after LPS injection in the body wall; in situ hybridization shows that unilocular and multilocular granulocytes contain the specific mRNAs.[132]

5.3 Cytokines

Various reports indicate the presence of molecules with immunomodulatory activity in ascidians,[133] and it is generally believed that they are produced by immunocytes.

In *B. schlosseri,* MCs are the main source of molecules recognized by antibodies raised against mammalian IL1α and TNFα; they are synthesized and released upon the recognition of foreign molecules.[86,107] The same molecules can induce the synthesis and the release in the medium of BsRBL by phagocytes[133]; conversely, BsRBL can stimulate MCs to release molecules immunopositive to anti-IL1α and anti-TNFα antibodies,[58] revealing the existence of a cross-talk between immunocytes.

In *B. schlosseri*, *B. leachii*, and *B. simodensis*, molecules immunopositive to anti-IL1α and anti-TNFα antibodies are produced and released by MCs during the inflammatory reaction due to contact among genetically incompatible colonies[89,112,134]; the same antibodies inhibit both the in vitro cytotoxicity, observed when hemocytes are exposed to cell-free hemolymph from incompatible colonies,[89] and the MC chemotaxis caused by the same hemolymph.[86]

Anti-IL1α and anti-TNFα antibodies can prevent, in vitro, the increase of yeast phagocytosis occurring when *B. schlosseri* hemocytes and yeast cells are incubated in a conditioned medium, that is, the supernatant of hemocyte cultures matched with yeast cells. Fractionation of hemocytes through discontinuous density-gradient centrifugation indicates that the increase in phagocytosis occurs when conditioned media come from hemocyte fractions rich in MCs.[135] The above observations suggest that MCs are the main sentinel cells in the organism, which, upon the recognition of nonself, release cytokines able to recruit other MCs and phagocytes, and stimulate the release of BsRBL by phagocytes, which, in turn, strengthen MC activity and favor phagocytosis of foreign material, allowing for its disposal.[58]

A similar cooperation between MCs and phagocytes has been reported in *C. intestinalis*.[136] In the same species, the synthesis of an inducible lectin with galectin features increases during the inflammation, following intratunic LPS injection. Its opsonizing and hemagglutinating activities are inhibited by anti-human IL1α antibodies.[137] In the *Ciona* genome, putative genes for IL-1 and TNF receptors are present,[54,138] and the analysis of a series of ESTs from *Ciona* hemocytes revealed the presence of transcripts for a putative protein similar to a mammalian IL17 receptor.[138] In addition, a gene for a TNFα homolog has been identified and cloned[54,139]; its transcription increases after LPS injection in the body wall, and its mRNA is located in hemocytes, in particular, granulocytes.[139] It probably exerts its role in recruiting hemocytes to the inflamed area; the same gene is active also during larval development, likely in relation to the migration of mesenchyme cells.[140]

5.4 Complement

Chapter 6: The Evolution of Complement System Functions and Pathways in Vertebrates treats in great detail the activation of a complement system, especially in vertebrates. In ascidians, both the alternative and lectin complement activation-pathways are present. In *H. roretzi*, transcripts for MASP-like proteins, C3, and Bf have been identified.[141–144] In the same species, integrin α and ß subunits are expressed on the surface of hemocytes, probably forming a C3 receptor.[145,146]

In *C. intestinalis*, two genes for C3 (CiC3-1 and CiC3-2) have been described. In situ hybridization indicates that transcription occurs in hemocytes (hyaline and granular amoebocytes, and compartment cells) and in ciliated cells bordering branchial stigmata.[147,148] The transcription of CiC3-1 by hemocytes and the quantity of the fragment CiC3-1a detected by immunohistochemistry increase after LPS injection in the tunic.[148] CiC3-1a exerts a chemotactic role toward hemocytes, recruiting them to the inflammation site[149] through its binding to a 100-kDa, G protein-coupled receptor, constitutively expressed in hyaline and granular amoebocytes.[150] In the same species, three genes (CiBf-1, CiBf-2, and CiBf-3) for complement Bf were described.[151] Moreover, a transcript for a collectins showing similarity for mammalian MBL, located in circulating granulocytes, has been reported: its expression increases after LPS injection in the tunic.[152] As described in more detail in chapter 11: Functions and Diversity of Fibrinogen-Related Domains, transcripts for MASP-like proteins and a ficolin were also identified.[54]

In *S. plicata*, a protein recognized by anti-C3 antibodies is secreted by phagocytes upon the exposure of hemocytes to molecules of bacterial, fungal, and algal origin.[153] In this species, a C-type lectin, similar to mammalian collectins, has been identified.[154]

Recently, in *B. schlosseri*, genes for C3 and Bf have been described: their transcription occurs in MCs, and the opsonic role of C3 was indirectly demonstrated.[155]

5.5 Antibacterial Activity

The involvement of hemocytes in the production of antimicrobial molecules has been demonstrated in *H. roretzi*, where two peptides, halocyamines A and B, are synthesized by MCs.[156] Their cytotoxic activity is probably related to the presence of diphenol rings, which can represent the natural substrate for PO, analogously to tunichromes.[92,157] In *S. clava*, MCs produce four histidine-rich, α-helix peptides, clavanins A–D,[158] which are 23 amino acids in size and isolated from hemocyte lysates.[158,159] In the same species, the transcripts for five putative cationic antimicrobial peptides, called styelins, later isolated from hemocyte lysates, have been identified.[160,161] In *C. intestinalis*, the presence of antibacterial activity in hemocyte lysates was described.[162] Transcriptome analysis allowed the identification of two families of α-helix antimicrobial peptides synthesized by hemocytes; their transcription is enhanced after the inoculum of nonself material in the body wall, and their microbicidal activity is related to their ability to permeabilize plasma membranes of target cells.[163,164]

6 ASCIDIAN HEMOCYTES AND OXIDATIVE STRESS RESPONSE

Phagocytes contain active antioxidant enzymes, such as glutathione S-transferase and glutathione peroxidase, protecting the cells from the ROS that they produce.[165]

In *C. intestinalis*, hemocytes are the site of synthesis of mRNAs coding for detoxifying molecules, such as metallothionein CiMT1, glutathione synthase, γ-glutamyl-cysteine ligase, and phytochelatin synthase. The extent of transcription increases after exposure to Cd.[166–168] *Ciona* hemocytes also represent the sole source, together with ovarian follicle cells, of mRNAs for the superoxide dismutases Ci-SODa and Ci-SODb.[169]

7 HEMOCYTES OF PELAGIC TUNICATES

Few data are currently available on the hemocytes of pelagic tunicates. Larvaceans lack hemocytes,[170,171] whereas some authors, in the past, have described the morphology of thaliacean hemocytes.[171] Recently, Cima et al.[171] have reported a morpho-functional and ultrastructural characterization of the circulating hemocytes of *Thalia democratica* oozooids. Four hemocyte types have been described: undifferentiated cells, phagocytes, granular cells, and storage cells. Phagocytes include amoeboid cells, with hyaline cytoplasm, and cells containing large vacuoles. Both phagocyte types share a similar content of hydrolytic enzymes, can migrate into the tunic and colonize it, and can be found outside of the animal body, adhering to the tunic that embeds the internal lumen of the oral siphon; it probably exerts an immunosurveillance role, similar to the one already described for immunocytes/phagocytic cells in *B. schlos*seri. Granular cells resemble vertebrate mast-cells in having heparin and histamine inside their granules; they do not show any similarity with ascidian cytotoxic cells. Storage cells are represented by nephrocytes, which, like in ascidians, have uric-acid crystals inside their vacuoles.

8 CONCLUDING REMARKS

Hemocytes represent an important constituent of tunicate hemolymph and play fundamental roles in the clearance of nitrogenous catabolites, the detoxification of toxic compounds, the storage of nutrients, and immunosurveillance, assuring the animal survival by coping with foreign, potentially pathogenic microbes entering the organism.

Today, the new sequencing and bioinformatic tools for genome and transcriptome analysis are opening new, interesting, and previously unimaginable perspectives on hemocyte research. The increasing amount of available sequences are shedding new light on hemocyte functions, their activation pathways, mutual cross-talk, and ontogenesis. The possibility of synthesizing (using chemical synthesis of recombinant technology) the gene products once the gene sequence is known, is rendering available a quantity of bioactive molecules produced by hemocytes, such as new antimicrobial peptides or anticancer compounds that could find interesting applications in biomedical and sanitary fields. In addition, future research on hemocytes will surely contribute to clarify unresolved aspects of hemocyte ontogeny and differentiation pathways, and their role in tunicate biology.

REFERENCES

1. Delsuc F, Brinkmann H, Chourrout D, Philippe H. Tunicates and not cephalochordates are the closest living relatives of vertebrates. *Nature* 2006;**439**:965–8.
2. Satoh N, Rokhsar D, Nishikawa T. Chordate evolution and the three-phylum system. *Proc R Soc* 2014;**281B** 20141729.
3. Burighel P, Cloney RA. Urochordata: Ascidiacea. In: Harrison FW, Ruppert EE, editors. *Microscopic anatomy of invertebrates*, vol. 15. Wiley-Liss: New York; 1997. p. 221–347.
4. Ruppert EE, Fox RS, Barnes RD. *Invertebrate zoology: a functional evolutionary approach.* 7th ed. Boston, MA: Thomson Learning Inc; 2004.
5. Satoh N. An advanced filter-feeder hypothesis for urochordate evolution. *Zool Sci* 2009;**26**: 97–111.
6. Swalla BJ, Cameron CB, Corley LS, Garey JR. Urochordates are monophyletic within the deuterostomes. *Syst Biol* 2000;**49**:52–64.
7. Nishino A, Satoh N. The simple tail of chordates: phylogenetic significance of appendicularians. *Genesis* 2001;**29**:36–45.
8. Stach T, Turbeville JM. Phylogeny of Tunicata inferred from molecular and morphological characters. *Mol Phylogenet Evol* 2002;**25**:408–28.
9. Swalla BJ, Smith AB. Deciphering deuterostome phylogeny: molecular, morphological and paleontological perspectives. *Philos Trans R Soc* 2008;**363B**:1557–68.
10. Tsagkogeorga G, Turon X, Hopcroft RR, Tilak MK, Feldstein T, Shenkar N, et al. An updated 18S rRNA phylogeny of tunicates based on mixture and secondary structure models. *BMC Evol Biol* 2009;**9**:187.
11. Goodbody I. The physiology of ascidians. *Adv Mar Biol* 1974;**12**:1–149.
12. Wright RK. Urochordates. In: Ratcliffe NA, Rowley AF, editors. *Invertebrate blood cells*, vol. 2. London: Academic Press; 1981. p. 565–626.
13. Hawkins CJ, Merefield PM, Parry DL, Biggs WR, Swinehart JH. Comparative study of the blood plasma of the ascidians *Pyurastolonifera* and *Ascidia ceratodes*. *Biol Bull* 1980;**159**:656–68.
14. Roman DA, Molina J, Rivera L. Inorganic aspects of the blood chemistry of ascidians. Ionic composition, and Ti, V, and Fe in the blood plasma of Pyurachilensis and Ascidia dispar. *Biol Bull* 1988;**175**:154–66.
15. Ballarin L, Cima F, Sabbadin A. Histoenzymatic staining and characterization of the colonial ascidian *Botryllus schlosseri* hemocytes. *Boll Zool* 1993;**60**:19–24.
16. Cima F, Perin A, Burighel P, Ballarin L. Morpho-functional characterisation of haemocytes of the compound ascidian *Botrylloides leachi* (Tunicata Ascidiacea). *Acta Zool* 2001;**82**:261–74.
17. Ballarin L, Cima F. Cytochemical properties of *Botryllus schlosseri* haemocytes: indications for morpho-functional characterisation. *Eur J Histochem* 2005;**49**:255–64.
18. Ermak TH. The hematogenic tissues of tunicates. In: Wright RK, Cooper EL, editors. *The phylogeny of thymus and bone marrow-bursa cells*. Amsterdam/North Holland: Elsevier; 1976. p. 45–56.

19. Wright RK, Ermak TH. Cellular defense systems of the Protochordata. In: Cohen N, Sigel MM, editors. *The reticuloendothelial system, a comprehensive treatise. Phylogeny and Ontogeny*, vol. 3. New York: Plenum Press; 1982. p. 283–320.

20. Cima F, Ballarin L. Undifferentiated cells in the blood of the colonial ascidian *Botryllus schlosseri*: a morpho-functional characterisation. *Invert Surviv J* 2007;**4**:29.

21. Kawamura K, Tachibana M, Sunanaga T. Cell proliferation dynamics of somatic and germ-line tissues during zooidal life span in the colonial tunicate *Botryllus primigenus*. *Dev Dyn* 2008;**237**:1812–25.

22. Voskoboynik A, Soen Y, Rinkevich Y, Rosner A, Ueno H, Reshef R, et al. Identification of the endostyle as a stem cell niche in a colonial chordate. *Cell Stem Cell* 2008;**3**:456–64.

23. Rinkevich Y, Voskoboynik A, Rosner A, Rabinowitz C, Paz G, Oren M, et al. Repeated, long-term cycling of putative stem cells between niches in a basal chordate. *Dev Cell* 2013;**24**:76–88.

24. De Leo G. Ascidian hemocytes and their involvement in defense reactions. *Boll Zool* 1992;**59**:195–213.

25. Pérès JM. Recherchessurle sang et les organesneuraux des Tuniciers. *Ann Inst Ocean (Monaco)* 1943;**21**:229–359.

26. Sabbadin A. Studio sulle cellule del sangue di *Botryllus schlosseri* (Pallas) (Ascidiacea). *Arch Ital Anat Embriol* 1955;**60**:33–67.

27. Ballarin L, Burighel P, Cima F. A tale of death and life: natural apoptosis in the colonial ascidian *Botryllus schlosseri* (*Urochordata Ascidiacea*). *Curr Pharm Des* 2008;**14**:138–47.

28. Ohtake S, Abe T, Shishikura F, Tanaka K. The phagocytes in hemolymph of *Halocynthia roretzi* and their phagocytic activity. *Zoolog Sci* 1994;**11**:681–91.

29. Lauzon RJ, Brown C, Kerr L, Tiozzo S. Phagocyte dynamics in a highly regenerative urochordate: insights into development and host defense. *Dev Biol* 2013;**374**:357–73.

30. Parrinello N, Cammarata M, Arizza V. Univacuolarrefractile hemocytes from the tunicate *Ciona intestinalis* are cytotoxic for mammalian erythrocytes *in vitro*. *Biol Bull* 1996;**190**:418–25.

31. Parrinello N, Arizza V, Chinnici C, Parrinello D, Cammarata M. Phenoloxidases in ascidian hemocytes: characterization of the prophenoloxidase activating system. *Comp Biochem Physiol* 2003;**135B**:583–91.

32. Arizza V, Parrinello D. Inflammatory hemocytes in *Ciona intestinalis* innate immune response. *Invert Surviv J* 2009;**6**:S58–66.

33. Ballarin L. Ascidian cytotoxic cells: state of the art and research perspectives. *Invert Surviv J* 2012;**9**:1–6.

34. Michibata H. New aspects of accumulation and reduction of vanadium ions in ascidians, based on concerted investigation from both a chemical and biological viewpoint. *Zoolog Sci* 1989;**6**:639–47.

35. Michibata H. The mechanism of accumulation of vanadium by ascidians: some progress towards an understanding of this unusual phenomenon. *Zool Sci* 1996;**13**:489–502.

36. Hirata J, Michibata H. Valency of vanadium in the vanadocytes of *Ascidia gemmata* separated by density-gradient centrifugation. *J Exp Zool* 1991;**257**:160–5.

37. Nette G, Scippa S, Genovese M, De Vincentiis M. Cytochemical localization of vanadium(III) in blood cells of ascidian *Phallusia mammillata* Cuvier, and its relevance to hematic cell lineage determination. *Comp Biochem Physiol* 1999;**122C**:231–7.

38. Sabbadin A, Tontodonati A. Nitrogenous excretion in the compound ascidian *Botryllus schlosseri* (Pallas) and *Botrylloides leachi* (Savigny). *Monit Zool Ital* 1967;**1**:185–90.

39. Milanesi C, Burighel P. Blood cell ultrastructure of the ascidian *Botryllus schlosseri* I. Hemoblast, granulocytes, macrophage, morula cell and nephrocyte. *Acta Zool* 1978;**59**:135–47.

40. Sabbadin A, Graziani G. New data on the inheritance of pigments and pigmentation patterns in the colonial ascidian *Botryllus schlosseri* (Pallas). *Riv Biol* 1967;**60**:559–98.
41. Burighel P, Milanesi C, Sabbadin A. Blood cell ultrastructure of the ascidian *Botryllus schlosseri* L II. Pigment cells. *Acta Zool* 1983;**64**:15–23.
42. Fujimoto H, Watanabe H. The characterization of granular amoebocytes and their possible roles in the asexual reproduction of the polystyelid ascidian Polyzoavesiculiphora. *J Morphol* 1976;**150**:623–38.
43. Sugino YM, Tsuji Y, Kawamura K. An ultrastructural study of blood cells in the ascidian Polyandrocarpamisakiensis: their classification and behavioral characteristics. *Mem Fac Sci Kochi Univ* 1993;**14**:33–41.
44. Ballarin L, Kawamura K. The hemocytes of *Polyandrocarpa misakiensis*: morphology and immune-related activities. *Invert Surviv J* 2009;**6**:154–61.
45. Ballarin L, Burighel P. RGD-containing molecules induce macropinocytosis in ascidian hyaline amoebocytes. *J Invertebr Pathol* 2006;**91**:124–30.
46. Ballarin L, Scanferla M, Cima F, Sabbadin A. Phagocyte spreading and phagocytosis in the compound ascidian *Botryllus schlosseri*: evidence for an integrin-like RGD-dependent recognition mechanism. *Dev Comp Immunol* 2002;**26**:39–48.
47. Sasaki N, Ogasawara M, Sekiguchi T, Kusumoto S, Satake H. Toll-like receptors of the ascidian *Ciona intestinalis*: prototypes with hybrid functionalities of vertebrate toll-like receptors. *J Biol Chem* 2009;**284**:27336–43.
48. Menin A, Ballarin L. Toll-like receptors in haemocytes of the colonial ascidian *Botryllus schlosseri*: preliminary results. *Invert Surviv J* 2007;**4**:31.
49. Menin A, Ballarin L. Exogenous IL-8 induces phagocyte activation in the compound ascidian *Botryllus schlosseri*. *Invert Surviv J* 2006;**3**:18–24.
50. Ballarin L. Immunobiology of compound ascidians, with particular reference to *Botryllus schlosseri*: state of the art. *Invert Surviv J* 2008;**5**:54–74.
51. Ballarin L, Cima F, Sabbadin A. Calcium homeostasis and yeast phagocytosis in hemocytes of the colonial ascidian *Botryllus schlosseri*. *Comp Biochem Physiol* 1997;**118A**:153–8.
52. Ishikawa G, Azumi K, Yokosawa H. Involvement of tyrosine kinase and phosphatidylinositol 3-kinase in phagocytosis by ascidian hemocytes. *Comp Biochem Physiol* 2000;**125A**:351–7.
53. Franchi N, Schiavon F, Betti M, Canesi L, Ballarin L. Insight on signal transduction pathways involved in phagocytosis in the colonial ascidian *Botryllus schlosseri*. *J Invertebr Pathol* 2013;**112**:260–6.
54. Azumi K, De Santis R, De Tomaso A, Rigoutsos I, Yoshizaki F, Pinto MR, et al. Genomic analysis of immunity in a Urochordate and the emergence of the vertebrate immune system: "waiting for Godot". *Immunogenetics* 2003;**55**:570–81.
55. Ballarin L, Cima F, Sabbadin A. Phagocytosis in the colonial ascidian *Botryllus schlosseri*. *Dev Comp Immunol* 1994;**18**:467–81.
56. Cima F, Ballarin L, Sabbadin A. New data on phagocytes and phagocytosis in the compound ascidian *Botryllus schlosseri*. *Ital J Zool* 1996;**63**:357–64.
57. Gasparini F, Franchi N, Spolaore B, Ballarin L. Novel rhamnose-binding lectins from the colonial ascidian *Botryllus schlosseri*. *Dev Comp Immunol* 2008;**32**:1177–91.
58. Franchi N, Schiavon F, Carletto M, Gasparini F, Bertoloni G, Tosatto SCE, et al. Immune roles of a rhamnose-binding lectin in the colonial ascidian *Botryllus schlosseri*. *Immunobiology* 2011;**216**:725–36.
59. Ballarin L, Menin A, Tallandini L, Matozzo V, Burighel P, Basso G, et al. Haemocytes and blastogenetic cycle in the colonial ascidian *Botryllus schlosseri*: a matter of life and death. *Cell Tissue Res* 2008;**331**:555–64.

60. Ballarin L, Schiavon F, Manni L. Natural apoptosis during the blastogenetic cycle of the colonial ascidian *Botryllus schlosseri*: a morphological analysis. *Zool Sci* 2010;**27**:96–102.
61. Cima F, Manni L, Basso G, Fortunato E, Accordi B, Schiavon F, et al. Hovering between death and life: natural apoptosis and phagocytes in the blastogenetic cycle of the colonial ascidian *Botryllus schlosseri*. *Dev Comp Immunol* 2010;**34**:272–85.
62. Cima F, Basso G, Ballarin L. Apoptosis and phosphatidylserine-mediated recognition during the take-over phase of the colonial life-cycle in the ascidian *Botryllus schlosseri*. *Cell Tissue Res* 2003;**312**:369–76.
63. Voskoboynik A, Rinkevich B, Weiss A, Moiseeva E, Reznick AZ. Macrophage involvement for successful degeneration of apoptotic organs in the colonial urochordate *Botryllus schlosseri*. *J Exp Biol* 2004;**207**:2409–16.
64. Cima F, Ballarin L, Gasparini F, Burighel P. External amoebocytes guard the pharynx entry in a tunicate (Ascidiacea). *Dev Comp Immunol* 2006;**30**:463–72.
65. Smith MJ. The blood cells and tunic of the ascidian *Halocynthia aurantium* (Pallas). I. Hematology, tunic morphology, and partition of cells between blood and tunic. *Biol Bull* 1970;**138**:354–78.
66. Smith MJ. The blood cells and tunic of the ascidian *Halocynthia aurantium* (Pallas) II. The histochemistry of blood cells and tunic. *Biol Bull* 1970;**138**:379–88.
67. Hirose E, Ishii T, Saito Y, Taneda Y. Phagocytic activity of tunic cells in the colonial ascidian *Aplidiumyamazii* (Polyclinidae Aplousobranchia). *Zool Sci* 1994;**11**:203–8.
68. Hirose E. Ascidian tunic cells: morphology and functional diversity of free cells outside the epidermis. *Invertebr Biol* 2009;**128**:83–96.
69. Bresciani J, Lützen J. *Gonophysema gullmarensis* (Copepodaparastica), an anatomical and biological study of an endoparasite living in the ascidian *Ascidiella aspersa*: 1. Anatomy. *Cah Biol Mar* 1960;**1**:157–83.
70. Monniot C. *Kystodelphysdrachi* n. g.n.sp., copepode enkystedans une branchie d'ascidie. *Vie Milieu* 1963;**14**:263–73.
71. Dudley PL. A light and electron microscopic study of tissue interactions between a parasitic copepod, *Scolecodeshuntsmani* (Henderson), and its host ascidian *Styela gibbsii* (Stimpson). *J Morphol* 1968;**124**:263–82.
72. Anderson RS. Cellular responses to foreign bodies in the tunicate *Molgula manhattensis* (DeKay). *Biol Bull* 1971;**141**:91–8.
73. Wright RK, Protochordate immunity. I. Primary immune response of the tunicate *Ciona intestinalis* to vertebrate erythrocytes. *J Invertebr Pathol* 1974;**24**:29–36.
74. De Leo G, Parrinello N, Parrinello D, Cassara G, Di Bella MA. Encapsulation response of *Ciona intestinalis* (Ascidiacea) to intratunical erythrocyte injection. I. The inner capsular architecture. *J Invertebr Pathol* 1996;**67**:205–12.
75. Parrinello N, De Leo G, Di Bella MA. Fine structural observations of the granulocytes involved in the tunic inflammatory-like reaction of *Ciona intestinalis* (Tunicata). *J Invertebr Pathol* 1990;**56**:181–9.
76. Shirae M, Hirose E, Saito Y. Behavior of hemocytes in the allorejection reaction in two compound ascidians *Botryllus scalaris* and *Symplegma reptans*. *Biol Bull* 1999;**197**:188–97.
77. Parrinello N, Arizza V, Cammarata M, Parrinello D. Cytotoxic activity of *Ciona intestinalis* (Tunicata) hemocytes: properties of the *in vitro* reaction against erythrocyte targets. *Dev Comp Immunol* 1993;**17**:19–27.
78. Parrinello N, Cammarata M, Lipari L, Arizza V. Sphingomyelin inhibition of *Ciona intestinalis* (Tunicata) cytotoxic hemocytes assayed against sheep erythrocytes. *Dev Comp Immunol* 1995;**19**:31–41.

79. Lipari L, Cammarata M, Arizza V, Parrinello D. Cytotoxic activity of *Styela plicata* hemocytes against mammalian cell targets: I. Properties of the in vitro reaction against erythrocytes. *Anim Biol* 1995;**4**:131–7.

80. Cammarata M, Candore G, Arizza V, Caruso C, Parrinello N. Cytotoxic activity of *Styela plicata* hemocytes against mammalian cell targets: II Properties of the in vitro reaction against human tumour cell lines. *Anim Biol* 1995;**4**:139–44.

81. Cammarata M, Arizza V, Parrinello N, Candore G, Caruso C. Phenoloxidase-dependent cytotoxic mechanism in ascidian (*Styela plicata*) hemocytes active against erythrocytes and K562 tumor cells. *Eur J Cell Biol* 1997;**74**:302–7.

82. Cammarata M, Arizza V, Cianciolo C, Parrinello D, Vazzana M, Vizzini A, et al. The prophenoloxidase system is activated during the tunic inflammatory reaction of *Ciona intestinalis*. *Cell Tissue Res* 2008;**333**:481–92.

83. Arizza V, Parrinello D, Cammarata M, Vazzana M, Vizzini A, Giaramita FT, et al. A lytic mechanism based on soluble phospholypases A2 (sPLA2) and β-galactoside specific lectins is exerted by *Ciona intestinalis* (ascidian) unilocularrefractile hemocytes against K562 cell line and mammalian erythrocytes. *Fish Shellfish Immunol* 2011;**30**:1014–23.

84. Ballarin L, Cima F, Sabbadin A. Morula cells and histocompatibility in the colonial ascidian *Botryllus schlosseri*. *Zool Sci* 1995;**12**:757–64.

85. Ballarin L, Menin A, Franchi N, Bertoloni G, Cima F. Morula cells and non-self recognition in the compound ascidian *Botryllus schlosseri*. *Invert Surviv J* 2005;**2**:1–5.

86. Cima F, Sabbadin A, Zaniolo G, Ballarin L. Colony specificity and chemotaxis in the compound ascidian *Botryllus schlosseri*. *Comp Biochem Physiol* 2006;**145A**:376–82.

87. Ballarin L, Cima F, Sabbadin A. Phenoloxidase and cytotoxicity in the compound ascidian *Botryllusschlosseri*. *Dev Comp Immunol* 1998;**22**:479–92.

88. Ballarin L, Cima F, Floreani M, Sabbadin A. Oxidative stress induces cytotoxicity during rejection reaction in the compound ascidian *Botryllus schlosseri*. *Comp Biochem Physiol* 2002;**133C**:411–8.

89. Cima F, Sabbadin A, Ballarin L. Cellular aspects of allorecognition in the compound ascidian *Botryllus schlosseri*. *Dev Comp Immunol* 2004;**28**:881–9.

90. De Barros CM, Emrich LC, Mello AdA, Da Fonseca RN, Allodi S. Regulation of nitric-oxide production in hemocytes of the ascidian *Phallusia nigra*. *Nitric Oxide Biol Ch* 2014;**38**:26–36.

91. Bruening RC, Oltz EM, Furukawa J, Nakanishi K, Kustin K. Isolation of tunichrome B-1, a reducing blood pigment of the sea squirt Ascidia nigra. *J Nat Prod* 1986;**49**:193–204.

92. Oltz EM, Bruening RC, Smith MJ, Kustin K, Nakanishi K. The tunichromes. A class of reducing blood pigments from sea squirts: isolation, structures, and vanadium chemistry. *J Am Chem Soc* 1988;**110**:6162–72.

93. Sugumaran M, Robinson WE. Structure, biosynthesis and possible function of tunichromes and related compounds. *Comp Biochem Physiol* 2012;**163B**:1–25.

94. García-García E, Gómez-González NE, Meseguer J, García-Ayala A, Mulero V. Histamine regulates the inflammatory response of the tunicate *Styela plicata*. *Dev Comp Immunol* 2014;**46**:382–91 2014.

95. Parrinello N. The reaction of *Ciona intestinalis* L (Tunicata) to subcuticular erythrocyte and protein injection. *Dev Comp Immunol* 1981;**5**(Suppl. 1):105–10.

96. Parrinello N, Patricolo E, Canicattì C. Inflammatory-like reaction in the tunic of *Ciona intestinalis* (Tunicata) I. Encapsulation and tissue injury. *Biol Bull* 1984;**167**:229–37.

97. Vizzini A, Pergolizzi M, Vazzana M, Salerno G, Di Sano C, Macaluso P, et al. FACIT collagen (1alpha-chain) is expressed by hemocytes and epidermis during the inflammatory response of the ascidian *Ciona intestinalis*. *Dev Comp Immunol* 2008;**32**:682–92.

98. Bonura A, Vizzini A, Salerno G, Parrinello D, Parrinello N, Longo V, et al. Cloning and expression of a novel component of the CAP superfamily enhanced in the inflammatory response to LPS of the ascidian *Ciona intestinalis*. *Cell Tissue Res* 2010;**342**:411–21.
99. Reddy AL, Bryan B, Hildemann WH. Integumentary allograft versus autograft reactions in *Ciona intestinalis*: a protochordate species of solitary tunicata. *Immunogenetics* 1975;**7**:584–90.
100. Raftos DA, Tait NN, Briscoe DA. Allograft rejection and alloimmune memory in the solitary urochordate *Styela plicata*. *Dev Comp Immunol* 1987;**11**:343–51.
101. Raftos DA, Tait NN, Briscoe DA. Cellular basis of allograft rejection in the solitary urochordate *Styela plicata*. *Dev Comp Immunol* 1987;**11**:713–25.
102. Parrinello N. Cytotoxic activity of tunicate hemocytes. In: Rinkevich B, Muller WEG, editors. *Invertebrate immunology*. Berlin: Springer-Verlag; 1996. p. 190–217.
103. Oka H. Colony specificity in compound ascidians. The genetic control of fusibility. In: Yukawa H, editor. *Profiles of Japanese science and scientists*. Tokyo: Kodanska; 1970. p. 196–206.
104. Sabbadin A. Le basi genetiche della capacità di fusione fra colonie in *Botryllus schlosseri* (Ascidiacea). *Rend Accad Naz Lincei* 1962;**32**:1021–35.
105. Katow H, Watanabe H. Fine structure of fusion reaction in the compound ascidian *Botryllus primigenus* Oka. *Dev Biol* 1980;**76**:1–14.
106. Zaniolo G, Manni L, Ballarin L. Colony specificity in *Botrylloides leachi*. I. Morphological aspects. *Invert Surviv J* 2006;**3**:125–36.
107. Ballarin L, Franchini A, Ottaviani E, Sabbadin A. Morula cells as the major immunomodulatory hemocytes in ascidians: evidences from the colonial species *Botryllus schlosseri*. *Biol Bull* 2001;**201**:59–64.
108. Hirose E, Saito Y, Watanabe H. A new type of the manifestation of colony specificity in the compound ascidian, *Botrylloides violaceus* Oka. *Biol Bull* 1988;**175**:240–5.
109. Hirose E, Saito Y, Watanabe H. Allogeneic rejection induced by cut surface contact in the compound ascidian, *Botrylloides simodensis*. *Invertebr Reprod Dev* 1990;**17**:159–64.
110. Hirose E, Saito Y, Watanabe H. Subcuticular rejection: an advanced mode of the allogeneic rejection in the compound ascidians *Botrylloides simodensis* and *B. fuscus*. *Biol Bull* 1997;**192**:53–61.
111. Shirae M, Ballarin L, Frizzo A, Saito Y, Hirose E. Involvement of quinones and phenoloxidase in the allorejection reaction in a colonial ascidian *Botrylloides simodensis*: histochemical and immunohistochemical study. *Mar Biol* 2002;**141**:659–65.
112. Ballarin L, Zaniolo G. Colony specificity in *Botrylloides leachi*. II. Cellular aspects of the non-fusion reaction. *Invert Surviv J* 2007;**4**:38–44.
113. Voskoboynik A, Newman AM, Corey DM, Sahoo D, Pushkarev D, Neff NF, et al. Identification of a colonial chordate histocompatibility gene. *Science* 2013;**341**:384–7.
114. Taketa DA, De Tomaso AW. *Botryllus schlosseri* allorecognition: tackling the enigma. *Dev Comp Immunol* 2015;**48**:254–65.
115. Rinkevich B, Douek J, Rabinowitz C, Paz G. The candidate Fu/HC gene in *Botryllus schlosseri* (Urochordata) and ascidians' historecognition—an oxymoron? *Dev Comp Immunol* 2012;**36**:718–27.
116. Rinkevich B. Rejection pattern in botryllid ascidian immunity: the first tier of allorecognition. *Can J Zool* 2005;**83**:101–21.
117. Saito Y, Hirose E, Watanabe H. Allorecognition in compound ascidians. *Int J Dev Biol* 1994;**38**:237–47.
118. Hirose E, Saito Y, Watranabe H. Surgical fusion between incompatible colonies of the compound ascidian *Botrylloides fuscus*. *Dev Comp Immunol* 1994;**18**:287–94.

119. Hirose E. Colonial allorecognition, hemolytic rejection, and viviparity in botryllid ascidians. *Zoolog Sci* 2003;**20**:387–94.
120. Shirae M, Saito Y. A comparison of hemocytes and their phenoloxidase activity among botryllid ascidians. *Zoolog Sci* 2000;**17**:881–91.
121. Okuyama M, Saito Y, Hirose E. Fusion between incompatible colonies of a viviparous ascidian *Botrylloides lentus*. *Invertebr Biol* 2002;**121**:163–9.
122. Chaga OY. Ortho-diphenoloxidase system of Ascidians. *Tsitologia* 1980;**22**:619–25.
123. Ballarin L, Franchi N, Schiavon F, Tosatto SC, Mičetić I, Kawamura K. Looking for putative phenoloxidases of compound ascidians: haemocyanin-like proteins in *Polyandrocarpamisakiensis* and *Botryllus schlosseri*. *Dev Comp Immunol* 2012;**38**:232–42.
124. Akita N, Hoshi M. Hemocytes release phenoloxidase upon contact reaction, an allogeneic interaction, in the ascidian *Halocynthia roretzi*. *Cell Struct Funct* 1995;**20**:81–7.
125. Hata S, Azumi K, Yokosawa H. Ascidian phenoloxidase: its release from hemocytes, isolation, characterisation and physiological roles. *Comp Biochem Physiol* 1998;**119B**:769–76.
126. Frizzo A, Guidolin L, Ballarin L, Sabbadin A. Purification and characterisation of phenoloxidase from the colonial ascidian *Botryllus schlosseri*. *Mar Biol* 1999;**135**:483–8.
127. Immesberger A, Burmester T. Putative phenoloxidase in the tunicate *Ciona intestinalis* and the origin of the arthropod hemocyanin superfamily. *J Comp Physiol* 2004;**174B**:169–80.
128. Cerenius L, Söderhäll K. The prophenoloxidase-activating system in invertebrates. *Immunolog Rev* 2004;**198**:116–26.
129. Ballarin L, Tonello C, Guidolin L, Sabbadin A. Purification and characterization of a humoral opsonin, with specificity for D-galactose, in the colonial ascidian *Botryllus schlosseri*. *Comp Biochem Physiol* 1999;**123B**:115–23.
130. Azumi K, Ozeki S, Yokosawa H, Ishii S. A novel lipopolysaccharide-binding hemagglutinin isolated from hemocytes of the solitary ascidian *Halocynthia roretzi*: it can agglutinate bacteria. *Dev Comp Immunol* 1991;**15**:9–16.
131. Houzelstein D, Gonçalves IR, Fadden AJ, Sidhu SS, Cooper DN, Drickamer K, et al. Phylogenetic analysis of the vertebrate galectin family. *Mol Biol Evol* 2004;**21**:1177–87.
132. Ballarin L, Cammarata M, Franchi N, Parrinello N. Routes in innate immunity evolution: galectins and rhamnose-binding lectins in ascidians. In: Kim S-W, editor. *Marine protein and peptides. Biological activities and applications.* Chichester: Wiley-Blackwell; 2013. p. 185–205.
133. Menin A, Ballarin L. Immunomodulatory molecules in the compound ascidian *Botryllus schlosseri*: evidence from conditioned media. *J Invertebr Pathol* 2008;**99**:275–80.
134. Franchi N, Hirose E, Ballarin L. Cellular aspects of allorecognition in the compound ascidian *Botrylloides simodensis*. *Invert Surviv J* 2014;**11**:219–23.
135. Menin A, Del Favero M, Cima F, Ballarin L. Release of phagocytosis-stimulating factor(s) by morula cells in a colonial ascidian. *Mar Biol* 2005;**148**:225–30.
136. Smith VJ, Peddie CM. Cell cooperation during host defense in the solitary tunicate *Ciona intestinalis* (L). *Biol Bull* 1992;**183**:211–9.
137. Parrinello N, Arizza V, Cammarata M, Giaramita FT, Pergolizzi M, Vazzana M, et al. Inducible lectins with galectin properties and human IL1α epitopes opsonize yeast during the inflammatory response of the ascidian *Ciona intestinalis*. *Cell Tissue Res* 2007;**329**:379–90.
138. Terajima D, Yamada S, Uchino R, Ikawa S, Ikeda M, Shida K, et al. Identification and sequence of seventy-nine new transcripts expressed in hemocytes of *Ciona intestinalis*, three of which may be involved in characteristic cell–cell communication. *DNA Res* 2003;**10**:203–12.
139. Parrinello N, Vizzini A, Arizza V, Salerno G, Parrinello D, Cammarata M, et al. Enhanced expression of a cloned and sequenced *Ciona intestinalis* TNFα-like (CiTNFα) gene during the LPS-induced inflammatory response. *Cell Tissue Res* 2008;**334**:305–17.

140. Parrinello N, Vizzini A, Salerno G, Sanfratello MA, Cammarata M, Arizza V, et al. Inflamed adult pharynx tissues and swimming larva of *Ciona intestinalis* share CiTNFα-producing cells. *Cell Tissue Res* 2010;**341**:299–311.

141. Ji X, Azumi K, Sasaki M, Nonaka M. Ancient origin of the complement lectin pathway revealed by molecular cloning of mannan binding protein-associated serine protease from a urochordate, the Japanese ascidian *Halocynthia roretzi*. *Proc Natl Acad Sci USA* 1997;**94**:6340–5.

142. Ji X, Namikawa-Yamada M, Nakanishi M, Sasaki M, Nonaka M. Molecular cloning of complement factor B from a solitary ascidian: unique combination of domains implicating ancient exon shuffling. *Immunopharmacology* 2000;**49**:43.

143. Nonaka M, Azumi K. Opsonic complement system of the solitary ascidian *Halocynthia roretzi*. *Dev Comp Immunol* 1999;**23**:421–7.

144. Nonaka M, Azumi K, Ji X, Namikawa-Yamada C, Sasaki M, Saiga H, et al. Opsonic complement component C3 in the solitary ascidian *Halocynthia roretzi*. *J Immunol* 1999;**162**:387–91.

145. Miyazawa S, Nonaka M. Characterization of novel ascidian ß integrins as primitive complement receptor subunits. *Immunogenetics* 2004;**55**:836–44.

146. Miyazawa S, Azumi K, Nonaka M. Cloning and characterization of integrin α subunits from the solitary ascidian *Halocynthia roretzi*. *J Immunol* 2001;**166**:1710–5.

147. Marino R, Kimura Y, DeSantis R, Lambris JD, Pinto MR. Complement in urochordates: cloning and characterization of two C3-like genes in the ascidian *Ciona intestinalis*. *Immunogenetics* 2002;**53**:1055–64.

148. Giacomelli S, Melillo D, Lambris JD, Pinto MR. Immune competence of the *Ciona intestinalis* pharynx: complement system-mediated activity. *Fish Shellfish Immunol* 2012;**33**:946–52.

149. Pinto MR, Chinnici CM, Kimura Y, Melillo D, Marino R, Spruce LA, et al. CiC3-1a-mediated chemotaxis in the deuterostome invertebrate *Ciona intestinalis* (Urochordata). *J Immunol* 2003;**171**:5521–8.

150. Melillo D, Sfyroera G, De Santis R, Graziano R, Marino R, Lambris JD, et al. First identification of a chemotactic receptor in an invertebrate species: structural and functional characterization of *Ciona intestinalis* C3a receptor. *J Immunol* 2006;**177**:4132–40.

151. Yoshizaki FY, Ikawa S, Satake M, Satoh N, Nonaka M. Structure and the evolutionary implication of the triplicated complement factor B genes of a urochordate ascidian, *Ciona intestinalis*. *Immunogenetics* 2005;**56**:930–42.

152. Bonura A, Vizzini A, Salerno G, Parrinello N, Longo V, Colombo P. Isolation and expression of a novel MBL-like collectin cDNA enhanced by LPS injection in the body wall of the ascidian *Ciona intestinalis*. *Mol Immunol* 2009;**46**:2389–94.

153. Raftos DA, Robbins J, Newton RA, Nair SV. A complement component C3a-like stimulates chemotaxis by hemocytes from an invertebrate chordate – the tunicate, *Pyura stolonifera*. *Comp Biochem Physiol* 2003;**134A**:377–86.

154. Nair SV, Pearce S, Green PL, Mahajan D, Newton RA, Raftos DA. A collectin-like protein from tunicates. *Comp Biochem Physiol* 2000;**125B**:279–89.

155. Franchi N, Ballarin L. Preliminary characterization of complement in a colonial tunicate: C3 Bf and inhibition of C3 opsonic activity by compstatin. *Dev Comp Immunol* 2014;**46**:430–8.

156. Azumi K, Yokosawa H, Ishii S. Halocyamines: novel antimicrobial tetrapeptide-like substances isolated from the hemocytes of the solitary ascidian *Halocynthia roretzi*. *Biochemistry* 1990;**29**:159–65.

157. Cai M, Sugumaran M, Robinson WE. The crosslinking and antimicrobial properties of tunichrome. *Comp Biochem Physiol* 2008;**151B**:110–7.

158. Menzel LP, Lee IH, Sjostrand B, Lehrer RI. Immunolocalization of clavanins in *Styela clava* hemocytes. *Dev Comp Immunol* 2002;**26**:505–15.

159. Lee IH, Zhao C, Cho Y, Harwig SSL, Cooper EL, Lehrer RI. Clavanins α-helical antimicrobial peptides from tunicate hemocytes. *FEBS Lett* 1997;**400**:158–62.
160. Zhao C, Liaw L, Lee IH, Lehrer RI. cDNA cloning of three cecropin-like antimicrobial peptides (Styelins) from the tunicate *Styela clava*. *FEBS Lett* 1997;**412**:144–8.
161. Taylor SW, Craig AG, Fischer WH, Park M, Lehrer RI, Styelin D. An extensively modified antimicrobial peptide from ascidian hemocytes. *J Biol Chem* 2000;**275**:38417–26.
162. Findlay C, Smith VJ. Antimicrobial factors in solitary ascidians. *Fish Shellfish Immunol* 1995;**5**:645–58.
163. Fedders H, Leippe M. A reverse search for antimicrobial peptides in *Ciona intestinalis*: Identification of a gene family expressed in hemocytes and evaluation of activity. *Dev Comp Immunol* 2008;**32**:286–98.
164. Fedders H, Michalek M, Grötzinger J, Leippe M. An exceptional salt-tolerant antimicrobial peptide derived from a novel gene family of haemocytes of the marine invertebrate *Ciona intestinalis*. *Biochem J* 2008;**416**:65–75.
165. Cima F, Dominici D, Ballarin L, Burighel P. Influence of tributyltin on activity of detoxifying enzyme from haemocytes of a colonial ascidian. *Fresenius Environ Bull* 2002;**11**:573–7.
166. Franchi N, Boldrin F, Ballarin L, Piccinni E. CiMT-1, an unusual chordate metallothionein gene in *Ciona intestinalis* genome: structure and expression studies. *J Exp Zool* 2011;**315A**:90–100.
167. Franchi N, Ferro D, Ballarin L, Santovito G. Transcription of genes involved in glutathione biosynthesis in the solitary tunicate *Ciona intestinalis* exposed to metals. *Aquat Toxicol* 2012;**114-115**:14–22.
168. Franchi N, Piccinni E, Ferro D, Basso G, Spolaore B, Santovito G, et al. Characterization and transcription studies of a phytochelatin synthase gene from the solitary tunicate *Ciona intestinalis* exposed to cadmium. *Aquat Toxicol* 2014;**152**:47–56.
169. Ferro D, Franchi N, Ballarin L, Cammarata M, Mangano V, Rigers B, et al. Characterization and metal-induced gene transcription of two new copper zinc superoxide dismutases in the solitary ascidian *Ciona intestinalis*. *Aquat Toxicol* 2013;**140–141**:369–79.
170. Seeliger O. Tunicata. *Bronn'sKlOrdTier* 1911;**3**.
171. Cima F, Caicci F, Sordino P. The haemocytes of the salp *Thalia democratica* (*Tunicata, Thaliacea*): an ultrastructural and histochemical study in the oozoid. *Acta Zool* 2014;**95**:375–91.

Chapter 3

Lymphocyte Populations in Jawless Vertebrates: Insights Into the Origin and Evolution of Adaptive Immunity

Yoichi Sutoh*, Masanori Kasahara**

*Emory Vaccine Center and Department of Pathology and Laboratory Medicine, Emory University, Atlanta, GA, United States; **Department of Pathology, Hokkaido University Graduate School of Medicine, Sapporo, Japan

1 INTRODUCTION

The human body is thought to have tens of millions of lymphocyte clones, each expressing antigen receptors with distinct specificities. When infected with pathogens, lymphocyte clones expressing specific receptors undergo proliferation and differentiate into effector lymphocytes. Most of these effector lymphocytes die by apoptosis shortly after the elimination of pathogens. Some lymphocytes, however, survive for a long time to build an immunological memory. These lymphocytes—known as memory lymphocytes—enable the host to mount a more prompt and vigorous immune response upon reexposure to the same pathogen. Although the adaptive immune system (AIS) is a complex biological system, its backbone is formed by highly diverse antigen receptors clonally expressed on lymphocytes.

The origin and evolution of the AIS and lymphocytes has attracted the interest of immunologists for a long time. Animals that have received particular attention in this regard are the jawless vertebrates represented by lampreys and hagfish. Studies conducted in the 1960s and 1970s showed that both lampreys and hagfish are capable of producing specific agglutinins against particulate antigens and rejecting skin allografts with immunological memory,[1–8] suggesting that the origin of adaptive immunity can be traced back to the emergence of jawless vertebrates. Consistent with this, jawless vertebrates have blood cells morphologically indistinguishable from mammalian lymphocytes. In lampreys, naive lymphocyte-like cells measure about 10 μm in diameter and have a round shape, with thin cytosol and a large nucleus.[9,10] In electron microscopy, thin

The Evolution of the Immune System. http://dx.doi.org/10.1016/B978-0-12-801975-7.00003-7

heterochromatin is found on the inside rim of the nuclear membrane.[9] After stimulation with particulate antigens such as sheep blood-cells and anthrax spore-coats, the lymphocyte-like cells undergo proliferation, differentiating into plasma cell-like cells with enlarged cytosol that contain well-developed rough endoplasmic reticulum.[11]

Transcriptome analysis revealed that lamprey and hagfish lymphocyte-like cells express many genes whose mammalian counterparts are expressed by lymphocytes, such as the genes coding for a homolog of Spi, B-cell receptor-associated protein (BCAP), GATA2/3, CXC chemokine receptor (CXCR) 4, and CD98.[12–14] However, the transcripts coding for major histocompatibility complex (MHC) molecules, T-cell receptors (TCRs), B-cell receptors (BCRs), or the RAG (recombination activating gene) enzymes were never identified from jawless vertebrates. This was puzzling because, at first glance, it contradicted the earlier studies that clearly demonstrated the ability of jawless vertebrates to reject skin allografts and to produce agglutinins specific for particulate antigens. Ultimately, this puzzle was resolved by the discovery that, instead of TCRs and BCRs, jawless vertebrates use a unique antigen receptor now known as variable lymphocyte receptors (VLR).[15–20]

2 OVERVIEW OF VLRs

2.1 Structure of VLR Proteins and Gene Assembly

VLR was discovered in lampreys as a gene coding for proteins with highly diverse sequences, through the analysis of a cDNA library, enriched for transcripts upregulated in antigen-stimulated lymphocyte-like cells.[21] Structurally, VLRs are a member of the leucine-rich repeat (LRR) family of proteins composed of a signal peptide (SP), an N-terminal LRR cassette (LRRNT), an 18-residue N-terminal LRR cassette (LRR1), a variable number of 24-residue LRR cassettes (LRRV), a 24-residue end LRRV cassette (LRRVe), a 13-residue truncated LRR cassette [also called the connecting peptide (CP)], a C-terminal LRR cassette (LRRCT), and an invariant domain containing a stalk region (Fig. 3.1A). The sequences of the regions ranging from the 3′-half of LRRNT (3′-LRRNT) to the 5′-half of LRRCT (5′-LRRCT) are highly diverse. By contrast, the sequences of the remaining regions—the SP, the 5′-half of LRRNT, the 3′-half of LRRCT, and the stalk region—are invariant.

Remarkably, the *VLR* gene has an incomplete structure incapable of encoding any protein in the genome of nonlymphoid cells, such as erythrocytes; this germline gene encodes only the invariant region of VLR proteins and lacks the sequences coding for the diversity region (Fig. 3.1B). Cassettes such as 3′-LRRNT, LRR1, LRRV, LRRVe, CP, and 5′-LRRCT, constituting the diversity region, are located in multiple copies (sometimes in several hundred copies) in the vicinity of the germline *VLR* gene. During lymphocyte development, the invariant intervening sequence of the

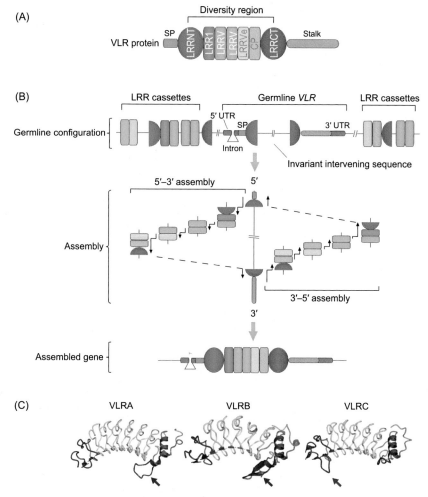

FIGURE 3.1   Domain organization, gene assembly, and tertiary structure of VLRs. (A) Domain organization of mature VLR protein. The diversity region is composed of the following LRR cassettes: the N-terminal LRR cap (LRRNT), LRR1, a variable number of LRRVs, LRRVe, a connecting peptide (CP), and the C-terminal LRR cap (LRRCT). SP, signal peptide. (B) Assembly of *VLR* genes. The germline *VLR* gene has an invariant intervening sequence instead of highly diverse LRR cassettes and is unable to encode functional proteins (top). During lymphocyte development, LRR cassettes, which are scattered around the germline *VLR*, replace the intervening sequence in a stepwise manner from either the 5′- or 3′-end (middle and bottom). This process, which resembles gene conversion, is thought to be mediated by cytidine deaminases of the AID-APOBEC family. (C) Tertiary structure of VLRs. VLR proteins have a horseshoe-shaped structure characteristic of LRR family proteins. The majority of variable amino acid residues are located on the β-sheet, facing the concave surface (shared by all three receptors), and the hypervariable loop in LRRCT (present only in VLRA and VLRB receptors; indicated by *red arrows*). Both ends of the β-sheet are capped by LRRNT and LRRCT (indicated by blue and red, respectively). Unlike VLRA or VLRB, lamprey VLRC has an invariable loop in LRRNT (indicated by a *blue arrow*). Like TCRs and BCRs, all three VLRs lack a signaling domain in the cytoplasmic region. Therefore, it is assumed that VLRs associate with signal transducers yet to be identified.

germline *VLR* gene is replaced by a gene conversion-like mechanism in a stepwise manner, beginning either from its 5′- or 3′-end, by adding flanking cassettes, and eventually forming a completely assembled *VLR* gene.[22-25] Short stretches of nucleotide homology (10–30 bps) are found between donor and acceptor sequences.[24,26,27] Therefore, the sequence located at the ends of the most newly copied cassette presumably determines which flanking LRR cassettes should be copied into the germline *VLR* gene in the next step. The sequences of LRR cassettes are highly variable and the number of copied LRRV cassettes is also variable. This enables assembled *VLR* genes to acquire sequence diversity comparable to that of TCRs and BCRs.[22,24] The assembly of *VLR* genes is mediated by cytidine deaminases (CDA) of the activation-induced cytidine deaminase (AID)-apolipoprotein B mRNA editing enzyme (APOBEC) family.[24] In lampreys, two CDAs named CDA1 and CDA2 have been identified.[24]

2.2   Both Lampreys and Hagfish Have Three *VLR* Genes

Initially, only one *VLR* gene was identified in lampreys.[21] Subsequent studies revealed that lampreys have two more *VLR* genes.[24,28] The three *VLR* genes are now known as *VLRA*, *VLRB*, and *VLRC*. Hagfish also have three *VLR* genes named *VLRA*, *VLRB*, and *VLRC*, thought to be orthologous to lamprey *VLRA*, *VLRB*, and *VLRC* genes,[29,30] indicating that these three genes already existed in a common ancestor of lampreys and hagfish.

Functional studies in lampreys demonstrated that the products of the three *VLR* genes are expressed on three distinct populations of lymphocyte-like cells[31,32] (Fig. 3.2). VLRA and VLRC, which are more closely related to each other in sequence than they are to VLRB, are membrane-bound receptors with no secretory form. VLRA+ cells and VLRC+ cells are T-cell-like and develop in the "thymoid," an organ assumed to be the equivalent of the gnathostome thymus.[33] On the other hand, VLRB is a glycosylphosphatidylinositol-anchored protein that also occurs in a secretory form. Secreted VLRB molecules form pentamers or tetramers of dimers and have 8–10 antigen binding sites.[34] This type of subunit organization resembles the subunit arrangement of gnathostome IgM antibodies and accounts for the strong agglutinating activities of VLRB antibodies. Interestingly, VLRB+ cells are B-cell-like, develop in hematopoietic organs, undergo clonal proliferation in response to antigen stimulation, and differentiate into plasma cell-like cells secreting VLRB antibodies.[11,22,31] Furthermore, similar to the allelic exclusion in *TCR* and *BCR* genes, each lymphocyte expresses only a single functional *VLR* allele, indicating that *VLR* assembly occurs in a monoallelic manner.[21,28,31] Collectively, these observations provided convincing evidence that lymphocyte-like cells in jawless vertebrates resemble gnathostome lymphocytes, not only morphologically, but also functionally, and hence should be regarded as authentic lymphocytes.

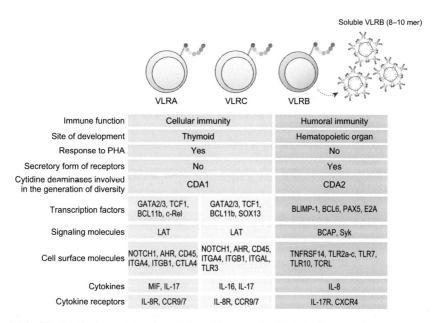

	VLRA	VLRC	VLRB
Immune function	Cellular immunity		Humoral immunity
Site of development	Thymoid		Hematopoietic organ
Response to PHA	Yes		No
Secretory form of receptors	No		Yes
Cytidine deaminases involved in the generation of diversity	CDA1		CDA2
Transcription factors	GATA2/3, TCF1, BCL11b, c-Rel	GATA2/3, TCF1, BCL11b, SOX13	BLIMP-1, BCL6, PAX5, E2A
Signaling molecules	LAT	LAT	BCAP, Syk
Cell surface molecules	NOTCH1, AHR, CD45, ITGA4, ITGB1, CTLA4	NOTCH1, AHR, CD45, ITGA4, ITGB1, ITGAL, TLR3	TNFRSF14, TLR2a-c, TLR7, TLR10, TCRL
Cytokines	MIF, IL-17	IL-16, IL-17	IL-8
Cytokine receptors	IL-8R, CCR9/7	IL-8R, CCR9/7	IL-17R, CXCR4

FIGURE 3.2 **Features of three populations of lamprey lymphocytes.** Lampreys have two lymphocyte lineages whose gene expression profiles resemble gnathostome T cells and B cells, respectively. VLRA and VLRC are membrane-bound receptors without any secretory form. VLRA+ cells and VLRC+ cells express molecules related to T-cell development and/or function. They also secrete IL-17, a pro-inflammatory cytokine released from immune cells, including Th17 cells in jawed vertebrates. VLRC+ cells specifically express genes such as *SOX13*, *ITGAL*, and *TLR3*, which are characteristically expressed in gnathostome γδ T cells. VLRB receptors occur in both membrane-bound and secretory forms. VLRB+ cells express molecules typically expressed in gnathostome B cells.

2.3 Crystal Structure of VLR Proteins and Antigen Recognition

Crystallographic analysis revealed that VLR proteins adopt a horseshoe-like solenoid structure characteristic of the LRR protein family, capped by LRRNT and LRRCT cassettes at N- and C-terminal ends, respectively (Fig. 3.1C).[35] The inner concave surface of the solenoid structure is formed from multiple β-strands (derived from LRRNT, LRR1, LRRV, LRRVe, and CP), which assemble into a continuous β-sheet. In VLRA and VLRB receptors, this β-sheet and a protruding loop formed in the 5′-LRRCT cap contain the majority of variable residues. Structural analysis of VLRB receptors in complex with antigens such as Type O blood antigen (H-trisaccharide) and hen egg-white lysozyme (HEL) demonstrated that VLRB binds antigens via the β-sheet and protruding loop in 5′-LRRCT.[36] Interestingly, the protrusion in 5′-LRRCT penetrated deeply into the catalytic cleft of HEL in the VLRB-HEL complex.[37] Immunoglobulins made up of V_H and V_L chains normally recognize epitopes exposed on the surface of molecules. The ability of VLRs to bind to residues hidden in the cleft is reminiscent of camel and shark V_H antibodies that preferentially target clefts.[38,39]

In one study, lampreys immunized with HEL produced not only specific VLRBs, but also specific VLRAs with binding affinity comparable to that of IgG.[40] The crystal structure of lamprey VLRA in a complex with HEL revealed that VLRA interacts with HEL through its concave surface and LRRCT.[41]

Unlike VLRA or VLRB receptors, VLRC lacks a protrusion in its LRRCT region[28,30,35] (Fig. 3.1C), and its LRRCT is semiinvariant. Also, unlike VLRA or VLRB receptors, the LRRNT of lamprey VLRC has a loop that protrudes into the concave surface.[42,43] This loop shows little sequence variation. These structural features of VLRC suggest that VLRC might recognize antigens in a unique manner. It is possible that VLRC interacts with putative antigen-presenting molecules through its invariant or semiinvariant LRRCT region and LRRNT loop.

2.4 *VLRA* and *VLRC* Genes are Tightly Linked in the Lamprey Genome

VLRA and *VLRC* loci are located close to each other in the lamprey genome.[26] Similar to the gnathostome *TCRA/TCRD* locus that shares some V segments, lamprey *VLRA* and *VLRC* genes often use the same LRR cassettes for their assembly.[44] Such sharing of LRR cassettes is also observed in assembled hagfish *VLRA* and *VLRC* genes, suggesting that *VLRA* and *VLRC* genes are also tightly linked in the hagfish genome. In contrast, neither lamprey nor hagfish VLRB receptors share identical LRR cassettes with the VLRA or VLRC receptors of respective species, suggesting that the germline *VLRB* gene is not situated close to the *VLRA/C* locus. Consistent with this, previous fluorescence in situ hybridization analysis showed that hagfish *VLRB* and *VLRC* (then known as *VLRA*) genes are physically well-separated, although they are on the same chromosome.[45] It appears that *VLR* genes increased their copy number by tandem duplication; subsequently, chromosomal inversion or intrachromosomal translocation presumably separated the *VLRB* gene from the *VLRA/C* genes, facilitating the functional specialization of the receptor genes.

3 THREE POPULATIONS OF AGNATHAN LYMPHOCYTES

3.1 VLRA⁺ Cells and VLRC⁺ Cells Resemble Gnathostome T Cells, Whereas VLRB⁺ Cells Resemble Gnathostome B Cells

VLRA⁺ cells and VLRC⁺ cells resemble gnathostome T cells in that they undergo proliferation in response to a T-cell mitogen such as phytohemagglutinin (PHA). They also resemble T cells in terms of gene expression profiles (Fig. 3.2). For instance, they express transcription factors involved in T-cell development, such as GATA2/3, B-cell CLL/lymphoma 11B (BCL11b), and T-cell factor 1 (TCF1), signaling molecules such as LAT (linker for activation of T cells), cell surface molecules such as NOTCH1, CD45, and aryl hydrocarbon receptor (AHR), cytokines such as IL-17, and cytokine receptors such as chemokine receptor 9/7 (CCR9/7), which regulate the migration of T-cell progenitors to the thymus.[31,32] VLRC$^+$ cells generally have a gene expression profile similar to that of VLRA$^+$ cells, but differ from VLRA$^+$ cells in that they express genes characteristically expressed in gnathostome γδ T cells, such as sex-determining region Y-box 13 (*SOX13*) coding for a fate-determining factor for the γδ T cell lineage, and Toll-like receptor 3 (TLR3).[32] VLRC$^+$ cells also express an integrin family of adhesion molecules involved in the epithelial localization of γδ T cells, such as integrins αL (ITGAL), α4 (ITGA4), and β1 (ITGB1).

On the other hand, VLRB$^+$ cells resemble gnathostome B cells, in that they differentiate into plasma cells and secrete specific VLRB molecules as antibodies, when challenged with particulate antigens.[11] Also, the gene expression profile of VLRB$^+$ cells is similar to that of gnathostome B cells; they express transcription factors such as B-lymphocyte-induced maturation protein 1 (BLIMP-1), B-cell CLL/lymphoma 6 (BCL6), and paired box protein 5 (PAX5), signal-transducing molecules such as spleen tyrosine kinase (Syk) and B-cell adaptor protein (BCAP), and Toll-like receptors such as TLR2a-c, TLR7, and TLR10.

Interestingly, T-cell-like VLRA$^+$ cells express the IL-8 receptor and IL-17, whereas B-cell-like VLRB$^+$ cells express IL-8 and the IL-17 receptor. This observation suggests that VLRA$^+$ and VLRB$^+$ cells may have a cross-talk via cytokines and possibly interact in a manner analogous to T–B cell collaboration[32] (Fig. 3.3).

In rodents, γδ T cells are a minor population of T lymphocytes in blood and peripheral lymphoid tissues; however, they occupy the majority of lymphocytes in epithelial layers of tissues such as skin, intestine, tongue, and the reproductive tract. These intraepithelial γδ T cells express TCRs with limited variability. Most notably, γδ T cells residing in the epidermis, known as dendritic epidermal T cells (DETC), express an invariant Vγ5Vδ1 (alternate nomenclature Vγ3Vδ1) TCR, lacking junctional diversity.[47,48] Interestingly, lamprey VLRC$^+$ cells are located predominantly in epithelial tissues and express restricted antigen receptor diversity, showing intriguing similarity to mouse DETCs and intraepithelial lymphocytes (Fig. 3.2).[49] When stimulated with poly I:C, a synthetic viral double-strand RNA (dsRNA) analog, VLRC$^+$ cells respond via their TLR3 and upregulate IL-16 expression. IL-16 is a chemoattractant recruiting CD4$^+$ leukocytes, such as T cells, monocytes, and eosinophils to the site of infection.[50] Therefore, similar to DETCs, epithelial VLRC$^+$ cells may perform a sentinel function in the epithelium.

3.2   Antigen Recognition by Agnathan T-Like Cells is Still Full of Mystery

When lampreys were immunized with anthrax spores, they generated VLRB$^+$ cells capable of binding to the spores, but VLRA$^+$ cells with such ability were

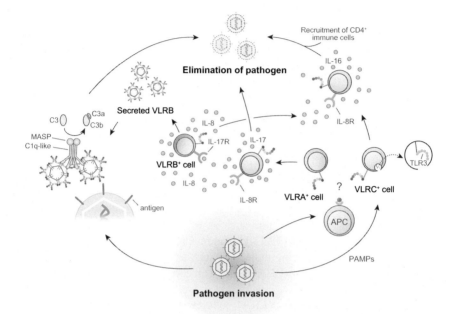

FIGURE 3.3   The presumed role of three populations of agnathan lymphocytes in eliminating pathogens. Invading pathogens are recognized by VLRs with specific binding specificities. VLRC⁺ cells also express TLR3 that recognizes viral double-stranded RNAs. Activated VLRA⁺ cells and VLRC⁺ cells secrete pro-inflammatory cytokines, such as IL-17, MIF, and IL-16, which presumably induce the migration of various immune cells to the site of infection. IL-17 released from VLRA⁺ cells may activate VLRB⁺ cells that express the IL-17 receptor and induce the secretion of VLRB antibodies into the serum. Secreted VLRB antibodies form an antigen–antibody complex that activates the complement pathway via binding to C1q-like protein and mannose-binding lectin-associated serine protease (MASP). VLRB⁺ cells might use IL-8 for cross-talk with VLRA⁺ cells and VLRC⁺ cells that express the IL-8 receptor. It is still uncertain whether jawless vertebrates have antigen-presenting molecules with functions equivalent to MHC molecules. Also unknown is whether VLRA and VLRC require antigen-presenting molecules for antigen recognition. This figure was modified from Sutoh and Kasahara.[46]

not detectable,[29] suggesting that VLRA receptors do not bind native bacterial surface epitopes and might recognize processed antigens in vivo similar to gnathostome αβ T cells. However, screening of a yeast display library resulted in the identification of lamprey VLRA molecules that directly bound to HEL.[40] Although this observation demonstrates that VLRA molecules are capable of binding unprocessed antigens, it is in contrast to the fact that αβ T cells, the presumed counterpart of agnathan VLRA⁺ cells, recognize only processed antigens bound to MHC class I or class II molecules. At present, it remains unknown whether VLRA receptors always recognize antigens without any requirement for antigen processing, or direct antigen recognition occurs only in some or exceptional cases. Also unknown is whether direct recognition occurs in vivo.

Currently, no information is available as to how VLRC$^+$ cells recognize antigens. If VLRC$^+$ cells are γδ T-cell-like, as discussed previously, they might recognize antigens directly in a manner similar to γδ T cells. This is, however, in apparent conflict with the speculation that lamprey VLRC receptors might interact with putative antigen-presenting molecules through their invariant loop in LRRNT and semiinvariant LRRCT. Much remains to be learned about antigen recognition by agnathan T-cell-like lymphocytes.

4 LYMPHOCYTE DEVELOPMENT IN JAWLESS VERTEBRATES

4.1 Development of VLRB$^+$ Cells

B cells develop in hematopoietic organs such as the bone marrow in mammals, the bursa of Fabricius in birds, the pronephros in bony fishes, and the spleen and spiral valves in cartilaginous fishes.[51–53] In adult lampreys, VLRB$^+$ cells are abundant in kidneys and blood. On the other hand, in lamprey larvae, VLRB$^+$ cells are abundant in the typhlosole, an invaginated spiral valve spanning the length of the intestine. Recent flow cytometric analysis showed that 26 and 41% of lymphocytes are VLRB$^+$ cells in typhlosoles and kidneys, respectively.[29] In both organs, cell proliferation was activated within 28 days after immunization by anthrax spore-coats. Moreover, in situ hybridization analysis detected CDA2 expression in VLRB$^+$ cells, in typhlosoles and kidneys supporting the idea that *VLRB* gene assembly occurs in these organs.[33] Although rigorous analysis with molecular markers remains to be conducted, available evidence indicates strongly that VLRB$^+$ cells develop in hematopoietic organs such as typhlosoles and kidneys, consistent with the idea that VLRB$^+$ cells represent B-lineage cells (Fig. 3.4).

4.2 Development of VLRA$^+$ Cells and VLRC$^+$ Cells

In jawed vertebrates, T-lineage progenitors generated in hematopoietic tissues migrate to the thymus. After successful V(D)J recombination of *TCR* genes, T cells are positively and negatively selected in the thymic cortex and medulla, respectively. As a result of thymic selection, only T cells expressing self-tolerant, MHC-restricted TCRs are allowed to survive and exit to the periphery. The thymus was histologically and/or functionally identified in all jawed vertebrates ranging from cartilaginous fish to mammals, consistent with the fact that they have MHC molecules and TCRs. In contrast, jawless vertebrates lack anatomical structures with discrete cortical and medullary regions resembling the thymus. Therefore, it was generally assumed until recently that the thymus emerged in a common ancestor of jawed vertebrates, concomitant with the emergence of TCR, BCR, MHC, and RAG molecules.[54,55] However, the discovery that VLRA$^+$ cells are T-cell-like,[31] and that jawless vertebrates have a genetic network involved in thymopoiesis,[54] initiated a renewed search for a thymus equivalent in lampreys, which led to the identification of the "thymoid"[33] (Fig. 3.4). "Thymoids" are located at the tips of the gill filaments in the gill basket, thus occurring, not

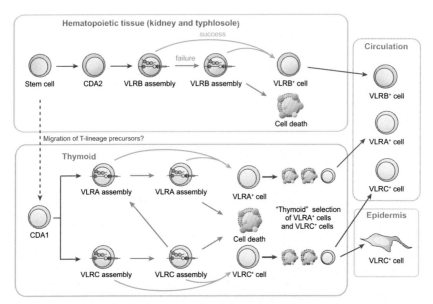

FIGURE 3.4   Lymphocyte development in jawless vertebrates. VLRB$^+$ cells are thought to develop in hematopoietic tissues such as kidneys and typhlosoles. Some lymphocytes in these tissues express a cytidine deaminase named CDA2, assumed to mediate *VLRB* gene assembly (top). On the other hand, VLRA$^+$ cells and VLRC$^+$ cells are thought to develop in an organ named "thymoid," located at the gill tip (bottom). Some lymphocytes in the "thymoid" express a cytidine deaminase named CDA1, assumed to mediate the assembly of *VLRA* and *VLRC* genes. Assembled VLRA and VLRC sequences incapable of encoding functional proteins are frequently observed in the "thymoid." Such nonfunctional gene assembly is rarely seen in circulating lymphocytes and other tissues, suggesting that the assembly of *VLRA* and *VLRC* genes occurs in the "thymoid" and that some sort of quality control mechanism is in operation in the "thymoid." It remains to be examined whether VLRA$^+$ cells and VLRC$^+$ cells are derived from the precursor cells that migrate from the hematopoietic tissue to the "thymoid" in a manner similar to gnathostome T cells. *Orange* and *green arrows* indicate unsuccessful and successful *VLR* gene assembly, respectively.

as a single organ, but as a constellation of specialized lymphoid tissues with no obvious corticomedullary differentiation. In "thymoids," VLRA$^+$ or VLRC$^+$ lymphocytes expressing CDA1 occur in close proximity to pharyngeal epithelial cells expressing FOXN1, a marker of the thymopoietic microenvironment in jawed vertebrates. Also, sequencing of *VLRA* and *VLRC* genes isolated from gill-tip tissues contained nonfunctionally assembled sequences over fourfold more frequently than in peripheral blood cells. Furthermore, VLRA$^+$ cells and VLRC$^+$ cells in peripheral blood, but not in "thymoids" underwent proliferation in response to PHA. These results suggest that the "thymoid" is a primary, rather than a secondary, lymphoid organ.[33] The thymus and the gill are both derived from the pharyngeal arch, and the thymus is located in the vicinity of the gill in cartilaginous and bony fishes. Therefore, the thymus and the "thymoid" appear to be homologous rather than analogous organs.

4.3   Cell Fate Determination of VLRA⁺ Cells and VLRC⁺ Cells

VLRB⁺ cells never express the *VLRA* gene nor the *VLRC* gene. Conversely, neither VLRA⁺ nor VLRC⁺ cells express the *VLRB* gene, consistent with the observation that the assembly of *VLRA/C* and *VLRB* genes occur in different primary lymphoid organs. In contrast, VLRA⁺ cells sometimes express incompletely assembled, nonfunctional *VLRC* transcripts. Likewise, a fraction of VLRC⁺ cells expresses incompletely assembled, nonfunctional *VLRA* transcripts, indicating that the assembly of *VLRA* and *VLRC* genes occurs concomitantly or sequentially. When analyzed by genomic PCR, the assembly of the *VLRA* gene was hardly found in VLRC⁺ cells. In contrast, the assembly of the *VLRC* gene was observed in the majority of VLRA⁺ cells, although 79% of assembly was nonproductive. The higher frequency of nonfunctional *VLRC* assembly in VLRA⁺ cells than nonfunctional *VLRA* assembly in VLRC⁺ cells suggests that the assembly of the *VLRC* gene precedes that of the *VLRA* gene, and that the germline *VLRA* gene undergoes assembly when both copies of the germline *VLRC* gene fail to undergo successful assembly.

4.4   Evidence for Selection in "Thymoids"

Accumulating evidence suggests that selection, somewhat similar to thymic selection, may be operating on VLRA⁺ cells and VLRC⁺ cells. On average, VLRB receptors have about 1.5 LRRV cassettes (excluding LRRVe), with the copy number of LRRV cassettes showing the binomial distribution.[56] In contrast, the average number of LRRV cassettes is about 3 in VLRA/VLRC receptors, and the copy number distribution of LRRV cassettes deviates from the binomial distribution, mainly because transcripts with two or fewer LRRV cassettes occur infrequently, thus suggesting that the VLRA/VLRC receptors with two or fewer LRRV cassettes may be selected against. Indeed, nonfunctional *VLRC* transcripts in VLRA⁺ cells shows greater variation in the copy number of LRRV cassettes than functional *VLRC* transcripts in VLRC⁺ cells.[42] Furthermore, the copy number of LRRV cassettes shows greater variation in *VLRC* transcripts isolated from the "thymoid" than in those isolated from the peripheral blood.[42] These observations suggest that VLRA/VLRC receptors expressed on the surface of lymphocytes are selected in the "thymoid". The observation that caspase-3 positive cells are frequently found in the "thymoid"[33] is also consistent with this suggestion. Interestingly, the second LRRV module in *VLRA/C*, but not *VLRB* transcripts, has distinctive sequence signatures. Therefore, the presumed selection in "thymoids" may influence not only the copy number of LRRV modules, but also the sequences in the second LRRV module.[56]

4.5   Evolution of Lymphocytes in Vertebrates

Jawless vertebrates have two major lineages of lymphocytes: one resembling gnathostome T cells and the other resembling gnathostome B cells.[31] Therefore, it is very likely that a common ancestor of jawed and jawless vertebrates had two lymphocyte lineages: one specialized for cellular immunity, and the other endowed with phagocytic activity but also oriented toward humoral immunity. It appears that jawless and jawed vertebrates then coopted different antigen receptors within the context of such lymphocyte lineages (Fig. 3.5). Because there is no evidence that urochordates (ascidians and other tunicates, described in chapter: Origin and Functions of Tunicate Hemocytes) or cephalochordates (amphioxus or lancelets) have lymphocytes, an ancestral lymphocyte appears to have emerged in the vertebrate lineage after it diverged from the invertebrate lineages of chordates. (For further discussion about the evolution of vertebrate lymphocytes, see chapter: The Evolution of Lymphocytes in Ectothermic Gnathostomata.)

Like jawed vertebrates, lampreys have two lineages of T-cell-like cells, with VLRA$^+$ cells and VLRC$^+$ cells resembling $\alpha\beta$ and $\gamma\delta$ T cells, respectively, in terms of gene expression profiles and tissue distribution.[32] Therefore, not only the separation of lymphocyte lineages into T-cell-like and B-cell-like cells, but also the separation of T-cell-like cells into $\alpha\beta$ T-like and $\gamma\delta$ T-like cells appears to have taken place in a common ancestor of vertebrates.

Searches for immunoglobulin superfamily proteins in jawless vertebrates identified potential evolutionary precursors of TCR/BCR, such as the lamprey "TCR-like gene" coding for an immunoreceptor tyrosine-based inhibition motif-bearing membrane protein, with one V-type and one C2-type immunoglobulin-like domain,[57] and "agnathan paired receptors resembling antigen receptors" (APAR) of hagfish, having a single extracellular V-type immunoglobulin-like domain with a canonical J segment.[58] The occurrence of these receptors in jawless vertebrates indicates that a common ancestor of jawed and jawless vertebrates had V-type immunoglobulin-like domains that could evolve into those of TCR/BCR.[59] On the other hand, VLR is assumed to have emerged from a glycoprotein Ibα (GPIbα)-like protein, a component of the platelet glycoprotein-receptor complex conserved in all vertebrates.[24] Therefore, it is likely that a common ancestor of jawed and jawless vertebrates possessed building blocks for both VLR-like and TCR/BCR-like receptors. Hence, it is reasonable to assume that a common ancestor of vertebrates had the potential for developing both VLR-based and TCR/BCR-based adaptive immunity. Then, what kind of receptors did a common ancestor of vertebrates use for antigen recognition?

A key observation in addressing this question is that both jawed and jawless vertebrates have cytidine deaminases of the AID/APOPEC family. In jawless vertebrates, two cytidine deaminases named CDA1 and CDA2 generate diversity of VLRs by a gene-conversion-like mechanism.[24] In jawed vertebrates, AID is involved in gene conversion, class switch recombination, and somatic hypermutation,[60] thus having functions overlapping with those of CDA1 and CDA2. Furthermore, in some animals, such as rabbits, sheep, and chickens, AID plays a major role in the diversification of antibody repertoire.[61] In contrast, the RAG enzymes involved in the V(D)J recombination of *TCR/BCR* genes are of transposon origin[62–64] and are present only in jawed vertebrates. These observations

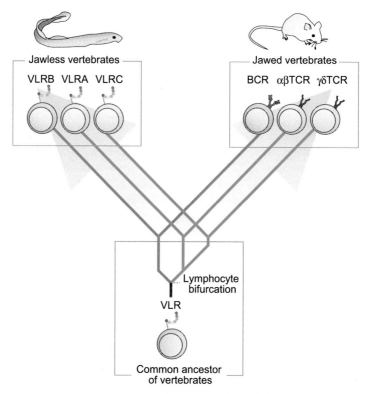

FIGURE 3.5 **Origin and evolution of lymphocytes in vertebrates.** Available evidence indicates that three lineages of lymphocytes (two T-cell-like and one B-cell-like lineage) emerged in a common ancestor of jawed and jawless vertebrates. This common ancestor most likely possessed cytidine deaminases (CDA) and VLR-like antigen receptors because CDA and GPIbα are present in both jawed and jawless vertebrate lineages. This ancestor also appears to have possessed potential precursors of TCRs/BCRs that became the targets of RAG insertion. Because the RAG enzymes are present only in the jawed vertebrate lineage, this insertion appears to have occurred only in a common ancestor of jawed vertebrates. Therefore, it is likely that a common ancestor of jawed and jawless vertebrates had an AIS based on VLRs and CDAs, and that this AIS was superseded by a more efficient TCR/BCR-based AIS in the jawed vertebrate lineage after the acquisition of RAG enzymes.

suggest that a common ancestor of jawed and jawless vertebrates probably used VLR-like receptors and employed the members of the AID/APOPEC family to generate the diversity of their antigen receptors. Presumably, VLRs were superseded by TCRs and BCRs in the jawed-vertebrate lineage because the acquisition of RAG transposons enabled the development of a more efficient and powerful antigen-recognition system.[16,65] The RAG transposon is thought to have been inserted into an ancestor of *TCR/BCR* genes. Therefore, the functional specialization of a gnathostome antigen-receptor into TCRs and BCRs, and then of the former into αβTCRs and γδTCRs, must have occurred under the strong functional constraint of the three lineages of specialized lymphocytes.

5 CONCLUSIONS

Despite the fact that jawed and jawless vertebrates use structurally unrelated receptors for antigen recognition, their AISs have much in common. Particularly striking is the conservation of lymphocyte lineages. Extant invertebrates, either protostomes or deuterostomes, lack lymphocytes. Therefore, it appears that T- and B-lymphocyte lineages specialized for cellular and humoral arms of adaptive immunity emerged in a common ancestor of jawed and jawless vertebrates.

Jawless vertebrates have neither MHC class I nor MHC class II molecules.[19,66,67] An important issue that remains unanswered is whether jawless vertebrates have antigen-presenting molecules with functions equivalent to gnathostome MHC molecules. The observation that VLRC+ cells (and presumably VLRA+ cells as well) undergo selection in the "thymoid"[42] suggests that jawless vertebrates have antigen-presenting molecules with functions equivalent to those of MHC molecules. The basic design of the AIS is well-conserved between jawed and jawless vertebrates, most likely because the lymphocyte lineages had been established in their common ancestor.[16,20] Given the overall similarity of the gnathostome and agnathan AISs, it seems likely that jawless vertebrates have antigen-presenting molecules that function as substitutes of gnathostome MHC molecules.

ACKNOWLEDGMENTS

This work has been supported by Grants-in-Aid for Scientific Research from The Ministry of Education, Culture, Sports, Science and Technology (MEXT) of Japan. We thank Dr Yukiko Miyatake for her kind help with the preparation of figures.

REFERENCES

1. Finstad J, Good RA. The evolution of the immune response III. Immunologic responses in the lamprey. *J Exp Med* 1964;**120**:1151–68.
2. Fujii T, Nakagawa H, Murakawa S. Immunity in lamprey II. Antigen-binding responses to sheep erythrocytes and hapten in the ammocoete. *Dev Comp Immunol* 1979;**3**:609–20.
3. Linthicum DS, Hildemann WH. Immunologic responses of Pacific hagfish III. Serum antibodies to cellular antigens. *J Immunol* 1970;**105**:912–8.
4. Litman GW, Finstad FJ, Howell J, Pollara BW, Good RA. The evolution of the immune response III. Structural studies of the lamprey immunoglobulin. *J Immunol* 1970;**105**:1278–85.
5. Marchalonis JJ, Edelman GM. Phylogenetic origins of antibody structure III. Antibodies in the primary immune response of the sea lamprey, petromyzon marinus. *J Exp Med* 1968;**127**:891–914.
6. Pollara B, Litman GW, Finstad J, Howell J, Good RA. The evolution of the immune response VII. Antibody to human "O" cells and properties of the immunoglobulin in lamprey. *J Immunol* 1970;**105**:738–45.
7. Acton RT, Weinheimer PF, Hildemann WH, Evans EE. Induced bactericidal response in the hagfish. *J Bacteriol* 1969;**99**:626–8.
8. Perey DY, Finstad J, Pollara B, Good RA. Evolution of the immune response VI. First and second set skin homograft rejections in primitive fishes. *Lab Invest* 1968;**19**:591–7.

9. Fujii T. Electron microscopy of the leucocytes of the typhlosole in ammocoetes, with special attention to the antibody-producing cells. *J Morphol* 1982;**173**:87–100.

10. Mayer WE, Uinuk-Ool T, Tichy H, Gartland LA, Klein J, Cooper MD. Isolation and characterization of lymphocyte-like cells from a lamprey. *Proc Natl Acad Sci USA* 2002;**99**:14350–5.

11. Alder MN, Herrin BR, Sadlonova A, Stockard CR, Grizzle WE, Gartland LA, et al. Antibody responses of variable lymphocyte receptors in the lamprey. *Nat Immunol* 2008;**9**:319–27.

12. Shintani S, Terzic J, Sato A, Saraga-Babic M, O'hUigin C, Tichy H, et al. Do lampreys have lymphocytes? The spi evidence. *Proc Natl Acad Sci USA* 2000;**97**:7417–22.

13. Suzuki T, Shin IT, Kohara Y, Kasahara M. Transcriptome analysis of hagfish leukocytes: a framework for understanding the immune system of jawless fishes. *Dev Comp Immunol* 2004;**28**:993–1003.

14. Uinuk-Ool T, Mayer WE, Sato A, Dongak R, Cooper MD, Klein J. Lamprey lymphocyte-like cells express homologs of genes involved in immunologically relevant activities of mammalian lymphocytes. *Proc Natl Acad Sci USA* 2002;**99**:14356–61.

15. Boehm T, McCurley N, Sutoh Y, Schorpp M, Kasahara M, Cooper MD. VLR-based adaptive immunity. *Annu Rev Immunol* 2012;**30**:203–20.

16. Kasahara M, Sutoh Y. Two forms of adaptive immunity in vertebrates: similarities and differences. *Adv Immunol* 2014;**122**:59–90.

17. Pancer Z, Cooper MD. The evolution of adaptive immunity. *Annu Rev Immunol* 2006;**24**:497–518.

18. Cooper MD, Alder MN. The evolution of adaptive immune systems. *Cell* 2006;**124**:815–22.

19. Flajnik MF, Kasahara M. Origin and evolution of the adaptive immune system: genetic events and selective pressures. *Nat Rev Genet* 2010;**11**:47–59.

20. Boehm T. Design principles of adaptive immune systems. *Nat Rev Immunol* 2011;**11**:307–17.

21. Pancer Z, Amemiya CT, Ehrhardt GR, Ceitlin J, Gartland GL, Cooper MD. Somatic diversification of variable lymphocyte receptors in the agnathan sea lamprey. *Nature* 2004;**430**:174–80.

22. Alder MN, Rogozin IB, Iyer LM, Glazko GV, Cooper MD, Pancer Z. Diversity and function of adaptive immune receptors in a jawless vertebrate. *Science* 2005;**310**:1970–3.

23. Nagawa F, Kishishita N, Shimizu K, Hirose S, Miyoshi M, Nezu J, et al. Antigen-receptor genes of the agnathan lamprey are assembled by a process involving copy choice. *Nat Immunol* 2007;**8**:206–13.

24. Rogozin IB, Iyer LM, Liang L, Glazko GV, Liston VG, Pavlov YI, et al. Evolution and diversification of lamprey antigen receptors: evidence for involvement of an AID-APOBEC family cytosine deaminase. *Nat Immunol* 2007;**8**:647–56.

25. Kishishita N, Nagawa F. Evolution of adaptive immunity: implications of a third lymphocyte lineage in lampreys. *Bioessays* 2014;**36**:244–50.

26. Das S, Hirano M, Aghaallaei N, Bajoghli B, Boehm T, Cooper MD. Organization of lamprey variable lymphocyte receptor C locus and repertoire development. *Proc Natl Acad Sci USA* 2013;**110**:6043–8.

27. Das S, Li J, Hirano M, Sutoh Y, Herrin BR, Cooper MD. Evolution of two prototypic T cell lineages. *Cell Immunol* 2015;**296**:87–94.

28. Kasamatsu J, Sutoh Y, Fugo K, Otsuka N, Iwabuchi K, Kasahara M. Identification of a third variable lymphocyte receptor in the lamprey. *Proc Natl Acad Sci USA* 2010;**107**:14304–8.

29. Pancer Z, Saha NR, Kasamatsu J, Suzuki T, Amemiya CT, Kasahara M, et al. Variable lymphocyte receptors in hagfish. *Proc Natl Acad Sci USA* 2005;**102**:9224–9.

30. Li J, Das S, Herrin BR, Hirano M, Cooper MD. Definition of a third *VLR* gene in hagfish. *Proc Natl Acad Sci USA* 2013;**110**:15013–8.

31. Guo P, Hirano M, Herrin BR, Li J, Yu C, Sadlonova A, et al. Dual nature of the adaptive immune system in lampreys. *Nature* 2009;**459**:796–802.

32. Hirano M, Guo P, McCurley N, Schorpp M, Das S, Boehm T, et al. Evolutionary implications of a third lymphocyte lineage in lampreys. *Nature* 2013;**501**:435–8.

33. Bajoghli B, Guo P, Aghaallaei N, Hirano M, Strohmeier C, McCurley N, et al. A thymus candidate in lampreys. *Nature* 2011;**470**:90–4.

34. Herrin BR, Alder MN, Roux KH, Sina C, Ehrhardt GR, Boydston JA, et al. Structure and specificity of lamprey monoclonal antibodies. *Proc Natl Acad Sci USA* 2008;**105**:2040–5.

35. Kim HM, Oh SC, Lim KJ, Kasamatsu J, Heo JY, Park BS, et al. Structural diversity of the hagfish variable lymphocyte receptors. *J Biol Chem* 2007;**282**:6726–32.

36. Han BW, Herrin BR, Cooper MD, Wilson IA. Antigen recognition by variable lymphocyte receptors. *Science* 2008;**321**:1834–7.

37. Velikovsky CA, Deng L, Tasumi S, Iyer LM, Kerzic MC, Aravind L, et al. Structure of a lamprey variable lymphocyte receptor in complex with a protein antigen. *Nat Struct Mol Biol* 2009;**16**:725–30.

38. Stanfield RL, Dooley H, Flajnik MF, Wilson IA. Crystal structure of a shark single-domain antibody V region in complex with lysozyme. *Science* 2004;**305**:1770–3.

39. De Genst E, Silence K, Decanniere K, Conrath K, Loris R, Kinne J, et al. Molecular basis for the preferential cleft recognition by dromedary heavy-chain antibodies. *Proc Natl Acad Sci USA* 2006;**103**:4586–91.

40. Tasumi S, Velikovsky CA, Xu G, Gai SA, Wittrup KD, Flajnik MF, et al. High-affinity lamprey VLRA and VLRB monoclonal antibodies. *Proc Natl Acad Sci USA* 2009;**106**:12891–6.

41. Deng L, Velikovsky CA, Xu G, Iyer LM, Tasumi S, Kerzic MC, et al. A structural basis for antigen recognition by the T cell-like lymphocytes of sea lamprey. *Proc Natl Acad Sci USA* 2010;**107**:13408–13.

42. Holland SJ, Gao M, Hirano M, Iyer LM, Luo M, Schorpp M, et al. Selection of the lamprey VLRC antigen receptor repertoire. *Proc Natl Acad Sci USA* 2014;**111**:14834–9.

43. Kanda R, Sutoh Y, Kasamatsu J, Maenaka K, Kasahara M, Ose T. Crystal structure of the lamprey variable lymphocyte receptor C reveals an unusual feature in its N-terminal capping module. *PLoS ONE* 2014;**9**:e85875.

44. Das S, Li J, Holland SJ, Iyer LM, Hirano M, Schorpp M, et al. Genomic donor cassette sharing during VLRA and VLRC assembly in jawless vertebrates. *Proc Natl Acad Sci USA* 2014;**111**:14828–33.

45. Kasamatsu J, Suzuki T, Ishijima J, Matsuda Y, Kasahara M. Two variable lymphocyte receptor genes of the inshore hagfish are located far apart on the same chromosome. *Immunogenetics* 2007;**59**:329–31.

46. Sutoh Y, Kasahara M. The immune system of agnathans (jawless vertebrates). In: Ratcliffe MJH, editor. *Encyclopedia of Immunobiology*. Cambridge (Massachusetts, USA): Academic Press, Elsevier; 2016.

47. Girardi M. Immunosurveillance and immunoregulation by γδ T cells. *J Invest Dermatol* 2006;**126**:25–31.

48. Hayday AC. γδ cells: a right time and a right place for a conserved third way of protection. *Annu Rev Immunol* 2000;**18**:975–1026.

49. Vantourout P, Hayday A, Six-of-the-best. Unique contributions of γδ T cells to immunology. *Nat Rev Immunol* 2013;**13**:88–100.

50. Cruikshank WW, Kornfeld H, Center DM. Interleukin-16. *J Leukoc Biol* 2000;**67**:757–66.

51. Cooper MD, Peterson RD, Good RA. Delineation of the thymic and bursal lymphoid systems in the chicken. *Nature* 1965;**205**:143–6.

52. Hansen JD, Zapata AG. Lymphocyte development in fish and amphibians. *Immunol Rev* 1998;**166**:199–220.

53. Glick G, Chang TS, Jaap RG. The bursa of Fabricius and antibody production. *Poultry Sci* 1956;**35**:224–34.
54. Bajoghli B, Aghaallaei N, Hess I, Rode I, Netuschil N, Tay BH, et al. Evolution of genetic networks underlying the emergence of thymopoiesis in vertebrates. *Cell* 2009;**138**:186–97.
55. Amemiya CT, Saha NR, Zapata A. Evolution and development of immunological structures in the lamprey. *Curr Opin Immunol* 2007;**19**:535–41.
56. Sutoh Y, Kasahara M. Copy number and sequence variation of leucine-rich repeat modules suggests distinct functional constraints operating on variable lymphocyte receptors expressed by agnathan T cell-like and B cell-like lymphocytes. *Immunogenetics* 2014;**66**:403–9.
57. Pancer Z, Mayer WE, Klein J, Cooper MD. Prototypic T. Cell receptor and CD4-like coreceptor are expressed by lymphocytes in the agnathan sea lamprey. *Proc Natl Acad Sci USA* 2004;**101**:13273–8.
58. Suzuki T, Shin IT, Fujiyama A, Kohara Y, Kasahara M. Hagfish leukocytes express a paired receptor family with a variable domain resembling those of antigen receptors. *J Immunol* 2005;**174**:2885–91.
59. Kasahara M, Kasamatsu J, Sutoh Y. Two types of antigen receptor systems in vertebrates. *Zoolog Sci* 2008;**25**:969–75.
60. Honjo T, Muramatsu M, Fagarasan S. AID: how does it aid antibody diversity? *Immunity* 2004;**20**:659–68.
61. Flajnik MF. Comparative analyses of immunoglobulin genes: surprises and portents. *Nat Rev Immunol* 2002;**2**:688–98.
62. Schatz DG, Swanson PC. V(D)J recombination: mechanisms of initiation. *Annu Rev Genet* 2011;**45**:167–202.
63. Kapitonov VV, Jurka J. RAG1 core and V(D)J recombination signal sequences were derived from transib transposons. *PLoS Biol* 2005;**3**:e181.
64. Kim MS, Lapkouski M, Yang W, Gellert M. Crystal structure of the V(D)J recombinase RAG1-RAG2. *Nature* 2015;**518**:507–11.
65. Kato L, Stanlie A, Begum NA, Kobayashi M, Aida M, Honjo T. An evolutionary view of the mechanism for immune and genome diversity. *J Immunol* 2012;**188**:3559–66.
66. Flajnik MF, Kasahara M. Comparative genomics of the MHC: glimpses into the evolution of the adaptive immune system. *Immunity* 2001;**15**:351–62.
67. Smith JJ, Kuraku S, Holt C, Sauka-Spengler T, Jiang N, Campbell MS, et al. Sequencing of the sea lamprey (*Petromyzon marinus*) genome provides insights into vertebrate evolution. *Nat Genet* 2013;**45**:415–21.

Chapter 4

The Evolution of Lymphocytes in Ectothermic Gnathostomata

Giuseppe Scapigliati, Francesco Buonocore
Department for Innovative Biology, Agro-Industry and Forestry, University of Tuscia, Viterbo, Italy

1 INTRODUCTION

Lymphocytes of vertebrates could be regarded as the direct successors of invertebrate immunocytes, in which the evolution shaped new functional defense activities coded by sets of new genes. This hypothesis can be drawn by observing the documented events that accompanied the origin of vertebrates.[1] A first whole-genome duplication occurred in chordates about 550 million years ago[2,3] and originated agnathan vertebrates that were provided with activation-induced cytidine deaminase (CDA) enzymes,[4] which were able to promote ordered shuffling of gene segments, known as somatic recombination, and also clonal cells that produce recombined antigen-recognizing molecules, or lymphocytes. The secreted or cell surface-associated antigen-recognizing molecules (antibodies) of agnathans are made of recombined peptides having leucine-rich repeats (LRR) motifs.[5]

A subsequent genome duplication event around 300 million years ago produced vertebrates with jaws, or gnathostomes, in which, by means of paralogous evolutionary mechanisms, the nonself recognition machinery is organized in a diverse assembly. Antigen and nonself sensing is based on immunocytes armed with receptors made of LRR motifs (Toll-like receptors, TLR), whereas effector lymphocytes use antibodies constituted by immunoglobulin (Ig)-based molecular motifs. These events have been reviewed more in detail in recent work,[6,7] and summarized in Fig. 4.1.

In gnathostomes, representing approximately 2% of extant metazoan species, immune defenses are based on innate-plus acquired systems, and, on the basis of available knowledge, it is henceforth conceivable to speculate on a difference between the "relative amounts" of innate and acquired responses in aquatic and terrestrial gnathostome species (GSP). Indeed, by analyzing cellular and molecular activities involved in antigen recognition, elimination, and memory, it

The Evolution of the Immune System. http://dx.doi.org/10.1016/B978-0-12-801975-7.00004-9

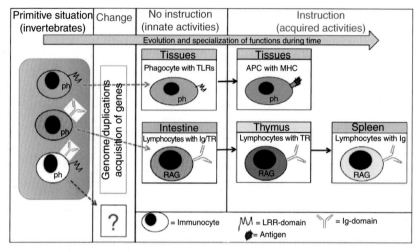

FIGURE 4.1 **Evolution of immunocytes.** In the primitive situation present in invertebrates, immunocytes are armed with antigen-sensing molecules composed of motifs based on LRR, Ig, or both. Genome duplications changed the situation in vertebrates, where immunocytes armed with LRR became phagocytes (ph) with TLRs, and lymphocytes armed with Ig/TRγδ became innate-type lymphocytes not requiring instruction from antigen-presenting cells (APC). By subsequent specializations, some phagocytes processed the antigen, and, together with MHC, became APC, whereas lymphocytes colonized lymphoid tissues and differentiated in Ig-retaining cells (T cells), or Ig-shedding cells (B cells).

appears that fishes rely on a predominance of innate responses, whereas avian and mammals have developed more finely tuned acquired-responses. A possible explanation of this observation might be found in the diverse exposure of aquatic and terrestrial GSP to their surrounding microbiomes because in a water environment the diffusion of pathogens can be easier and faster than in an aerial (terrestrial) environment. As a consequence of this, fishes are armed with a mucosa-associated innate system capable of fast antigen-recognition and elimination. In addition, recent evidence has shown that some fish species lack of fundamental component of acquired responses such as IgM genes,[8] specific IgM production,[9] or an entire subset of T-helper responses or MHC$_{II}$ genes.[10,11]

A "big event" in the evolutionary history of vertebrates was the acquisition of jaws, which permitted in early GSP the swallowing of large-sized food, with possible consequent injuries to the intestinal tract. It can be speculated that these possible injuries could have permitted the entry of pathogens through the intestinal mucosa, and that, in turn, gut-associated immunocytes faced this new situation with novel Gnathostome-associated genes. Among these genes, the recombination-activating genes (RAG) coded for enzymes were able to shuffle Ig-based antigen receptors, and thus, continuing the speculation, RAG-containing immunocytes in intestine could have become precursors of intra-epithelial lymphocytes (IEL). On the other hand, immunocytes armed with LRR-based receptors maintained the ancient function of antigen sensing and phagocytosis. Subsequently, the lymphocytes acquired specialization either by retaining the Ig-based antigen receptor on their surface (T cells), or shedding it in body fluids (B cells). These speculations (reassumed in Fig. 4.1) could be useful to discuss the presence of innate-type lymphocytes originating in the intestine,[12] not requiring MHC-driven antigen presentation, and of MHC-instructed T cells originated in the thymus, as previously postulated.[13]

In support of this hypothesis, it should be remembered that invertebrates have an intestinal recognition-system that may discriminate between pathogenic and beneficial microbes[14,15]; this feature has been conserved in GSP in innate-type lymphocyte subpopulations.

A GSP lymphocyte could be defined in the simplest way as an immunocyte expressing Ig domain-based antigen receptors and having RAG enzymes. The Ig domain is as old as unicellular metazoans,[16] and has been rearranged during evolution as a recognition mechanism in multicellular species. The GSP Ig domain-based antigen receptors are B-cell receptors (BR), or Ig, and T-cell receptors (TR). The BR and BR coreceptors are inserted into the outer membrane of B lymphocytes, and thus function as an antigen–receptor complex; alternatively the BR can be secreted as an antibody-effector molecule in body fluids by plasma B cells. The TR and TR coreceptors are permanently inserted into the plasma membrane of T cells, and the cells must have a physical contact with the antigen to perform their functions. Each lymphocytic cell carries one type of somatically rearranged BR or TR, and thus may originate a clone of cells upon induction.

2 FISHES

Fishes are a taxonomically heterogeneous group of chordates in the subphylum of Vertebrata, included in the supraclasses of Agnatha and Gnathostomata. Fish Gnathostomata classes are Condrychthyes (cartilaginous fish; eg, sharks/skates), Actinopterygii (ray-finned fish; eg, trout/tuna), and Sarcopterygii (lobe-finned fish; eg, coelacanths), and constitute more than 50% of the extant vertebrate species.

Fishes are the most ancient vertebrate group in which "classical" features of acquired immune responses have originated, namely, RAG enzymes driving somatic recombination, cell-bound and soluble BR and TR, and long-lasting memory for antigens. Lymphocytes of fish are cells showing the main morphological and functional adaptations that have been conserved during the evolution of jawed vertebrates, and that are specialized with diverse adaptation strategies in the various clades, as shown in Fig. 4.2. For the similarities among the basic features of the immune system in vertebrates, the importance of studying the fish immune-system is clear for evolutionary and applicative studies. Indeed, some fish species, and in particular the zebrafish *Danio rerio*, are actually employed as models for vertebrate physiology studies, including animal and human health.

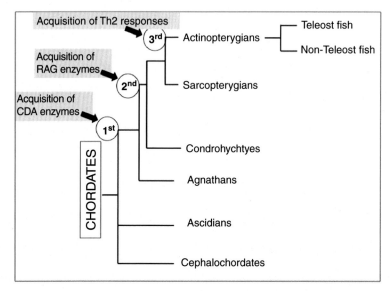

FIGURE 4.2 **Acquisition of master genes.** The figure is part of a phylogenetic tree of chordates, showing main genetic modification events that originated cytidine deaminase (CDA) enzymes involved in agnathans, in somatic recombination of LRR-based motifs and VLR-based lymphocytes, or RAG genes recombining Ig-based motifs that originate lymphocytes, and acquisition of Th2 T-cell responses.

After early speculations, more than 60 years of investigation on fish immunology has established that jawed fish species are endowed with a lymphocyte configuration that is conserved in the following orders, and include B-cell co-receptors and accessory molecules, TRαβ/γδ with accessory molecules, and a complete set of T-cell subpopulations.[17]

2.1 B Cells

B lymphocytes are characterized by two physiological stages: a resting state, where the cell surface-bound Ig serves as a receptor antigen and can receive input from other cells; and an activated state, where B cells secrete Ig of various classes. Activated B cells expand clonally, undergo dramatic morphological changes, and start to produce and secrete soluble antigen-specific Ig in body fluids. This feature had allowed for the early detection of antigen-specific antibodies in the blood of trout about 70 years ago.[18]

2.1.1 Cartilaginous Fish

The most ancient extant gnathostomes are cartilaginous fish, and much information is available on the molecular immunobiology of skates, and, principally, sharks. The B lymphocytes of sharks were deduced by the presence of a clear antibody response against bovine albumin in 1967,[19] and subsequently, by the first quantitation in skates of Ig-bearing cells with an antiserum.[20] Lymphocytes had been first described microscopically in the blood and intestines of sharks for their morphological similarity to their mammalian counterparts,[21,22] but the possible presence of B-cell subpopulations was only deduced by the identification of diverse Ig-heavy chain genes. Cartilaginous fish express genes coding for IgM (monomeric and pentameric), IgW,[23] and IgNAR.[24,25] The IgNAR is particular to cartilaginous species, distinct from Ig- and TR- rearranging gene systems, and it is diversified by somatic mutation at a higher frequency than IgM and IgW. However, it is intriguing to observe that, despite the availability of much literature on the molecular and genetic features of cartilaginous fish Ig, there is a lack of information on immuno-morphology features of B cells and of their in vitro activities, with the exception of a work describing IgM-mediated cytotoxicity in a shark species.[26]

In summary, little information is available on the cell biology properties of B lymphocytes of cartilaginous fish species, whereas much knowledge is accumulated on the B cells of bony fish.

2.1.2 Bony Fish

The possible presence of antibody-secreting cells in bony fish was discovered around 70 years ago, when a salmonid species was immunized against an antigen.[18] Following that, antigen-induced antibody production with biochemical features similar to mammalian IgM was reported in 1966.[27,28] The identification of a bony fish IgM-type antibody was done in sera and mucus,[29,30] and was followed much later by the discovery of genes coding for IgD in 1997,[31] and for IgZ/IgT in 2005.[32,33] The immunobiology of B cells and antibody production in response to pathogens has been the subject of much research, boosted by the increasing demand of information for fish vaccination in aquaculture.

The IgM-secreting B cells are the predominant class of B lymphocytes, and the kinetic of IgM production in response to antigens appears to be conserved in all vertebrates, with the exception of coelacanth fish,[8] the only vertebrate species where IgM genes are missing.

By using specific antibodies, the number of IgM-bearing lymphocytes have been determined in a number of fish species; their percentages range from 10 to 20% of leukocytes in nonmucosal tissues (head, kidney, spleen, and blood), to 1–5% in mucosal tissues (intestine, gills, and skin). This striking difference reflects the antigen route inside an organism: uptake through mucosa, recognition of nonself nature, molecule processing and triggering of responses, and delivery of information to B cells for systemic immunity and long-term effects.

The capability of IgM-B cells to secrete antigen-specific antibodies has been employed for many years to evaluate B-cell activity, by stimulating "in vitro" leukocytes from an immunized fish with an antigen and measuring the number of IgM-producing cells by ELISPOT,[34] or the amount of IgM produced by memory B cells.[35] The ELISPOT technology has reached an exquisite sensitivity, with the possibility of detecting single IgM-producing B cells.[36] Molecular-biology data have elucidated many aspects of immunogenetics of Ig heavy- and light-chain rearrangement, and recent investigations have described the extreme diversity between the Ig classes and B-cell repertoire of clonal responses in fish,[6] and complex IgM and IgT responses during viral infections in trout.[37] However, despite the amount of information describing molecular features of Ig genes, the knowledge of cell biology features of fish B lymphocytes is limited and mostly related to IgM-producing cells. The distribution of B cells in fish is prominently related to the tissue because mucosal surfaces have a low number of IgM B cells, whereas internal lymphoid tissues such as spleen and kidney show higher percentages.[38,39] On the other hand, mucosa-associated IgT-B cells can be found in the intestine,[40] in the skin,[41] and in nasal epithelium.[42] Regarding the mucosal epithelium of gills, a substantial expression of the IgD gene and a low expression of IgM and IgT has been recently observed in trout,[43] suggesting a role for IgD-producing B cells in this tissue. The teleost-related molecule CCR7, which defined the presence of B lymphocytes that produce IgM, IgD, and IgT, has been preliminarily shown by ISH in mandarin fish.[44]

From available data, it can be speculated that in teleost fish the amount of expressed Ig genes may follow a gradient IgM > IgT > IgD, but it is not clear whether this gradient is related to a similar number of B cells producing these Ig.

A striking feature of fish B cells is their phagocytic capability reported in trout, cod, and salmon[45,46]; this capability led us to speculate about the evolution of this feature. By assuming that B cells inherited from invertebrate immunocytes the capability of phagocytosing particles also for food, then, by using novel vertebrate-associated features (eg, proteasome-associated genes), they can use phagocytosis also for reprocessing the nonself in the form of membrane-exposed antigens to perform antigen-presenting cell functions. Indeed, to support this hypothesis it should be remembered that lymphocytes from amphibians and reptiles also have phagocytic activity.[45,47,48] Human B cells are not phagocytic (with the exclusion of B cell lymphomas[49]), but they may act as antigen-presenting cells.[50] Recently, an interesting work showed the possible presence of innate-type B lymphocytes in zebrafish with similarities to mammalian B-1 and B7 B-cell subpopulations.[51]

Some knowledge is available on the ontogenesis and development of B cells in fish. This aspect was investigated in more detail in carp and sea bass, and what appears evident in all species investigated is the late appearance of B cells with respect to T cells.[52]

2.1.3   Amphibians

Amphibians are terrestrial animals characterized by having a physiological dependence on the water environment, mainly related to reproduction and development. For this feature, amphibians are subjected to environmental stressors deriving from either terrestrial or water origin, and these stressors may induce immunodepression, which is considered to be a condition linked to severe global amphibian decline.[53] Amphibians, and, in particular, the clawed frog *Xenopus laevis*, have been the subject of investigations that had added impressive knowledge to vertebrate lymphocyte biology from 50 years ago. The first reports on antibody activity and the presence of plasma cells from amphibians were in 1968,[54,55] followed years later by papers on lymphoctyes.[56–58] Since then, the distribution of IgM in splenic lymphocytes,[59] the identification of two different types of B cell populations,[60] and the first preparation of mAb against B cells able to separate these cells from other leukocytes were described.[61] Subsequently, the preparation and use of mAb allowed for the first identification in *Axolotl* of different B-cell populations[62] and of different Ig heavy-chain isotypes.[63] As in fish, however, most of the work on amphibian B cells has been done by analyzing data from molecular biology experiments that showed the presence of four diverse Ig light chains[64]; the sequencing of the *Xenopus* genome allowed for the definition of Ig heavy-chain classes of amphibians, namely, IgM, IgX, IgY, and IgF.[65] The IgY appears to be present in mucosal tissues during larval development, then substituted by IgX,[66] and the IgY gene is considered to be the ancestor of mammalian IgG and IgE.[67,68] The data on characterization of B cells are scarce and mostly restricted to IgM-producing cells, where it was shown the in vitro proliferation induced by anti-IgM antibodies,[69,70] and the distribution of IgM-positive cells in tadpoles and adult *Xenopus*. More recently, ELISA data employing antibodies specific for IgX showed the modulation of this Ig mucosal class after oral immunization of *Xenopus*.[71] With respect to B cells, a more extensive literature on amphibian T cells is available (see further).

2.1.4 Reptiles

Among the Vertebrata classes, the reptile immunology is the least investigated for unclear reasons, but likely due to reptiles minor use as farmed or domestic animals, or as animal models in general. However, some knowledge is available on gene sequences of Ig classes present in reptiles (IgM, IgD, IgY, IgA),[72] and the genome cloning of a lizard species (*Anolis carolinensis*) sheds light on the immunogenetics of reptiles.[73] At present, little information is available in the literature describing lymphocytes in reptiles, although their presence can be deduced by a discrete amount of knowledge of the molecular biology of immunoglobulin genes.[74–76] First data on the reptile acquired immune-system date back to 1963, with the determination of serological antibody responses in a turtle.[77] Then, immune responses in the Tuatara were reported, without a characterization of effector cells.[78] Following that, investigations were reported on Ig structure[79] and Ig classes.[80] The presence of cell-surface-associated IgM was demonstrated in a snake species,[81] followed by revealing the percentages of B cells in tissues of a lizard (*Calotes versicolor*), employing rabbit antisera against IgM and IgY. These data showed B-cell percentages in lizard tissues in a range similar to that of other vertebrates. The presence of a cell-mediated antibody response, obtained through cooperation of B and T cells, was shown in reptiles by immunizing turtles against a proteic antigen, and then measuring specific antibody responses and in vitro proliferation of lymphocytes.[82]

The phagocytic activity of B cells has also been shown in nonadherent PBL leukocytes from the turtle *Trachemys scripta*,[83] thus showing the conservation of this "ancient" lymphocyte feature in reptiles.

2.2 T Cells

T cells of vertebrate species are responsible for cell-mediate immunity and for regulation of lymphocyte responses; they perform these activities by expressing in their surface TR and associated coreceptors for nonself recognition, and by producing families of cytokines that act as regulators of immune responses. T lymphocytes originate in the thymus—although there is a debate on the possible origin of some subpopulations in the intestine[13]—and are considered to have preceded B cells in evolution, as supposed by functional and developmental data.[7] Diverse subpopulations of T cells have been identified in mammals and classified on the basis of associated physiological activities, namely cytotoxic, helper, regulators, and IL-17-producing; all the genes associated with these activities have been found in ectothermic vertebrates.[17] A common molecular feature grouping T-cell subpopulations is the presence of a CD3 coreceptor, despite these subpopulations very diverse behavior with respect to nonself recognition because some T cells that are mostly concentrated in mucosal tissues are spontaneously cytotoxic without MHC-mediated antigen presentation.[84] In addition, it is interesting to observe that in some species the evolution allowed for unconventional assets of T lymphocyte physiology, such as the lacking of expressed MHC_{II} genes in pipefish[11] or the lacking of CD4 and MHC_{II} genes in the genome of cod.[85]

2.2.1 Cartilaginous Fish

Extant cartilaginous fish can be considered the oldest representatives of jawed vertebrates having TR gene systems,[86] and T lymphocytes were supposed to be present in cartilaginous fish because of the proliferation induced by lectins in lemon shark.[87] Interestingly, first speculations on TR of cartilaginous species reported that the Ig molecule was the TR of sharks,[88] until complete TR sequences had been identified sometime later, with typical signatures of TR genes present in jawed vertebrates.[89] Subsequently, RAG1 and RAG2 genes were discovered in sharks, demonstrating that cartilaginous species may somatically rearrange Ig and TR, and that the physiological plan of acquired immune-responses present in all jawed vertebrates is assumed to be as old as sharks and skates.[90]

As reported previously, most of the knowledge of cartilaginous-fish lymphocytes has been achieved on molecular assets of Ig and TR genes and on their expression; moreover, a gap exists with regard to functional studies on "in vivo" and "in vitro" lymphocyte responses, as these studies are still at an initial stage.

The anatomical localization of T cells in the shark thymus has been investigated in situ by using riboprobes for TRαβ, TRγδ, RAG-1, and TdT,[91] and results showed a T-cell topography generally similar to that of other vertebrates, but with a higher number of thymocytes expressing TRγδ. By northern blotting analysis, the expression of TRγδ resulted similarly with TRαβ in examined tissues, suggesting a possible contribution of innate immune lymphocytes to lymphocyte activities in sharks. However, putative functional features of T lymphocytes in sharks and skates can only be deduced by the presence of functional TR transcripts, and thus much work is required to investigate in vitro and in vivo immunophysiology of T cells.

Recently, the sequencing of elephant shark genomes provided interesting insights into the evolution of cartilaginous fish T-cell responses.[10] This work provided molecular evidence for the presence of CD8- and Th1-related master gene regulators, and the lacking of Th2-related master gene regulators, thus hypothesizing the presence of complete sets of T lymphocytes, including CD4/Th cells from Osteichthyes onward, as shown in a recent study.[17]

2.2.2 Bony Fish

First investigations on T-cell activities in bony fish reported transplant rejection by T cells,[92] and B–T-cell cooperation by the hapten–carrier effect in secondary in vitro stimulation.[93] However, these activities were only deduced in the absence of specific lymphocyte markers. The use of monoclonal antibodies and the obtainment of IgM-purified cells tested in vitro with LPS and lectins, established the presence of lymphocyte subpopulations homologous to mammalian B and T cells.[94] Subsequently, the presence of an immunological memory and B–T-cell cooperation was assessed by the analysis of an in vitro secondary antibody-response from an antigen-sensitive precursor cell pool.[95] In contrast to B lymphocytes, specific markers for T cells of teleosts have been obtained in 1995 (mAb DLT15, which recognizes pan-T cells in sea bass[96]), and in 1998 (mAb WCL38, which recognizes carp mucosal T cells[97]). Descriptions of these T-cell markers have been previously reported in detail.[98,99] Historically, the first direct in vivo observation of a functional T-cell activity in fish, namely an allograft rejection, was reported in sea bass, using the DLT15 mAb.[100] More recently, specific mAbs for salmonids CD3ε and CD8α,[101–103] CD8α and CD4 for ginbuna carp,[104–106] have been obtained.

An interesting model to investigate in vitro cellular activities of T cells has been achieved through the development of T-cell lines from carp.[107] These T-cell clones express both CD8- and CD4- related genes, may proliferate in vitro, and represent an interesting model to investigate functional in vitro properties of cyprinid T cells.[108]

The obtainment of molecular and cellular markers for T-cell molecules boosted the knowledge of functional in vivo and in vitro activities in bony fish. In rainbow trout, it was shown the typical T-cell recombination profiles already known in mammals by spectra-typing analysis of somatic recombination of TRβ and of TRγ CDR3 sequences, induced in vitro and in vivo by viral stimulants.[109,110] The presence of cytotoxic T cells (CTL) was shown in trout and carp through the expression of TRβ and CD8α,[111,112] and in sea bass by in situ hybridization with TRβ mRNA riboprobes in effector T cells involved in allograft rejection.[113] The activities of T cells against viruses are a hallmark in vertebrate immunity, and there is extensive literature on antiviral activities in fish; of particular mention are studies on the in vitro production of ginbuna carp CTL clones specific for viral antigens,[114,107,108] and studies on T-cell proliferation induced by nodavirus infection in Atlantic halibut.[115]

Bony fish express all the sets of genes coding for T-cell activities as they are known in mammals, and a recent review summarized in detail the knowledge of functional activities of CD8- and CD4-bearing T cells.[7] In the sea bass, a recent study showed that the gills express all master genes for cytotoxic and helper activities of T cells, leukocytes proliferated in response to lectins, and proliferating cells contained T cells.[17] Interestingly, and in contrast to the intestine, the gills showed little expression of RAG genes, suggesting different pathways of T-cell differentiation and activities between the intestine and gills. The antigen-induced differentiation of lymphocytes and the maintenance of a memory are pathways in which dendritic cells (DC) play a fundamental role; a recent study described in zebrafish conserved immunophenotypes for DC, with cell activities showing antigen-specific CD4(+) T-cell activation similar to mammalian counterparts.

2.2.3 Amphibians

As for B cells, most of the knowledge regarding amphibian T lymphocytes has been achieved in *Xenopus*. Early reports on identification of T cells in *Rana* by mitogen-induced proliferation date back to 1978,[116] and by using agglutination and rosetting technologies the presence of T- and B-lymphocytes was later confirmed.[117] Cytotoxic and helper T cells were identified in *Xenopus* through involvement of IL-2 stimulation.[118] First mAbs against thymocytes and T cells were reported soon after,[119] whereas a mAb for the T cell-specific marker molecule CD3 was only available much later.[120] The production of IL-2 by T cells stimulated with mitogens was later confirmed,[121] together with the expression of MHC_{II} antigens on T cells,[122] and MHC-restrictions of T-cell proliferative responses.[123] The metamorphosis in amphibians, largely investigated in *Xenopus*, is a process involving extensive remodeling of lymphoid tissues and of the thymus, with the persistence of thymus-originated T cells in adult frogs,[124] the in vitro culturing of CD4/CD8 thymocytes,[125] and the development of T cells and natural killer-cells in thymectomized animals.[126] Regarding functional activities of T cells in *Xenopus*, the presence of primary- and memory-CD8 responses against viral infections has been reported,[127] along with the restricted diversity of TCR delta chains in Axolotl.[128]

2.2.4 Reptiles

Although the information on reptilian T cells is scarce, for the possible reasons already outlined in Section 2.4, it can be easily argued that T cells have been found in all of the reptile species investigated.[129] An early study on a lizard species reported on the possible presence of cytotoxic and regulatory T cells[130]; subsequent investigations on T cells were reported for a lizard,[131] and a T cell-mediated allograft rejection was described in a skink species.[132] Most available information on T-cell responses in reptiles is on mitogenic responses related to seasonal variations in lizards.[133–135] Basic T-cell functions such as mitogen-stimulated proliferation and mixed leucocyte reaction (MLR) have been investigated in Tuatara, the only extant species of an ancient order,[129] and found similar to other vertebrates. By employing a commercially available rabbit antihuman CD3 marker immunoreactive against a green turtle after an in-vivo injection of PHA, it has been demonstrated that these injections had activated T lymphocytes in reptiles in a manner similar to mammals.[136]

3 CONCLUSIONS

Studies on the developmental appearance of lymphocytes in ectothermic vertebrates revealed the precedence of T lymphocytes with respect to B lymphocytes, and this could reflect the origin of these cells, with T cells evolutionary older than B cells.[7] Also, the sites of lymphopoiesis are more evident for T cells, being the thymus and/or the intestine, whereas the sites for B-cell lymphopoiesis are less clear. In cartilaginous fish, the spleen, Leydig's organ, and the spiral valve may be a site for B-cell development. In teleosts, the kidney is the principal source of B-cell development, and amphibians appear to use several different sites (spleen, bone marrow, and/or kidney).

Importantly, emerging functional and morphological evidence suggests the presence of innate-type lymphocytes in fish that display spontaneous antibacterial activity (CD4+-T cells) and spontaneous killing without antigen presentation (TRγδ/CD8α-T cells). In addition, TRγδ T cells are important effectors in mucosal tissues, and they have been shown to be functionally active in fish,[110] whereas in mammals they have been considered to be a bridge between the innate and adaptive immune-systems.[137]

Last but not least, an important but poorly investigated feature in the physiology of vertebrate lymphocytes is the relationship between the nervous system and immune system. It should be remembered that the intestine of all vertebrate classes contains high percentages of lymphocytes, which are mainly T cells, and studies in fish showed the expression of receptors for serotonin (5-HT3), which has been found to be implicated in T-cell proliferation.[138]

REFERENCES

1. Litman GW, Rast JP, Fugmann SD. The origins of vertebrate adaptive immunity. *Nat Rev Immunol* 2010;**10**:543–53.
2. Ohno S. Patterns in genome evolution. *Curr Opin Genet Dev* 1993;**3**:911–4.
3. Cañestro C, Albalat R, Irimia M, Garcia-Fernàndez J. Impact of gene gains, losses and duplication modes on the origin and diversification of vertebrates. *Semin Cell Dev Biol* 2013;**24**:83–94.

4. Mariuzza RA, Velikovsky CA, Deng L, Xu G, Pancer Z. Structural insights into the evolution of the adaptive immune system: the variable lymphocyte receptors of jawless vertebrates. *Biol Chem* 2010;**391**:753–60.

5. Pancer Z, Cooper MD. The evolution of adaptive immunity. *Annu Rev Immunol* 2006;**24**:497–518.

6. Fillatreau S, Six A, Magadan S, Castro R, Sunyer JO, Boudinot P. The astonishing diversity of Ig classes and B cell repertoires in teleost fish. *Front Immunol* 2013;**13**(4) 28.

7. Scapigliati G. Functional aspects of fish lymphocytes. *Dev Comp Immunol* 2013;**41**:200–8.

8. Amemiya CT, Alföldi J, Lee AP, Fan S, Philippe H, MacCallum I, et al. Analysis of the African coelacanth genome sheds light on tetrapod evolution. *Nature* 2013;**496**:311–6.

9. Lund V, Børdal S, Kjellsen O, Mikkelsen H, Schrøder MB. Comparison of antibody responses in Atlantic cod (*Gadus morhua* L) to Aeromonas salmonicida and Vibrio anguillarum. *Dev Comp Immunol* 2006;**30**:1145–55.

10. Venkatesh B, Lee AP, Ravi V, Maurya AK, Lian MM, Swann JB, Ohta Y, et al. Elephant shark genome provides unique insights into gnathostome evolution. *Nature* 2014;**505**:174–9.

11. Haase D, Roth O, Kalbe M, Schmiedeskamp G, Scharsack JP, Rosenstiel P, Reusch TB. Absence of major histocompatibility complex class II mediated immunity in pipefish Syngnathus typhle: evidence from deep transcriptome sequencing. *Biol Lett* 2013;**27**:20130044.

12. Eberl G. Development and evolution of RORγt+ cells in a microbe's world. *Immunol Rev* 2012;**245**:177–88.

13. Matsunaga T, Rahman A. In search of the origin of the thymus: the thymus and GALT may be evolutionarily related. *Scand J Immunol* 2001;**53**:1–6.

14. Spencer VN, Joerg G. Knowing your friends: invertebrate innate immunity fosters beneficial bacterial symbioses. *Nature Rev Microbiol* 2012;**10**:815–27.

15. Liberti A, Melillo D, Zucchetti I, Natale L, Dishaw LJ, Litman GW, De Santis R, Pinto MR. Expression of *Ciona intestinalis* variable region-containing chitin-binding proteins during development of the gastrointestinal tract and their role in host-microbe interactions. *PLoS One* 2014;**9** e94984.

16. Gauthier ME, Du Pasquier L, Degnan BM. The genome of the sponge *Amphimedon queenslandica* provides new perspectives into the origin of Toll-like and interleukin 1 receptor pathways. *Evol Dev* 2010;**12**:519–33.

17. Nuñez Ortiz N, Gerdol M, Stocchi V, Marozzi C, Randelli E, Bernini C, Buonocore F, Picchietti S, Papeschi C, Sood N, Pallavicini A, Scapigliati G. T cell transcripts and T cell activities in the gills of the teleost fish sea bass (*Dicentrarchus labrax*). *Dev Comp Immunol* 2014;**47**:309–18.

18. Duff DCB. The oral immunization of trout against *Bacterium Salmonicida*. *J Immunol* 1942;**44**:87–94.

19. Clem LW, Small Jr PA. Phylogeny of immunoglobulin structure and function. I. Immunoglobulins of the lemon shark. *J Exp Med* 1967;**125**:893–920.

20. Ellis AE, Parkhouse RM. Surface immunoglobulins on the lymphocytes of the skate *Raja naevus*. *Eur J Immunol* 1975;**5**:726–8.

21. Hyder SL, Cayer ML, Pettey CL. Cell types in peripheral blood of the nurse shark: an approach to structure and function. *Tissue Cell* 1983;**15**:437–55.

22. Hart S, Wrathmell AB, Harris JE. Ontogeny of gut-associated lymphoid tissue (GALT) in the dogfish *Scyliorhinus canicula* L. *Vet Immunol Immunopathol* 1986;**12**:107–16.

23. Berstein RM, Schluter SF, Shen S, Marchalonis JJ. A new high molecular weight immunoglobulin class from the carcharhine shark: implications for the properties of the primordial immunoglobulin. *Proc Natl Acad Sci USA* 1996;**93**:3289–93.

24. Greenberg AS, Avila D, Hughes M, Hughes A, McKinney EC, Flajnik MF. A new antigen receptor gene family that undergoes rearrangement and extensive somatic diversification in sharks. *Nature* 1995;**374**:168–73.

25. Dooley H, Flajnik MF. Antibody repertoire development in cartilaginous fish. *Dev Comp Immunol* 2006;**30**:43–56.
26. McKinney EC, Flajnik MF. IgM-mediated opsonization and cytotoxicity in the shark. *J Leukoc Biol* 1997;**61**:141–6.
27. Everhart DL, Shefner AM. Specificity of fish antibody. *J Immunol* 1966;**97**:231–4.
28. Marchalonis J, Edelman GM. Polypeptide chains of immunoglobulins from the smooth dogfish (*Mustelus canis*). *Science* 1966;**154**:1567–8.
29. Acton RT, Weinheimer PF, Hall SJ, Niedermeier W, Shelton E, Bennett JC. Tetrameric immune macroglobulins in three orders of bony fishes. *Proc Natl Acad Sci USA* 1971;**68**:107–11.
30. Bradshaw CM, Richard AS, Sigel MM. IgM antibodies in fish mucus. *Proc Soc Exp Biol Med* 1971;**136**:1122–4.
31. Wilson M, Bengtén E, Miller NW, Clem LW, Du Pasquier L, Warr GW. A novel chimeric Ig heavy chain from a teleost fish shares similarities to IgD. *Proc Natl Acad Sci USA* 1997;**94**:4593–7.
32. Hansen JD, Landis ED, Phillips RB. Discovery of a unique Ig heavy-chain isotype (IgT) in rainbow trout: implications for a distinctive B cell developmental pathway in teleost fish. *Proc Natl Acad Sci USA* 2005;**102**:6919–24.
33. Savan R, Aman A, Nakao M, Watanuki H, Sakai M. Discovery of a novel immunoglobulin heavy chain gene chimera from common carp (*Cyprinus carpio* L). *Immunogenetics* 2005;**57**:458–63.
34. Siwicki A, Dunier M. Quantification of antibody secreting cells to *Yersinia ruckeri* by ELISPOT assay after in vivo and in vitro immunization of rainbow trout (*Oncorhynchus mykiss*). *Vet Immunol Immunopathol* 1993;**37**:73–80.
35. Meloni S, Scapigliati G. Evaluation of immunoglobulins produced in vitro by head kidney leucocytes of sea bass *Dicentrarchus labrax* by immunoenzymatic assay. *Fish Shellfish Immunol* 2000;**10**:95–9.
36. Bromage E, Stephens R, Hassoun L. The third dimension of ELISPOTs: quantifying antibody secretion from individual plasma cells. *J Immunol Meth* 2009;**346**:75–9.
37. Castro R, Jouneau L, Pham HP, Bouchez O, Giudicelli V, Lefranc MP, Quillet E, Benmansour A, Cazals F, Six A, Fillatreau S, Sunyer O, Boudinot P. Teleost fish mount complex clonal IgM and IgT responses in spleen upon systemic viral infection. *PLoS Pathog* 2013;**9** e1003098.
38. Romano N, Abelli L, Mastrolia L, Scapigliati G. Immunocytochemical detection and cytomorphology of lymphocyte subpopulations in a teleost fish *Dicentrarchus labrax* (L). *Cell Tissue Res* 1997;**289**:163–71.
39. Salinas I, Zhang YA, Sunyer JO. Mucosal immunoglobulins and B cells of teleost fish. *Dev Comp Immunol* 2011;**35**:1346–65.
40. Zhang YA, Salinas I, Li J, Parra D, Bjork S, Xu Z, LaPatra SE, Bartholomew J, Sunyer JO. IgT, a primitive immunoglobulin class specialized in mucosal immunity. *Nat Immunol* 2010;**11**:827–35.
41. Xu Z, Parra D, Gómez D, Salinas I, Zhang YA, von Gersdorff Jørgensen L, Heinecke RD, Buchmann K, LaPatra S, Sunyer JO. Teleost skin, an ancient mucosal surface that elicits gut-like immune responses. *Proc Natl Acad Sci USA* 2013;**110**:13097–102.
42. Tacchi L, Musharrafieh R, Larragoite ET, Crossey K, Erhardt EB, Martin SAM, LaPatra SE, Salinas I. Nasal immunity is an ancient arm of the mucosal immune system of vertebrates. *Nat Commun* 2014;**5** 5205.
43. Castro R, Bromage E, Abós B, Pignatelli J, González Granja A, Luque A, Tafalla C. CCR7 is mainly expressed in teleost gills, where it defines an IgD + IgM- B lymphocyte subset. *J Immunol* 2014;**192**:1257–66.
44. Tian J, Sun B, Luo Y, Zhang Y, Nie P. Distribution of IgM, IgD and IgZ in mandarin fish Siniperca chuatsi lymphoid tissues and their transcriptional changes after Flavobacterium columnare stimulation. *Aquaculture* 2009;**288**:14–21.

45. Li J, Barreda DR, Zhang YA, Boshra H, Gelman AE, Lapatra S, Tort L, Sunyer JO. B lymphocytes from early vertebrates have potent phagocytic and microbicidal abilities. *Nat Immunol* 2006;**7**:1116–24.

46. Øverland HS, Pettersen EF, Rønneseth A, Wergeland HI. Phagocytosis by B-cells and neutrophils in Atlantic salmon (*Salmo salar* L) and Atlantic cod (*Gadus morhua* L.). *Fish Shellfish Immunol* 2010;**28**:193–204.

47. Zimmerman LM, Vogel LA, Edwards KA, Bowden RM. Phagocytic B cells in a reptile. *Biol Lett* 2010;**6**:270–3.

48. Muñoz FA, Franco-Noguez SY, Gonzalez-Ballesteros E, Negrete-Philippe AC, Flores-Romo L. Characterisation of the green turtle's leukocyte subpopulations by flow cytometry and evaluation of their phagocytic activity. *Vet Res Commun* 2014;**38**:123–8.

49. Utsinger PD, Yount WJ, Fuller CR, Logue MJ, Orringer EP. Hairy cell leukemia: B-lymphocyte and phagocytic properties. *Blood* 1977;**49**:19–27.

50. Stockinger B. Capacity of antigen uptake by B cells, fibroblasts or macrophages determines efficiency of presentation of a soluble self antigen (C5) to T lymphocytes. *Eur J Immunol* 1992;**22**:1271–8.

51. Zhu LY, Lin AF, Shao T, Nie L, Dong WR, Xiang LX, Shao JZ. B cells in teleost fish act as pivotal initiating APCs in priming adaptive immunity: an evolutionary perspective on the origin of the B-1 cell subset and B7 molecules. *J Immunol* 2014;**192**:2699–714.

52. Rombout JHWM, Huttenhuis HBT, Picchietti S, Scapigliati G. Phylogeny and ontogeny of fish leucocytes. *Fish Shellfish Immunol* 2005;**19**:441–55.

53. McMahon TA, Sears BF, Venesky MD, Bessler SM, Brown JM, Deutsch K, et al. Amphibians acquire resistance to live and dead fungus overcoming fungal immunosuppression. *Nature* 2014;**511**:224–7.

54. Lykakis JJ, Cox FE. Immunological responses of the toad, *Xenopus laevis*, to the antigens of the ciliate *Tetrahymena pyriformis*. *Immunology* 1968;**15**:429–37.

55. Cowden RB, Dyer RF, Gebhardt BM, Volpe EP. Amphibian plasma cells. *J Immunol* 1968;**100**:1293–5.

56. Du Pasquier L, Weiss N. The thymus during the ontogeny of the toad *Xenopus laevis*: growth, membrane-bound immunoglobulins and mixed lymphocyte reaction. *Eur J Immunol* 1973;**3**:773–7.

57. Steiner LA, Mikoryak CA, Lopes AD, Green C. Immunoglobulins in ranid frogs and tadpoles. *Adv Exp Med Biol* 1975;**64**:173–83.

58. Du Pasquier L, Wabl MR. The ontogenesis of lymphocyte diversity in anuran amphibians. *Cold Spring Harb Symp Quant Biol* 1977;**2**:771–9.

59. Azimi IH. Distribution of immunoglobulin determinants on the surface of *Xenopus laevis* splenic lymphocytes. *J Exp Zool* 1977;**201**:115–26.

60. Mattes MJ, Steiner LA. Surface immunoglobulin on frog lymphocytes Identification of two lymphocyte populations. *J Immunol* 1978;**121**:1116–27.

61. Bleicher PA, Cohen N. Monoclonal anti-IgM can separate T cell from B cell proliferative responses in the frog *Xenopus laevis*. *J Immunol* 1981;**127**:1549–55.

62. Tournefier A, Guillet F, Ardavin C, Charlemagne J. Surface markers of axolotl lymphocytes as defined by monoclonal antibodies. *Immunology* 1988;**63**:269–76.

63. Tournefier A, Fellah S, Charlemagne J. Monoclonal antibodies to axolotl immunoglobulins specific for different heavy chains isotypes expressed by independent lymphocyte subpopulations. *Immunol Lett* 1988;**18**:145–8.

64. Criscitiello MF, Flajnik MF. Four primordial immunoglobulin light chain isotypes, including lambda and kappa, identified in the most primitive living jawed vertebrates. *Eur J Immunol* 2007;**37**:2683–94.

65. Hellsten U, Harland RM, Gilchrist MJ, Hendrix D, Jurka J, Kapitonov V, et al. *Science* 2010;**328**:633–6.

66. Schaerlinger B, Bascove M, Frippiat JP. A new isotype of immunoglobulin heavy chain in the urodele amphibian *Pleurodeles waltl* predominantly expressed in larvae. *Mol Immunol* 2008;**45**:776–86.

67. Warr GW, Magor KE, Higgins DA. IgY: clues to the origins of modern antibodies. *Immunol Today* 1995;**16**:392–8.

68. Mashoof S, Goodroe A, Du CC, Eubanks JO, Jacobs N, Steiner JM, Tizard I, Suchodolski JS, Criscitiello MF. Ancient T-independence of mucosal IgX/A: Gut microbiota unaffected by larval thymectomy in *Xenopus laevis*. *Mucosal Immunol* 2013;**6**:358–68.

69. Schwager J, Hadji-Azimi I. Anti-immunoglobulin M induces both B-lymphocyte proliferation and differentiation in *Xenopus laevis*. *Differentiation* 1985;**30**:29–34.

70. Hadji-Azimi I, Coosemans V, Canicatti C. B-lymphocyte populations in *Xenopus laevis*. *Dev Comp Immunol* 1990;**14**:69–84.

71. Du CC, Mashoof SM, Criscitiello MF. Oral immunization of the African clawed frog (*Xenopus laevis*) upregulates the mucosal immunoglobulin IgX. *Vet Immunol Immunopathol* 2012;**145**:493–8.

72. Pettinello R, Dooley H. The immunoglobulins of cold-blooded vertebrates. *Biomolecules* 2014;**4**:1045–69.

73. Eckalbar WL, Hutchins ED, Markov GJ, Allen AN, Corneveaux JJ, Lindblad-Toh K, Di Palma F, Alföldi J, Huentelman MJ, Kusumi K. Genome reannotation of the lizard *Anolis carolinensis* based on 14 adult and embryonic deep transcriptomes. *BMC Genomics* 2013;**23**(14) 49.

74. Das S, Hirano M, Tako R, McCallister C, Nikolaidis N. Evolutionary genomics of immunoglobulin-encoding Loci in vertebrates. *Curr Genomics* 2012;**13**:95–102.

75. Li L, Wang T, Sun Y, Cheng G, Yang H, Wei Z, Wang P, Hu X, Ren L, Meng Q, et al. Extensive diversification of IgD-, IgY-, and truncated IgY(deltaFc)-encoding genes in the red-eared turtle (*Trachemys scripta elegans*). *J Immunol* 2012;**189**:3995–4004.

76. Gambon DF, Sanchez EC, Magadan MS. The immunoglobulin heavy chain locus in the reptile *Anolis carolinensis*. *Mol Immunol* 2009;**46**:1679–87.

77. Grey H. Phylogeny of the immune response: studies on some physical, chemical, and serologic characteristics of antibody produced in the turtle. *J Immunol* 1966;**91**:819–25.

78. Marchalonis JJ, Ealey EH, Diener E. Immune response of the tuatara Sphenodon punctatus. *Aust J Exp Biol Med Sci* 1969;**47**(3):367–80.

79. Leslie GA, Clem LW. Phylogeny of immunoglobulin structure and function VI. 17S, 7. 5S and 5. 7S anti-DNP of the turtle, Pseudemys scripta. *J Immunol* 1972;**108**:1656–64.

80. Natarajan K, Muthukkaruppan VR. Immunoglobulin classes in the garden lizard *Calotes versicolor*. *Dev Comp Immunol* 1984;**8**:845–54.

81. Kawaguchi S, Hiruki T, Harada T, Morikawa S. Frequencies of cell-surface or cytoplasmic IgM-bearing cells in the spleen, thymus and peripheral blood of the snake *Elaphe quadrivirgata*. *Dev Comp Immunol* 1980;**4**:559–63.

82. Work TM, Balazs GH, Rameyer RA, Chang SP, Berestecky J. Assessing humoral and cell-mediated immune response in Hawaiian green turtles *Chelonia mydas*. *Vet Immunol Immunopathol* 2000;**74**:179–94.

83. Zimmerman LM, Vogel LA, Edwards KA, Bowden RM, Phagocytic B. Cells in a reptile. *Biol Lett* 2010;**6**:270–3.

84. Van Kaer L, Algood HM, Singh K, Parekh VV, Greer MJ, Piazuelo MB, Weitkamp JH, Matta P, Chaturvedi R, Wilson KT, Olivares-Villagómez D. CD8αα⁺ innate-type lymphocytes in the intestinal epithelium mediate mucosal immunity. *Immunity* 2014;**41**:451–64.

85. Star B, Nederbragt AJ, Jentoft S, Grimholt U, Malmstrom M, et al. The genome sequence of Atlantic cod reveals a unique immune system. *Nature* 2011;**477**:207–10.

86. Litman GW, Anderson MK, Rast JP. Evolution of antigen binding receptors. *Annu Rev Immunol* 1999;**17**:109–47.

87. Lopez DM, Sigel MM, Lee JC. Phylogenetic studies on T cells I. Lymphocytes of the shark with differential response to phytohemagglutinin and concanavalin A. *Cell Immunol* 1974;**10**:287–93.

88. Warr GW, Decker JM, Marchalonis JJ. Evolutionary and developmental aspects of T-cell recognition. *Immunol Commun* 1976;**5**:281–301.

89. Rast JP, Litman GW. T-cell receptor gene homologs are present in the most primitive jawed vertebrates. *Proc Natl Acad Sci USA* 1994;**91**:9248–52.

90. Schluter SF, Marchalonis JJ. Cloning of shark RAG2 and characterization of the RAG1/RAG2 gene locus. *FASEB J* 2003;**17**:470–2.

91. Criscitiello MF, Ohta Y, Saltis M, McKinney EC, Flajnik MF. Evolutionarily conserved TCR binding sites, identification of T cells in primary lymphoid tissues, and surprising trans-rearrangements in nurse shark. *J Immunol* 2010;**184**:6950–60.

92. Hildemann WH. Transplantation reactions of two species of Osteichthyes (Teleostei) from South Pacific coral reefs. *Transplantation* 1972;**14**:261–7.

93. Yocum D, Cuchens M, Clem LW. The hapten–carrier effect in teleost fish. *J Immunol* 1975;**114**:925–7.

94. DeLuca D, Wilson M, Warr GW. Lymphocyte heterogeneity in the trout, *Salmo gairdneri*, defined with monoclonal antibodies to IgM. *Eur J Immunol* 1983;**13**:546–51.

95. Arkoosh MR, Kaattari SL. Development of immunological memory in rainbow trout (*Oncorhynchus mykiss*) I. An immunochemical and cellular analysis of the B cell response. *Dev Comp Immunol* 1991;**15**:279–93.

96. Scapigliati G, Mazzini M, Mastrolia L, Romano N, Abelli L. Production and characterisation of a monoclonal antibody against the thymocytes of the sea bass *Dicentrarchus labrax* L. (Teleostea Percicthydae). *Fish Shellfish Immunol* 1995;**5**:393–405.

97. Rombout JHWM, Joosten PH, Engelsma MY, Vos AP, Tarvene N, Taverne-Thiele JJ. Indications for a distinct putative T cell population in mucosal tissue of carp (*Cyprinus carpio* L). *Dev Comp Immunol* 1998;**22**:63–77.

98. Rombout JHWM, Huttenhuis HBT, Picchietti S, Scapigliati G. Phylogeny and ontogeny of fish leucocytes. *Fish Shellfish Immunol* 2005;**19**:441–55.

99. Randelli E, Buonocore F, Scapigliati G. Cell markers and determinants in fish immunology. *Fish Shellfish Immunol* 2008;**25**:326–40.

100. Abelli L, Baldassini MR, Mastrolia L, Scapigliati G. Immunodetection of lymphocyte subpopulations involved in allograft rejection in a teleost (*Dicentrarchus labrax* L.). *Cell Immunol* 1999;**191**:152–60.

101. Liu Y, Moore L, Koppang EO, Hordvik I. Characterization of the CD3zeta CD3gammadelta and CD3epsilon subunits of the T cell receptor complex in Atlantic salmon. *Dev Comp Immunol* 2008;**32**:26–35.

102. Takizawa F, Dijkstra JM, Kotterba P, Korytář T, Kock H, Köllner B, et al. The expression of CD8α discriminates distinct T cell subsets in teleost fish. *Dev Comp Immunol* 2011;**35**:752–63.

103. Boardman T, Warner C, Ramirez-Gomez F, Matrisciano J, Bromage E. Characterization of an anti-rainbow trout (*Oncorhynchus mykiss*) CD3ε monoclonal antibody. *Vet Immunol Immunopathol* 2012;**145**:511–5.

104. Toda H, Saito Y, Koike T, Takizawa F, Araki K, Yabu T, et al. Conservation of characteristics and functions of CD4 positive lymphocytes in a teleost fish. *Dev Comp Immunol* 2011;**35**:650–60.

105. Toda H, Yabu T, Shiba H, Moritomo T, Nakanishi T. Evaluating antigen-specific cyto-toxicity of CD8+ T cells in fish by granzyme B-like activity. *Vet Immunol Immunopathol* 2011;**141**:168–72.
106. Marozzi C, Bertoni F, Randelli E, Buonocore F, Timperio AM, Scapigliati G. A monoclonal antibody for the CD45 receptor in the teleost fish *Dicentrarchus labrax*. *Dev Comp Immunol* 2012;**37**:342–53.
107. Yamaguchi T, Katakura F, Shitanda S, Niida Y, Toda H, Ohtani M, Yabu T, Suetake H, Moritomo T, Nakanishi T. Clonal growth of carp (*Cyprinus carpio*) T cells in vitro. *Dev Comp Immunol* 2011;**35**:193–202.
108. Yamaguchi T, Katakura F, Someya K, Dijkstra JM, Moritomo T, Nakanishi T. Clonal growth of carp (*Cyprinus carpio*) T cells in vitro: long-term proliferation of Th2-like cells. *Fish Shellfish Immunol* 2013;**34**:433–42.
109. Boudinot P, Boubekeur S, Benmansour A. Rhabdovirus infection induces public and private T cell responses in teleost fish. *J Immunol* 2001;**167**:6202–9.
110. Buonocore F, Castro R, Randelli E, Lefranc MP, Six A, Kuhl H, Reinhardt R, Facchiano A, Boudinot P, Scapigliati G. Diversity, molecular characterization and expression of T cell receptor γ in a teleost fish, the sea bass (*Dicentrarchus labrax* L). *PLoS One* 2012;**7**:1–11 e47957.
111. Fischer U, Utke K, Ototake M, Dijkstra JM, Köllner B. Adaptive cell-mediated cytotoxic-ity against allogeneic targets by CD8-positive lymphocytes of rainbow trout (*Oncorhynchus mykiss*). *Dev Comp Immunol* 2003;**27**:323–37.
112. Somamoto T, Yoshiura Y, Sato A, Nakao M, Nakanishi T, Okamoto N, Ototake M. Expression profiles of TCRbeta and CD8alpha mRNA correlate with virus-specific cell-mediated cyto-toxic activity in ginbuna crucian carp. *Virology* 2006;**348**:370–7.
113. Romano N, Baldassini MR, Buonocore F, Picchietti S, Mastrolia L, Abelli L. In vivo allograft rejection in a bony fish *Dicentrarchus labrax* (L): characterisation of effector lymphocytes. *Cell Tissue Res* 2005;**321**:353–63.
114. Somamoto T, Okamoto N, Nakanishi T, Ototake M, Nakao M. In vitro generation of viral-antigen dependent cytotoxic T-cells from ginbuna crucian carp Carassius auratus langsdorfii. *Virology* 2009;**389**:26–33.
115. Overgård AC, Nerland AH, Fiksdal IU, Patel S. Atlantic halibut experimentally infected with nodavirus shows increased levels of T-cell marker and IFNγ transcripts. *Dev Comp Immunol* 2012;**37**:139–50.
116. Wright RK, Cooper EL. Leopard frog (*Rana pipiens*) spleen lymphocyte responses to plant lectins: kinetics and carbohydrate inhibition. *Dev Comp Immunol* 1978;**2**:95–107.
117. Klempau AE, Cooper EL. T-lymphocyte and B-lymphocyte dichotomy in anuran amphibians: I. T-lymphocyte proportions, distribution and ontogeny, as measured by E-rosetting, nylon wool adherence, postmetamorphic thymectomy, and non-specific esterase staining. *Dev Comp Immunol* 1983;**7**:99–110.
118. Efrat S, Kaempfer R. A qualitative difference in the interleukin 2 (IL-2) requirement of helper and cytotoxic T lymphocytes. *Cell Immunol* 1984;**88**:207–12.
119. Nagata S. Development of T lymphocytes in *Xenopus laevis*: appearance of the antigen recog-nized by an anti-thymocyte mouse monoclonal antibody. *Dev Biol* 1986;**114**:389–94.
120. Dzialo RC, Cooper MD. An amphibian CD3 homologue of the mammalian CD3 gamma and delta genes. *Eur J Immunol* 1997;**27**:1640–7.
121. Watkins D, Cohen N. Mitogen-activated *Xenopus laevis* lymphocytes produce a T-cell growth factor. *Immunology* 1987;**62**:119–25.
122. Rollins-Smith LA, Blair P. Expression of class II major histocompatibility complex antigens on adult T cells in Xenopus is metamorphosis-dependent. *Dev Immunol* 1990;**1**:97–104.

123. Harding FA, Flajnik MF, Cohen N. MHC restriction of T-cell proliferative responses in *Xenopus*. *Dev Comp Immunol* 1993;**17**:425–37.

124. Rollins-Smith LA, Needham DA, Davis AT, Blair PJ. Late thymectomy in *Xenopus* tadpoles reveals a population of T cells that persists through metamorphosis. *Dev Comp Immunol* 1996;**20**:165–74.

125. Robert J, Cohen N. In vitro differentiation of a CD4/CD8 double-positive equivalent thymocyte subset in adult *Xenopus*. *Int Immunol* 1999;**11**:499–508.

126. Horton JD, Horton TL, Dzialo R, Gravenor I, Minter R, Ritchie P, Gartland L, Watson MD, Cooper MD. T-cell and natural killer cell development in thymectomized *Xenopus*. *Immunol Rev* 1998;**166**:245–58.

127. Morales HD, Robert J. Characterization of primary and memory CD8 T-cell responses against ranavirus (FV3) in *Xenopus laevis*. *J Virol* 2007;**81**:2240–8.

128. André S, Kerfourn F, Affaticati P, Guerci A, Ravassard P, Fellah JS. Highly restricted diversity of TCR delta chains of the amphibian Mexican axolotl (*Ambystoma mexicanum*) in peripheral tissues. *Eur J Immunol* 2007;**37**:1621–33.

129. Burnham DK, Keall SN, Nelson NJ, Daugherty CH. T cell function in tuatara (*Sphenodon punctatus*). *Comp Immunol Microbiol Infect Dis* 2005;**28**:213–22.

130. Cuchens MA, Clem LW. Phylogeny of lymphocyte heterogeneity IV. Evidence for T-like and B-like cells in reptiles. *Dev Comp Immunol* 1979;**3**:465–75.

131. Manickasundari M, Selvaraj P, Pitchappan RM. Studies on T-cells of the lizard *Calotes versicolor*: adherent and non-adherent populations of the spleen. *Dev Comp Immunol* 1984;**8**:367–74.

132. Afifi A, Mohamed ER, El Ridi R. Seasonal conditions determine the manner of rejection in reptiles. *J Exp Zool* 1993;**265**:459–68.

133. El Ridi R, Wahby AF, Saad AH, Soliman MAW, Concanavalin A. Responsiveness and interleukin 2 production in the snake *Spalersophis diadema*. *Immunobiology* 1987;**174**:177–89.

134. el Masri M, Saad AH, Mansour MH, Badir N. Seasonal distribution and hormonal modulation of reptilian T cells. *Immunobiology* 1995;**193**:15–41.

135. Muñoz FJ, De la Fuente M. The effect of the seasonal cycle on the splenic leukocyte functions in the turtle *Mauremys caspica*. *Physiol Biochem Zool* 2001;**74**:660–7.

136. Muñoz FA, Estrada-Parra S, Romero-Rojas A, Work TM, Gonzalez-Ballesteros E, Estrada-Garcia I. Identification of CD3+ T lymphocytes in the green turtle *Chelonia mydas*. *Vet Immunol Immunopathol* 2009;**131**:211–7.

137. Holtmeier W, Kabelitz D, Gammadelta T. Cells link innate and adaptive immune responses. *Chem Immunol Allergy* 2005;**86**:151–83.

138. Meyniel JP, Khan NA, Ferrière F, Deschaux P. Identification of lymphocyte 5-HT3 receptor subtype and its implication in fish T-cell proliferation. *Immunol Lett* 1997;**55**:151–60.

Chapter 5

Vertebrate Cytokines and Their Evolution

Christopher J Secombes*, Tiehui Wang*, Steve Bird**

*Scottish Fish Immunology Research Centre, University of Aberdeen, Zoology Building, Tillydrone Avenue, Aberdeen, United Kingdom; **Molecular Genetics, Department of Biological Sciences, University of Waikato, Hamilton, New Zealand

1 INTRODUCTION

This review will outline what we know about cytokines and their evolution within vertebrates. It will focus on the interleukins, as key cytokines involved in the regulation of adaptive immunity, but will also include the TNF family of cytokines. It will not cover the evolution of interferons, which is described in chapter: Antiviral Immunity: Origin and Evolution in Vertebrates, or the chemokines, which have had many recent reviews (eg, Refs. [1–6]). It will build upon our recent reviews of fish cytokines,[7–10] to update on the latest fish discoveries and discuss, in the context of cytokine evolution, within the other—mostly nonmammalian—vertebrate classes.

2 THE IL-1 CYTOKINE FAMILY

Interleukin-1β was the first family member discovered within mice and humans, and has been characterized within a wide variety of mammalian species.[11] The interleukin-1 (IL-1) family of cytokines has four main members: IL-1α (IL-1F1), IL-1β (IL-1F2), IL-1RN (IL-1F3), and IL-18 (IL-1F4), with a number of molecules showing clear homology to this group: FIL-1δ or IL-36RN (IL-1F5), FIL-1ε or IL-36α (IL-1F6), IL-1H4 or IL-37 (IL-1F7), IL-1H2 or IL-36β (IL-1F8), IL-1ε or IL-36γ (IL-1F9), IL-1Hy2 or IL-38 (IL-1F10), and IL-33 (IL-1F11). These are encoded at three separate loci within the human genome, with IL-1F4 and IL-1F11 lying on chromosomes 11 and 9, respectively, and the remaining nine present at a single locus on chromosome 2.[12] All members of the IL-1 family belong to the β-trefoil superfamily, as β-sheets are present within their tertiary structure, which fold to form a trefoil-like structure.[13,14] In addition, each member contains an IL-1 family signature pattern or motif, taken from a selected conserved region in the C-terminal section, with the following consensus pattern: [FC]-x-S-[ASLV]-x(2)-P-x(2)-[FYLIV]-[LI]-[SCA]-T-x(7)-[LIVM],

The Evolution of the Immune System. http://dx.doi.org/10.1016/B978-0-12-801975-7.00005-0

as found in the PROSITE database.[15] To date, only IL-1F2, IL-1F3, IL-1F4, and IL-1F5 homologs have been discovered outside of mammals, which are discussed later in the chapter.

2.1 Vertebrate IL-1F2

In mammals, IL-1 is a major mediator of inflammation, and in general initiates and/or increases a wide variety of nonstructural, function-associated genes that are characteristically expressed during inflammation, particularly other cytokines. It is one of the key mediators of the body's response to microbial invasion, inflammation, immunological reactions, and tissue injury. Both in vivo and in vitro experiments have shown that IL-1α and β have similar, if not identical, multiple biological effects which have been well-cataloged,[16–20] with both forms affecting nearly every cell type and sharing a common receptor on target cells. Work, however, has shown that the endogenous roles of IL-α and IL-1β are different where IL-1β, but not IL-1α, is a potent activator of the humoral immune response, and has been shown more recently to induce local inflammation in delayed-type hypersensitivity responses.[21,22] IL-1α and IL-1β are produced by a wide range of cell types,[17] including neutrophils, natural killer-cells, B-lymphocytes, T-lymphocytes, and cells of the central nervous system, but are made in the largest amounts by blood monocytes and tissue macrophages.[13,21] These cells act as an important source because of their strategic locations, ability to synthesize large amounts of IL-1, and ability to process the IL-1 precursor more effectively than other cells.

IL-1α and IL-1β also differ substantially in relation to localization, maturation, and secretion. Both forms are translated into pro-IL-1α and pro-IL-1β (both of which are 31 kDa), which have no signal peptide, and thus remain in the cytosol and do not accumulate in any organelles.[23] Enzymes are then involved which cleave them, to produce mature forms, which then augments the activity of these peptides. Pro-IL-1α, but not pro-IL-1β, is cleaved by calcium-dependent membrane proteases called calpains,[24] to give a 17 kDa mature peptide. IL-1α is rarely found in the circulation or extracellular biological fluids, and is generally associated with the plasma membrane of the producing cells, acting locally.[25] Pro-IL-1α is just as active as the mature form, and appears to remain intracellular and act at this level.[26] Pro-IL-1β remains primarily cytosolic and is only active once proteolytically cleaved and transported out of the cell; several mechanisms control this. A cysteine protease, IL-1β converting enzyme (ICE) or caspase-1, is the enzyme responsible for this cleavage of pro-IL-1β,[26] and requires an exogenous source of adenosine 5′-triphosphate (ATP) to trigger it.[27] Both ICE and pro-IL-1β can coexist without mature IL-1β being formed, suggesting ICE activity must be regulated (Schonbeck et al., 1997). In humans, to generate mature IL-1β, ICE specifically cleaves the bond between the aspartate amino acid (aa) at position 116 and alanine aa at position 117.[28] Cleavage of pro-IL-1β seems an obligatory step for IL-1β release, as treatment with ICE inhibitors fails to cause detectable levels of extracellular pro-IL-1β, although some ICE inhibitors cause pro-IL-1β to be secreted instead of the mature form.[29] In addition, there are alternative mechanisms present for the processing of the pro-IL-1β, and several sites in pro-IL-1β have been shown to be vulnerable to cleavage by enzymes in the vicinity of alanine 117. Proteolytic enzymes, including chymase, elastase, cathepsin G, collagenase, and matrix metalloproteinases,[30,31] as well as neutrophil- and macrophage-derived serine proteases,[32] have been shown to cleave pro-IL-1β into a form similar in size and specific activity to the ICE-processed IL-1β.

Due to the importance of IL-1 in the immune system of mammals, and evidence suggesting its biological activity in the immune system of nonmammalian vertebrates, work has focused on isolating this gene in selected species. To date, no homolog of IL-1F1 has been found in nonmammalian vertebrates, however, IL-1F2 has been characterized within a wide range of organisms.

2.1.1 Nonmammalian IL-1F2

IL-1β has been cloned from selected species within each nonmammalian vertebrate group, which include birds,[33] reptiles,[34] amphibians,[35] bony fishes,[8] including representatives from Salmoniformes,[36,37] Cypriniformes,[38–40] Gadiformes,[41] Percomorpharia,[42–45] Elopomorpha,[46] Carangimorphariae,[47,48] Osmeriformes,[49] Scombriformes,[50] and cartilaginous fish.[51] Overall, aa identities of these molecules with their mammalian homologs are generally low, however, early studies showed that features such as the IL-1 family signature are reasonably well-conserved, and that highest aa homology was generally found where β-sheets were predicted to form, providing evidence that each protein had a similar folding pattern indicative of a β-trefoil family member.[52] Subsequently, the crystal structure of chicken IL-1β[53] and the 3D modeling of selected fish IL-1β[54–56] has supported this conclusion. Interestingly, although there is conservation of a 12 β-sheets structure, when the chicken[57] and fish ligands are modeled while interacting with their respective receptors, there is a high level of variability of positions involved in receptor binding. However, the mode of binding and overall shape of the ligand–receptor complex appears to be maintained, implying that each species has evolved its own unique interleukin-1 signaling system through ligand–receptor coevolution.

The involvement of IL-1β in the nonmammalian vertebrate immune response is supported by expression studies in chicken, Chinese soft-shelled turtle, *Xenopus*, numerous bony fish, and cartilaginous fish. In chicken, IL-1β is quickly induced in blood monocyte derived macrophages, reaching optimal levels within 1 h after LPS treatment,[33] and is upregulated in Sertoli cells exposed to LPS.[58] The Chinese soft-shelled turtle IL-1β was significantly increased within the spleen and intestine that had undergone acute cold stress after *Aeromonas hydrophilia* infection.[34] Within *Xenopus*, the IL-1β transcript was inducible in vivo, either following injection with LPS,[35] or after exposure to immunotoxins.[59,60] For bony fish IL-1β, many studies have investigated its expression in vitro and in vivo, where it has been shown to be significantly enhanced in immune tissues, primary cultures of head kidney (HK) cells, isolated macrophage cultures, or available fish cell-lines, in response to immunostimulants and immune-response modifiers, such as LPS, PMA, and imiquimod[36,41,43,44,61–64] or disease-causing agents, such as viruses, bacteria, or parasites[45,47,49,65,66] IL-1β expression has also been shown to be modulated in fish in response to tissue damage, UV exposure, herbicides, and diet.[67–71] In addition, incomplete spliced variants of the IL-1β gene have been identified in a number of fish, which are generally expressed at lower levels, relative to the mature transcript, and are not universally present in all tissues that express IL-1β.[61,63,72] It is thought that these incompletely spliced forms may be involved in the regulation of the mature transcript, as has been seen in mammals in certain situations.[73] Lastly, expression studies in *Scyliorhinus caniculus* have also shown that the IL-1β molecule is biologically relevant within cartilaginous fish immune responses.[51] IL-1β could be induced using LPS in vivo in the spleen and testes, and in vitro in splenocytes.

2.1.2 Multiple IL-1F2 Genes in Fish

Within trout, carp, and the channel catfish, more than one IL-1β gene was found to be present,[39,74,75] with each copy sharing a high level of aa identity. In trout, the second gene (IL-1β2) has a similar intron–exon organization to the first IL-1β gene (IL-1β1) sequenced,[36] except for small differences in the sizes of the introns and exons. Induction of IL-1β2 expression has also been observed, where a clear dose-dependent induction of the trout IL-1β2 is seen in cultured trout leucocytes in response to LPS. In carp, along with IL-1β1, there were two different IL-1β2 sequences identified, and IL-1β2 mRNA expression was upregulated in HK cells in vivo, similar to carp IL-1β1, after infection with *Trypanoplasma borreli* and in vitro by stimulation with LPS.[39] At the time of their discovery, the existence of two IL-1β copies in the trout and carp genome came as no surprise, due to the tetraploid nature of these species.

More recently, additional copies of the IL-1β gene have been discovered in trout and salmon, called IL-1β3,[76] and in diploid species, such as the Japanese flounder, called nIL1β-L1,[77] and in gilt-head seabream, called IL-1Fm2.[78] Although clearly related to IL-1β genes already discovered in fish, these copies share low aa identity to them, which is clearly shown within phylogenetic analysis, where they form their own distinct group. Furthermore, where gene organization has been determined, this is different between each IL-1β gene. From this, it has been clearly shown that fish have two very clear types of IL-1β that can be found within a wide variety of fish species, using available genomes and sequence databases.[76,78] In addition, investigating where each of these genes are found within genomes has shown that they are located in different regions; however, there is conservation of gene synteny around them, which suggests that they may have arisen from a fish-specific genome duplication event.[79] Although a lot remains to be done, in order to understand the role of each type of IL-1β gene in fish, preliminary investigations have been carried out. In flounder and trout, clear differences in the constitutive expression of the two groups of IL-1β genes in tissues, such as the gills and spleen, can be seen. In trout, IL-1β3 was upregulated in primary macrophage cultures, in response to pathogen-associated molecular patterns (PAMPs), proinflammatory cytokines, and viral infection, suggesting that it also has a role in inflammation and host defense.[76] In sea bream, although IL-1Fm2 could be slightly upregulated in a variety of tissues following exposure to PAMPs or bacterial infection, the combination of PAMPs with the recombinant IL-1Fm2 was able to significantly upregulate expression in macrophages and granulocytes.[78] Lastly, recombinant IL-1Fm2 could also activate the respiratory burst of sea-bream phagocytes, and synergistically induce the expression of IL-1β, TNF-α, IL-8, and IL-10 when combined with PAMPs.

2.1.3 Processing of Nonmammalian IL-1F2

Functional studies with the recombinant (r)IL-1 protein have been carried out in nonmammalian vertebrates, based on predictions of a possible start of the mature peptide from alignments with mammalian species. It is clear from the proteins that have been produced for chicken and a wide range of bony fish, that they are active,[33,43,44,57,80–85] and even peptides from the mature peptide region can elicit some responses.[54,86] In chicken, the rIL-1β-induced expression of a CXC chemokine in chicken fibroblasts[33] and plasma cortisol levels were significantly upregulated upon injection with IL-1β, in a similar fashion as that seen in mice and rats.[57] In fish, early studies in trout showed that IL-1β induces the expression of itself, COX2, and MHC II in macrophages in vitro, and when injected into the peritoneal cavity of fish it significantly enhances peritoneal leucocyte phagocytosis and resistance to challenge with the bacterium *Aeromonas salmonicida*.[80,81] More recent studies in the grass carp have found that grass carp rIL-1β can simultaneously upregulate grass carp IL-1β and TGF-β1 expression via NF-κB and MAPK6, signaling in grass carp HK leukocytes; moreover, its use as an adjuvant within flounder[84] can enhance the antibody titer against the antigens, bovine serum albumin, or green fluorescent protein.

Despite proven activity of these recombinants, how nonmammalian IL-1β is processed into its mature form and the location of the actual cut site, is still in question. Analysis of nonmammalian vertebrate IL-1β genes shows that no apparent signal peptide is present,[52] indicating that these molecules are secreted through a nonclassical pathway not involving the golgi/endoplasmic reticulum route. In fish, evidence exists showing that IL-1 is made as a precursor that is subsequently cleaved,[87,88] as seen in mammals, but the mechanism of cleavage is less clear. In mammals, ICE cleaves immediately after an aspartic acid,[89] however, analysis of this region in known nonmammalian vertebrates typically reveals no clear ICE cut site. Recent investigations within sea bass have provided evidence that IL-1β is cleaved by ICE at a phylogenetically conserved aspartic acid present in all known sequences.[90] Interestingly, in chicken a different phylogenetically conserved aspartic acid appears to be the preferred cleavage site, which could mean processing may be class- and/or species-specific. Further evidence of the involvement of ICE in the processing of mature IL-1β has been shown in studies using the zebrafish model. Primary leucocytes from adult zebrafish display caspase-like activity that results in processing of IL-1β during *Francisella noatunensis* infection,[91] which can be considerably reduced with the use of caspase-1 or pancaspase inhibitors. Similarly, tissue injury of larvae induces leucocyte expression of IL-1β, which was shown to activate leucocytes throughout the embryo,[92] with the response drastically reduced with ICE or pancaspase inhibitors.

It is important to note that mammalian studies have also shown that the precursor IL-1β can be cleaved at different aa residues and by different cleavage enzymes to obtain a biologically active molecule. These include proteases that can be found in inflammatory fluids, at sites of neutrophil, lymphocyte, or macrophage infiltration, and can therefore participate in the generation of active IL-1β. Examples include granzyme A, elastase, trypsin, and chymotrypsin, producing biologically active IL-1β.[93,94] In addition, a mast-cell chymase and various extracellular matrix metalloproteinases (MMP) have also been shown to produce biologically active IL-1β.[31,95,96] Evidence of ICE-independent mechanisms have also been shown to exist in fish, where the stimulation or infection of sea-bream macrophages could induce ICE-independent processing and release of IL-1β.[78]

2.2   Vertebrate IL-1F4

IL-1F4, also known as IFN-γ inducing factor (IGIF) or IL-18, was initially cloned in mice from a partial aa sequence, deduced from the purified protein[97] and then later in humans.[98] Analysis of the primary aa sequence of both human and mouse IL-18 indicated the presence of an IL-1 signature-like sequence, and it was proposed that IL-18 contained 12 strands of β-sheets, forming the β-trefoil fold, typical of the IL-1 family.[99] IL-18 exists as an inactive pro-IL-18 molecule until it is cleaved by ICE to generate the mature active form of IL-18.[100,101] It appears that the correct folding of IL-18 occurs prior to processing with ICE, at the level of pro-IL-18.[102] The structure and processing of this molecule suggest that IL-18 and IL-1 originate from a common ancestor, although the target specificities and the receptor systems are completely different. It has also been reported that the IL-1 receptor-related protein is the functional component of the IL-18 receptor.[103] In contrast to what is observed with IL-1β, constitutive gene expression of IL-18 has been seen within various cell types, including unstimulated, freshly isolated human PBMC and murine splenocytes,[104] and hematopoietic cell lines of myelomonocytic origin.[105] It has been shown that the promoter for IL-18 does not contain a TATA box, and that promoter activity upstream of exon-2 acts constitutively.[106] It is also found that the 3′−UTR of human IL-18 lacks the AUUUA destabilization sequence, allowing for more sustained levels of the polyadenylated species and translation into protein. The presence of preformed pro-IL-18 in the cell would allow for a very rapid production of the mature, active molecule once the cell is activated.

Currently, within nonmammalian vertebrates, IL-18 has only been cloned within birds and bony fish. It was first isolated from chicken,[107] but has also been discovered in turkey,[108] duck,[109] trout, and fugu.[110] In addition, an analysis of available genomes and sequences available within the databases has identified that this gene can be found within each major vertebrate group (Fig. 5.1A). Highest

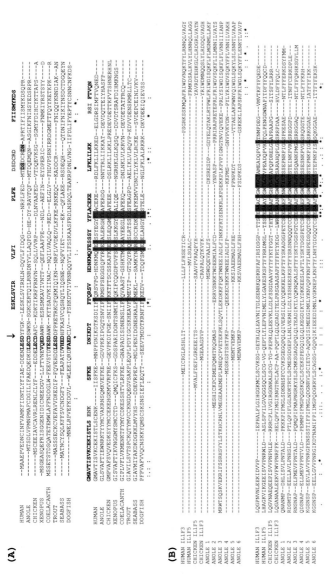

FIGURE 5.1 Multiple alignment of selected vertebrate IL-18 (A) and IL-1ra and IL-1F5 (B) amino-acid sequences, generated using ClustalX. Highlighted in red are the IL-1 family signatures. Above the human IL-18 sequences are the regions that contain the 12 β-sheets and the potential ICE cut site is indicated (↓). Accession numbers for IL-18 are: human, AAK95950.1; anole, FG762485.1; chicken, CX789574.1; Xenopus, NP989939.1; Xenopus, XP002942520.2; coelacanth, AHG59335.1; trout, CAD89352.2; sea bass, FM014619.1; dogfish, CX789574.1. Accession numbers for IL-1F3 are: human, CAA36262.1; chicken, CCD83122.1. Accession numbers for IL-1F5 are: human, NP775262.1; chicken, CCE26532.1. Anole IL-1RN/IL-1F5-like sequences are all predicted from a genomic scaffold sequence, accession number GL343238.1.

identity is seen within the areas encoding the 12 β-strands, involved in the β-trefoil structure, and there is good conservation of a variation on the IL-1 signature, F-x(12)-F-x-S-x(6)-F-L.[111] However, unlike IL-1F2, sequence comparison does reveal a possible site for cleavage by ICE, at an aspartic acid, indicating that it may be processed in a similar way as its mammalian counterpart. Using this predicted cut site, a chicken[107] and duck[109] mature rIL-18 has been produced that stimulates the synthesis of IFN-γ in cultured primary chicken spleen-cells and proliferation of duck lymphocytes. More investigations into the bioactivity of chicken IL-18 have also revealed it as a major growth factor for CD4+ T-cells, and can stimulate IFN-γ release in these cells, indicating the conservation of a Th1-like response in this vertebrate group.[112] This has prompted many investigations looking at its use as an adjuvant alongside viral vaccines toward infectious bronchitis virus,[113] infectious laryngotracheitis virus,[114,115] fowlpox virus,[116–118] infectious bursal disease virus,[119] avian influenza,[118,120–124] and Newcastle disease virus.[124–126] In many cases, beneficial effects have been seen, which include higher protection, and an enhancement in the immune response in the form of significantly higher levels of antibodies and lymphocyte proliferation.

Although no functional studies exist for fish IL-18, expression studies in trout do show high constitutive expression in immune and nonimmune tissue, but no modulation of expression in HK cells stimulated with LPS, polyI:C, or trout rIL-1β, similar to what is seen in mammalian studies, where IL-18 is stored as an inactive precursor in the cytoplasm of cells and its processing by ICE stimulates release.[127] Lastly, in trout, an alternatively spliced form of IL-18 mRNA was also identified, with a 17 aa deletion in the precursor region, which is also widely expressed, but at much lower levels than the unspliced form. Interestingly, expression is upregulated by LPS and polyI:C in HK cells, which suggests alternative splicing could be regulating IL-18 activities in trout.

2.3 Bird and Reptile IL-1F3 and IL-1F5

Other than the family members previously discussed, the question of which IL-1F homologs exist outside of mammals requires investigation. Recent work in chickens has uncovered the existence of gene sequences that encode for homologs of IL-1F3 and IL-1F5.[128,129] IL-1F3, also known as IL-1 receptor antagonist (IL-1RN), is a specific antagonist of IL-1, binding to the IL-1 receptor without transmitting any signal into the cell.[130] Unlike IL-1α/β, IL-1RN has only one binding site for IL-1RI, which explains the absence of signal transmission.[131] The IL-1RN cDNA encodes a 177 aa protein containing a 25 aa signal peptide, allowing the protein to be secreted into the extracellular environment, named secretory IL-1RN (sIL-1RN). Upon LPS stimulation, human blood monocytes initially express this gene,[23,132] but after 24 h the primary transcript in these cells is an intracellular form of IL-1RN (icIL-1ra), which arises due to alternative splicing of the sIL-1RN mRNA, which modifies the exon encoding for the signal peptide.[133] A second form of icIL-1RN is also generated by alternative splicing of the mRNA, and has been termed icIL-1RN type 2,[134] and these two intracellular isoforms may represent a reservoir of IL-1RN, released upon cell death, whose function is to limit the proinflammatory action of cell debris. Within chicken, two novel chicken IL-1 family sequences have been identified,[128] representing sIL-1ra and icIL-1ra structural variants of the IL-1RN gene. In addition, both structural variants had two further putative splice variants (SVs), which is different in humans, where alternative splicing of icIL-1RN gives three different transcripts, and no known SVs for sIL-1RN exist. In functional studies using the full length sIL-1RN and icIL-1RN, inhibition of chicken IL-1F2 activity was shown within a macrophage cell line, however the four SVs did not show inhibition.

IL-1F5, also known as IL-36 receptor antagonist (IL-36RN), shows a strong relationship to IL-1RN, sharing 44% aa identity. It is a receptor antagonist of the receptor named IL-1 receptor related protein (IL-1Rrp2), and inhibits the multiple stimulatory effects induced by the agonists, IL-1F6, IL-1F8, and IL-1F9.[135] Both IL-1F2- and LPS-induced inflammation has been shown to be antagonized by IL-1F5 in the brain of mice and rats, leading to an antiinflammatory response.[136] Within chicken, a sequence representing a putative IL-1F5 homolog has been identified with high similarity to both chicken IL-1F2 and IL-1F3.[129] Although it exhibits low homology with its mammalian orthologs, high conservation is observed in the areas that are predicted to encode the β-strands, important for the β-trefoil structure. Similar to what is found in humans, neither a prodomain nor a signal peptide appears to exist in the N-terminal of the predicted protein sequence; however, a putative nuclear export sequence (NES) that is involved in the controlled transport of proteins across a nuclear membrane, is present, which is absent in mammalian IL-1F5. Unlike the human gene, this gene showed high constitutive expression in all tissues and cell subsets examined. Expression was shown to be significantly upregulated following bacterial infection, but significantly downregulated by infectious bursal disease virus (IBDV) in a line of birds which are susceptible to this disease.[129] Functional activity of the protein was attempted, and inhibition of LPS-mediated upregulation of IL-1F2 and iNOS expression in a chicken macrophage cell line was shown. However, it is not known whether homologs of IL-1F6, IL-1F8, and IL-1F9 exist in chickens, so the mechanism of action remains unclear.

How each of the chicken IL-1F members are arranged in the genome is of great interest because in humans IL-1F3 and IL-1F5 are grouped with a number of other members, including IL-1F2. It is known in chickens that neither IL-1F3 nor IL-1F5 are found near IL-1F2 in the genome, however, it is unclear if both of these newly discovered family members are close to each other, as the region where IL-1F3 is located has not yet been sequenced, and IL-1F5 is located on unfinished contigs. However, evidence from the reptile genome suggests that these two family members may exist together in the genome, as within a scaffold (Accession no. GL343238.1) up to six individual sequences with strong homology to mammalian IL-1F3 and IL-1F5 can be identified (Fig. 5.1B), although their exact identity is uncertain.

2.4 Novel Fish IL-1F

Although only IL-1F2 and IL-F4 have been discovered in fish, candidate genes have been characterized in a few fish species that are related to the already characterized fish IL-1F genes, but that have no direct homolog in mammals. This was first discovered in trout,[137] where the unique gene organization, together with its location in the genome and low homology to known family members, suggested that this was a novel IL-1F (nIL-1F) member. However, the predicted aa sequence was found to contain an IL-1F signature region, a potential IL-1 converting enzyme cut site, and by building a 3D model, predicted to have a β-trefoil structure and be able to bind to the IL-1RI receptor protein. In addition, expression levels were increased either following infection or stimulation of macrophages with LPS or trout rIL-1β. Interestingly, although not a direct homolog of mammalian IL-1F3, the functional activity of the recombinant protein could antagonize the effects of trout recombinant IL-1β by changing inflammatory gene expression in a trout macrophage cell line, suggesting it could be a novel antagonist of fish IL-1β. More recently, a homolog to this novel gene has been isolated from Japanese flounder, where its expression can be increased in PBL following LPS stimulation,[77] and in grass carp, where the rnIL-1F can bind the type I IL-1β receptor and attenuate rIL-1β activity, confirming that it is a receptor antagonist.[138]

3 THE IL-2 CYTOKINE FAMILY (γC CYTOKINES)

The IL-2 cytokine family (also known as γ-chain (γC) cytokines) are those that signal through a receptor containing the γC (CD132). This family consists of IL-2, IL-4, IL-7, IL-9, IL-15, and IL-21, which have been well-studied in mammals, in addition to IL-2-Like (IL-2L), IL-15L, and IL-4/13 molecules, which have been identified recently.

3.1 IL-2 and IL-2L

IL-2 genes have been described in mammals, birds, and recently in teleost and cartilaginous fish.[8,139] The homology of IL-2 protein sequences between lineages is low, for example, avian IL-2 shares 18.4–27.3% aa identity to mammalian IL-2, and the trout IL-2 shares 17.8–23.2% aa identity with avian and mammalian IL-2.[140] The identity of IL-2 in different lineages is supported by the conserved synteny and gene organization. IL-2 and IL-21 are closely related cytokines that are next to each other, not only in mammals, but also in birds, teleost fish, and the elephant shark.[139,141,142]

Mammalian IL-2 is a pleiotropic cytokine produced after antigen activation. It drives T-cell growth, augments NK cytolytic activity, induces the differentiation of regulatory T cells, and mediates activation-induced cell death.[143] Bird IL-2 has effects comparable to mammals, including lymphocyte proliferation, activation of NK cells, and clearance of intracellular pathogens.[144] The bioactivity of fish rIL-2 has only been described in rainbow trout. The trout rIL-2 protein increases the expression of at least two transcription factors, STAT5 and Blimp-1, as well as IFN-γ, γIP, and IL-2 itself.[140]

An IL-2-Like gene (IL-2L) has also been discovered in several teleost fish genomes, for example, fugu, tetraodon, and stickleback. The fugu IL-2 and IL-2L molecules share only 20.5% aa identity. The fish IL-2 and IL-2L are located next to each other and may have arisen from a local gene duplication.[8] No functional studies have been performed to date.

3.2   IL-4 and IL-4/13

IL-4 was initially identified as a T cell-derived B cell growth factor[145] and an immunoglobulin switch factor for IgG1 and IgE, and was later found to also act on T cells, mast cells, and other cells.[146] Although they only share low aa sequence identity to IL-4 (eg, 23% in humans and 22% in cows), IL-13 was found to mediate virtually all of the IL-4 actions on nonhematopoietic cells, and to some degree on hematopoietic cells.[147] IL-4 and IL-13 are present in mammals and birds, where they are gene neighbors linked to KIF3A and RAD50, respectively. This locus contains several other cytokines, including IL-3, IL-5, and granulocyte-macrophage colony-stimulating factor, and forms the type 2 cytokine gene-cluster.[148] Mammalian IL-4 and IL-13 are Th2-type cytokines with pleiotropic functions in immunity. They mediate resistance to many gastrointestinal parasites, but also promote allergic inflammation, asthma, and fibrosis.[146] In chicken, coadministration of the DNA vaccine against Newcastle disease with the IL-4 gene resulted in highest IgY levels and increased protection.[149]

IL-4 and IL-13 can bind to a common receptor composed of the IL-4Rα and IL-13Rα1 subunits (type II receptor), although they can individually bind to the type I receptor composed of the IL-4Rα and γC subunits (IL-4), or to the IL-13Rα2 receptor (IL-13).[10] All of the receptor subunits have been cloned in fish, with two copies of each in salmonids, due to the 4R whole genome duplication (WGD).[150] However, clear orthologs of IL-4 or IL-13 are missing in other vertebrates. The first IL-4/IL-13 related gene, IL-4/13A, was identified in the teleost pufferfish (*Tetraodon nigroviridis*) genome, next to RAD50.[151] A second IL-4/IL-13-like gene, IL-4/13B, was later discovered at a different locus, next to KIF3A.[152,153] More recently a single IL-4/13 gene was identified in the genome between KIF3A and RAD50 in the 2R bony fish, spotted gar *Lepisosteus oculatus,*[10] and at least two IL-4/13 genes between KIF3A and RAD50 in the 2R cartilaginous fish, elephant shark *Callorhinchus milii.*[142,154] Three IL-4/13 genes, IL-4/13A, IL-4/13B1, and IL-4/13B2, have been characterized in salmonids, with the last two having arisen from the salmonid 4R WGD.[155] It seems likely that a single IL-4/IL-13 gene existed in ancestral gnathostomes, which has been duplicated in different lineages by WGD and/or tandem gene-duplication events.[10]

Functional studies of IL-4/13A have been performed in zebrafish and rainbow trout. Zebrafish injected with rIL-4/13A showed increased numbers of DC-SIGN+ (CD209) cells (a possible dendritic cell-marker) in PBL 5 days postinjection[156] and increased numbers of IgZ-2+ B cells in PBL 2 days postinjection.[157] In salmonids, the IL-4/13A was highly and broadly expressed constitutively, but the IL-4/13B paralogs are highly inducible by the T-cell mitogen PHA and the cytokines IL-2 and IL-21. Recombinant rainbow trout IL-4/13A and B isoforms showed overlapping but also distinct functions. They both increase IgM secretion by B cells, but cannot induce B-cell proliferation in vitro. They induce an early expression of acute-response proteins and antimicrobial peptide genes. They also modulate the expression of receptors for IL-4/13, IFN-γ, and IL-6 family cytokines, cellular markers for T cells, macrophages, dendritic cells, and pro- and antiinflammatory genes, suggesting a pleiotropic role of these molecules in fish immunity.[155]

3.3 IL-7

Mammalian IL-7 is a nonhematopoietic cell-derived cytokine with a central role in the adaptive immune system. It promotes lymphocyte development in the thymus and maintains survival of naive and memory T-cell homeostasis in the periphery.[158] The IL-7 gene is present in mammals and birds (chicken IL-7, ENSGALG00000022798). A fish IL-7 gene that shares limited homology to mammalian IL-7 has been described in fugu. The organization of the fugu IL-7 gene is the same as in the mouse, and consists of five exons and four introns, but differs from the human gene, where six exons and five introns are present. Comparison of the fugu and human genomes shows that some synteny exists around the IL-7 gene, with the presence of both the protein kinase inhibitor-a and chromosome 8 ORF 70 (C8orf70) genes, with IL-7 and C8orf70 having the same transcriptional orientation.[159] IL-7 is also present in the elephant shark genome.[160]

3.4 IL-9

IL-9 is a pleiotropic cytokine that has several effects on numerous hematopoietic cells. It stimulates the proliferation of activated T cells, promotes the proliferation and differentiation of mast cells, and increases production of IgE by B cells. It also promotes expression of mast cell proteases, upregulates the high-affinity IgE receptor, and induces IL-6 production.[161] One source of IL-9 production is Th9 cells that might contribute to both protective immunity and immunopathological disease.[162] IL-9 has only been described in mammals, but sequences are present in the database for birds (eg, chicken IL-9, ENSGALG00000006329) and amphibians (eg, *Xenopus tropicalis* IL-9, DQ221744). No IL-9 has been identified in the genomes of teleost and cartilaginous fish.

3.5 IL-15 and IL-15L

IL-15 has been described in mammals, birds, teleosts, and cartilaginous fish.[8,163,142] IL-15 is also present in the genome of amphibians (eg, *Xenopus* IL-15, XP_012812039) and reptiles (eg, lizard IL-15, ENSACAG00000028882). Two genes with homology to IL-15 have been discovered in fish. One of the genes shows a similar gene organization and gene synteny with mammalian and chicken IL-15, and has been also termed IL-15.[164–166] The second gene has a four-exon structure and is in a different genome location, and has been termed IL-15-like (IL-15L).[167,168] IL-15L genes have also been found recently in cattle, horses, sheep, pigs, and rabbits, but is a pseudogene in humans and mice.[169] IL-15L shares only ~21% aa identity with IL-15, however, IL-15L possesses many of the IL-15 residues important for binding to IL-15Rα; moreover, bovine rIL-15L can interact with IL-15Rα. IL-2 and IL-15 are closely related γC cytokines that share an additional receptor chain IL-2Rβ with their private, but related, IL-2Rα and IL-15Rα chains. It seems that three similar cytokines, IL-2, IL-15, and IL-15L were present in early vertebrates, and IL-15L had been lost in several, but not all, groups of mammals.[169]

Mammalian IL-15 is a proinflammatory cytokine involved in the development, survival, proliferation, and activation of multiple lymphocyte lineages. It is not expressed in T cells, but is abundantly produced by a large variety of tissues and cell types: (1) tissues include the placenta, skeletal muscle, kidney, lung, and heart tissue; and (2) cell types include epithelial cells, fibroblasts, keratinocytes, nerve cells, monocytes, macrophages, and dendritic cells.[170] In agreement with this, there is no increase in IL-15 expression in HK leucocytes after treatment with the T-cell mitogen PHA, or with PMA, CI, or a combination of the latter two, whereas the expression of other γC cytokines, including IL-2 and IL-21, is highly induced.[171] The expression of the trout IL-15 gene is induced by rIFN-γ and polyI:C, but is refractory to LPS in cell lines (RTS-11 and RTG-2).[165] IL-15 signaling is well-known to evoke a Th1-type immune response by inducing release of IFN-γ and TNF-α.[170] Trout rIL-15 can also upregulate IFN-γ expression in splenic leucocytes.[165] To date there are no functional reports on IL-15L.

3.6 IL-21

IL-21 genes have been described in mammals, birds, amphibians, and recently in teleost and cartilaginous fish. Although the gene synteny is clearly conserved at this locus in mammals, birds, and teleost fish,[141] the IL-21 gene organization shows some interesting features. In mammals and birds the gene has 5 exons/4 introns, as does the fugu gene; however, the other fish genes show a 6 exon organization. It appears that all of the fish genes have an extra intron that splits exon 3 of mammals.[171,172]

Mammalian IL-21 is predominantly produced by T follicular helper (Tfh) cells, Th17 cells, and NKT cells.[173] Chicken IL-21 is expressed in most lymphoid tissues, predominantly by CD4+ TCRαβ+ T cells.[174] The IL-21 gene in fugu and tetraodon shows low constitutive expression but can be induced by stimulation in vivo with LPS or polyI:C.[141,172] The expression of trout IL-21 is relatively high in gills, intestine, skin, HK, and spleen, and is induced in vivo by bacterial and viral infection.[171] In HK cells, trout IL-21 expression is rapidly induced by the T-cell mitogen PHA, suggesting that trout IL-21 may be produced in activated T cells, as seen in mammals.

Mammalian IL-21 has potent effects on all lymphocytes. IL-21 can contribute to the generation of murine Th2, Th17, and Tfh cells, whereas it impedes development of Th1 and Treg cells. It synergizes with other γC cytokines (eg, IL-15 and IL-7) to induce proliferation and expression of effector molecules (eg, IFN-γ, granzyme, and perforin) in CD8+ T cells, and the production of IFN-γ and IL-10 in NK and NKT cells. IL-21 also induces B cells to differentiate into memory and plasma cells, hallmarks of long-lived humoral immunity.[173] Chicken IL-21 synergistically enhances T cell proliferation and inhibits maturation of dendritic cells as in mammals.[174] Fish IL-21 bioactivity has been reported in rainbow trout. Trout rIL-21 rapidly induces the expression of IFN-γ, IL-10, IL-17A/F1 and 3, IL-22 and IL-4/13B paralogs in HK cells, and marker genes of Th1, Th2, and Th17 cells.[170,175,154] It also increases the expression of the Th cell markers CD4, T-bet, and GATA3, and maintains the expression of CD8α, CD8β, and IgM at a late stage of stimulation. The activation of JAK/STAT3, Akt1/2, and PI3K pathways were shown to be responsible for trout rIL-21 action. Intraperitoneal injection of trout rIL-21 increased the expression of IFN-γ, IL-10, IL-21, IL-22, CD8, and IgM.[171] These results suggest that IL-21 is likely a key regulator of T and B cell function in fish.

4   IL-6/IL-12 SUPERFAMILY

The IL-6 family in mammals includes IL-6, IL-11, leukemia inhibitory factor (LIF), oncostatin M (OSM), ciliary neurotrophic factor (CNTF), cardiotrophin-1 (CT1), cardiotrophin-2 (CT2; also known as neuropoietin, NP) and cardiotrophin-like cytokine (CLC). These cytokines signal through receptor complexes consisting of the common signal-transducing receptor protein, glycoprotein 130 (gp130), which is combined with another signal-transducing β receptor (LIFRβ or OSMRβ), or with a nonsignaling α receptor (IL-6Rα, IL-11Rα, or CNTFRα).[176] A recent addition to the IL-6 family is IL-31 that signals through a unique receptor complex, composed of the IL-31Rα and OSMR without gp130.[177] Human IL-31Rα and gp130 share 28% aa identity and are located head-to-head on chromosome 5q11.2, suggesting that these two genes are likely the product of a gene duplication, with IL-31Rα replacing gp130 in the IL-31 receptor complex.[178] IL-31 plays an important role in the functioning of skin and of airway and intestinal epithelia, but to date it has been reported only in mammals.

The mammalian IL-12 cytokine family consists of four heterodimeric cytokines, IL-12, IL-23, IL-27, and IL-35, that signal through unique pairings of five cytokine receptor chains: IL-12Rβ1, IL-12Rβ2, IL-27R (WSX-1), IL-23R, and gp130. Each cytokine consists of an α-chain (p19, p28, and p35) and a β-chain (p40 and Ebi3). The α subunits are structurally homologous to IL-6 family cytokines that are characterized by a unique up-up-down-down four-helix bundle conformation. The β subunits are homologous to the extracellular domains of the α receptors for IL-6 cytokines (eg, IL-6Rα and CNTFR), but lack a transmembrane domain, and are therefore secreted as soluble α/β heterodimers. Thus, the IL-6 and IL-12 families are structurally related, forming the IL-6/IL-12 superfamily.[179,180]

4.1 IL-6 Family

4.1.1 IL-6

Mammalian IL-6 is a pleiotropic cytokine produced by various cells to regulate hematopoiesis, inflammation, immune responses, and bone homeostasis.[181] Mammalian IL-6 can signal by binding to the membrane-bound IL-6Rα that subsequently associates with membrane-bound gp130, and initiates intracellular signaling (classic signaling). IL-6 can also bind to the soluble (s)IL-6Rα that can be generated by proteolytic cleavage or alternative splicing. The complex of IL-6 and the sIL-6Rα, which is structurally similar to IL-12 cytokines, binds to membrane-bound gp130, which initiates signaling (trans-signaling).[182] IL-6 genes are present in mammals, birds, reptiles, amphibians, teleost, and cartilaginous fish (Fig. 5.2).

In the mammalian paradigm, the classic signaling of IL-6 is important for the protection against bacterial infection, and the proinflammatory activities of IL-6 are mainly mediated by the trans-signaling mechanism. Chicken rIL-6 induces proliferation of the IL-6-dependent murine hybridoma cell-line 7TD1 and increases serum corticosterone levels in vivo.[187] Trout rIL-6 induced the expression of the antimicrobial peptide genes cathelicidin-2 and hepcidin in macrophages.[181] Fish rIL-6 also promotes antibody production, as seen in mammals.[188,189]

4.1.2 IL-11

Mammalian IL-11 exerts pleiotropic activities by stimulating hemopoiesis and thrombopoiesis, regulating macrophage differentiation, and conferring mucosal protection in the intestine.[186] In addition to mammals, IL-11 genes are present in reptiles and amphibians, but they are missing in the current chicken genome. However, an IL-11Rα has been reported.[190]

The first nonmammalian IL-11 gene was discovered in fish by EST-type analysis in rainbow trout.[191] Further studies in other species, for which genomes are available, have now discovered that in fact two IL-11 genes exist in 3R fish, termed IL-11a and IL-11b, due to the fish-wide 3R WGD[192,193]; (Fig. 5.2). Trout IL-11a is highly upregulated in spleen, HK, and liver by bacterial infection in vivo and by LPS, polyI:C, and rIL-1β in vitro in the macrophage-like RTS-11 cell line.[191] No bioactivity analysis has been reported for fish IL-11 to date.

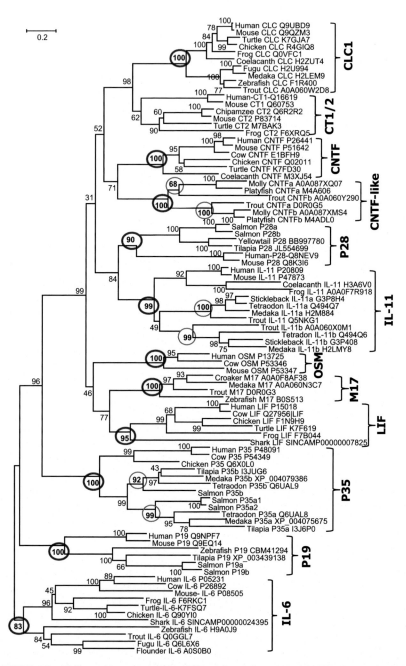

FIGURE 5.2 Phylogenetic tree analysis of the alpha chains of the IL-6/IL-12 superfamily.
Sequences were chosen from representative species of mammals, birds, reptiles, amphibians, and fish. The phylogenetic tree was constructed using amino-acid multiple alignments and the neighbor-joining method within the MEGA6 program. Node values represent percent bootstrap confidence derived from 10,000 replications. The accession number for each sequence is given after the common species/molecule names. The Atlantic salmon molecules are from Wang et al.,[183] Husain et al.,[184] and Jiang et al.[185] The bootstrap values of highly supported molecular types are indicated by *red circles*, and that of the paralogs due to the 3R (fish) WGD are indicated by *blue circles*.

4.1.3   LIF, OSM, and M17

In mammals, LIF and OSM are closest in the IL-6 family, located on the same genomic locus in the same direction, and can signal via a receptor complex of LIFR and gp130 that is used by three other cytokines (CNTF, CT1, and CLC). OSM can also signal via gp130 and OSMR, where the OSMR sits tail-to-tail with LIFR on the same chromosome in mammals. Both LIF and OSM have a very broad range of overlapping activities on almost all organ systems, including the hemopoietic, bone remodeling, and nervous systems.[70,194] However, LIF knockout mice have a rather restricted set of developmental defects, including loss of female fertility and defects in some neurons and glial populations,[194] whereas OSM knockout mice have reduced thymocytes and neurons, and abnormal thymus structure (Richards, 2015).

LIF genes are present in birds, reptiles, and amphibians (Fig. 5.2) in the syntenic genomic loci of mammals that contain LIF and OSM, with OSM missing in these lineages. A LIF/OSM-related gene, named M17, has also been reported in a few teleosts, which is also present in a syntenic region and has the same gene organization as mammalian LIF and OSM.[195–197] A LIF gene has also been identified in the shark genome.[160] It is likely that an ancestral LIF/M17 gene had been present in early vertebrates and then was expanded to LIF and OSM in mammals by local gene duplication.

Trout M17 is highly expressed in immune tissues, including gills, spleen, and HK, as well as in the brain. Furthermore, trout M17 expression is upregulated by stimulation of RTS-11 cells by LPS, polyI:C, and rIL-1β, and by bacterial infection in vivo.[197] Zebrafish M17 (LIF) is upregulated after nerve injury, and the M17 knockdown delayed functional recovery after optic nerve injury in vivo.[198] Goldfish rM17 induces the production of nitric oxide in goldfish macrophages, and stimulates the proliferation of macrophage progenitor cells when added in combination with cell-conditioned medium.[199] These results suggest roles of M17 in the fish immune and nervous systems.

4.1.4   CNTF and CNTF-Like

CNTF is a pluripotent neurotrophic factor originally isolated from chick-embryo ciliary neurons. It has potent effects on the development and maintenance of the nervous system, as well as on cardiomyocytes, osteoblasts, immune cells, adipocytes, and skeletal muscle cells.[200] The CNTF genes are present in tetrapods, including coelacanth, amphibians, birds, reptiles, and mammals (Fig. 5.2). Two CNTF-like genes (CNTFa and CNTFb) are present in several teleost fish genomes, likely due to the 3R WGD. The fish CNTF share limited aa identities (21–24%) with tetrapod CNTF molecules, and have a three-exon/two-intron structure, whereas the tetrapod CNTF gene has a two-exon gene organization. Furthermore, the genomic loci of fish CNTF-like genes lack conserved synteny to tetrapod CNTF loci. These data suggest that the fish CNTF-like genes are not orthologs of tetrapod CNTF.[197]

The trout CNTFa gene is highly expressed in brain and muscle, and does not respond positively to immune stimulation and infection.[197] The medaka

CNTFb gene is located in the Y-chromosome-specific region containing the sex-determining gene, and its expression is male-biased prior to the onset of sexual maturity.[201] The comparative analysis of CNTF paralogs has yet to be performed.

4.1.5   CLC, CT1, and CT2

The cardiotrophin-like cytokine (CLC) (also known as neurotrophin-1/B cell-stimulating factor-3) has been demonstrated to have potent neurotrophic effects and B-cell stimulatory properties, and to act as a modulator of pituitary cortico-troph POMC gene expression and ACTH secretion.[202] CLC contains a putative signal peptide and so should enter the classical secretory pathway; however, it is retained within the cell by a mechanism that is unknown as of yet. For cellular secretion of CLC, heteromeric complex formation with other factors (eg, cytokine receptor-like factor-1 or soluble CNTFRα) seems to be required.[202] In addition to mammals, CLC genes are predicted in birds, reptiles, amphibians, and teleost fish (Fig. 5.2). No functional analysis has been reported in lower vertebrates.

Mammalian CT1 and CT2 are closely located in the genome, with a head-to-head transcriptional orientation, and have a conserved three-exon gene structure, suggesting that they arose from a gene duplication event.[203] Both genes are active in mammals, with the exception of humans, where the CT2 gene has been pseudogenized. A CT2-like sequence is present in amphibians and reptiles, but is apparently missing in birds and fish (Fig. 5.2).

4.2   The IL-12 Family

4.2.1   IL-12

IL-12, the prototypical heterodimeric cytokine, was purified as an NK cell stimulatory factor (NKSF). When added to human PBL, NKSF induces IFN-γ production, augments NK cell-mediated cytotoxicity, and enhances the mitogenic response of T cells. NKSF activity was associated with a 70-kDa anionic glycoprotein that could be reduced to two peptides with a molecular mass of 40 (p40) and 35 (p35) kDa, suggesting that this cytokine is a heterodimer.[204] IL-12 cDNA cloning revealed that the p35 and p40 subunits in human and mouse are encoded by two independent genes located on different chromosomes.

4.2.1.1   p35, p35a, and p35b

A single p35 gene has been reported in mammals and birds. Fish p35 was discovered, along with p40, by analysis of the fugu genome.[205] The cloning of p35 in other fish species revealed that two p35, p35a, and p35b are present in teleost fish, due to the 3R WGD. Furthermore, the salmonids possess four p35 loci, with three active p35 genes—p35a1, p35a2, and p35b—due to the 4R WGD in this lineage.[206] Lineage-specific gene organizations of p35 genes are apparent. Whereas the exons of all p35 genes are separated by a phase I intron in the signal peptides and phase 0 introns in the mature peptide regions, exon duplication and intron insertion events appear to have happened in different lineages. Human and mouse p35 genes have 7 exons, with exons 4 and 5 the same size. However, only one equivalent exon is present in birds and teleost fish, suggesting a mammalian-specific exon duplication. Fish p35b genes have a 7 exon/ 6 intron structure, with the sum of exons 5 and 6 equivalent to the second-to-last exon in salmonid p35a and tetrapod p35 genes, suggesting an intron-insertion event early after the 3R WGD[206] P35 is also found in the elephant shark genome.[142]

4.2.1.2 p40, p40a, p40b, and p40c

A single p40 gene has been reported in tetrapods, including mammals, birds, reptiles, amphibians, and coelacanth. The fish p40 chain was first found in the fugu genome along with p35.[205] Remarkably, multiple isoforms of this gene are present in fish. Thus, in carp, zebrafish, and pufferfish three isoforms are known, with p40a and p40b more similar, and p40c more distantly related, in phylogenetic tree and homology analysis. For example, in carp, p40a and p40b have 32% aa identity, but 24–26% to p40c.[207] The salmonids also have three p40 paralogs (p40b1, p40b2, and p40c), with p40a missing, and p40b1 and p40b2 derived from the 4R WGD.[206] All the p40 genes have the 8 exon/7 intron structure, except for salmonid p40b genes, which have an extra intron in the 3′-UTR, and tilapia p40b that has an intron insertion in exon 3. One difference of note, however, is that the last intron of fish p40c genes is phase 0, in contrast to phase II in fish p40a and p40b, and mouse p40.[206] Partial sequences of two p40-like genes have also been predicted in the elephant shark genome.[160]

Teleost p40c molecules are divergent from p40a, p40b, and mammalian p40 in terms of identities/similarities, disulphide bond potential, and gene organization. They branch from the root of the p40 group in phylogenetic tree analysis, where teleost p40a and p40b group first to the tetrapod p40 clade. The loci of teleost p40a, p40b, and mammalian p40 show considerable gene synteny that is largely missing in the teleost p40c loci. Such evidence suggests that teleost p40a and p40b molecules are indeed coorthologs of tetrapod p40, likely due to the 3R WGD, whereas teleost p40c perhaps emerged in a different way.[206]

In general, fish p40 isoforms are highly expressed in most tissues compared to that of p35. The lower level of constitutive expression of p35 paralogs relative to p40 paralogs in most tissues in many different fish species suggests that the fish p35 subunit may be a rate-limiting factor for heterodimeric IL-12 production in fish.[208] Although differentially expressed in most tissues, the comparable and high-level expression of p35a1, p35a2, and p40c in salmonid blood suggests that the IL-12 isoforms, p35a1/p40c and p35a2/p40c, may be constitutively produced and have a homeostatic role. In salmonids, the p40c expression is dominant in the major immune organs (ie, spleen, HK, thymus, gills, and blood), whereas the p40b1 and/or p40b2 are highly expressed in integumentary tissues (eg, intestine, gills, tail fins, and scales). This could indicate a differential tissue-specific distribution of

TABLE 5.1 The Expanding IL-12 Family in 3R Teleosts and 4R Salmonids

	Molecules	2R Mammals	3R Teleosts	4R Salmonids
α-chain	p35	p35	p35a, p35b	p35a1, p35a2, p35b
	p28	p28	p28	p28a, p28b
	p19	p19	p19	p19a, p19b
β-chain	p40	p40	p40a, p40b, p40c	p40b1, p40b2, p40c
	EBI3	EBI3	EBI3	EBI3
Cytokine isoforms	IL-12 (p35/p40)	1	6	9
	IL-23 (p19/p40)	1	3	6
	IL-27 (p28/EBI3)	1	1	2
	IL-35 (p35/EBI3)	1	2	3
	Total	4	12	20

different IL-12 isoforms that could have some bearing on their differential roles in fish immunity.[180,206]

4.2.1.3 Fish IL-12 Isoforms

It seems that IL-12 has been present from early vertebrates (cartilaginous and teleost fish) to mammals. The presence of multiple divergent p40 and p35 subunits means multiple IL-12 isoforms may exist in teleost fish that could have different functions. Thus, up to nine IL-12 isoforms could be produced in salmonids, and up to six IL-12 isoforms in other 3R teleosts (Table 5.1). The evaluation of the bioactivities of each of these putative fish IL-12 isoforms will be a challenge because of the dimeric nature of IL-12 and the potential presence of other isoforms. Two isoforms of trout rIL-12 containing the same p35a1 and different p40 (p40b1 or p40c) has been produced in CHO cells as single chains. Both isoforms induce IFN-γ expression, but only one isoform upregulates IL-10 expression, suggesting functional differentiation of different isoforms.[180] A single-chain rIL-12 has also been described in Grouper (*Epinephelus coioides*) that had a modest impact on gene expression (eg, less than 2.5-fold for TNF-α) and stimulated PBL proliferation at high concentrations (>125 pM, equivalent to 8 μg/ml).[209] The bioactivity of p40c has also been investigated in rock bream (*Oplegnathus fasciatus*) and has been shown to stimulate respiratory burst activity of PBL at high concentrations (>10 μM, equivalent to 400 μg/ml).[210] The biological relevance of these studies remains to be clarified, as the concentrations used are unlikely to be within the physiological range.

4.2.2 IL-23

IL-23 is comprised of the unique p19 α-chain linked by disulphide bonding to the p40 β-chain that is shared by IL-12. Human and mouse p19 genes were discovered by a computational approach,[211] and have no biological activity unless combined with p40 to form IL-23. IL-23 activates STAT4 in PHA-activated T-cell blasts and induces strong proliferation of mouse memory (CD4 + CD45Rb^low) T cells, a unique activity of IL-23 versus IL-12, which has no effect on this cell population.[211] IL-23 is also a central cytokine controlling Th17 development, but can contribute to autoimmune diseases.[212]

Using a synteny approach, fish p19 genes were first cloned in zebrafish,[213] and later in salmonids.[185] Only one p19 gene is present in zebrafish, but two (p19a and p19b) in salmonids, with trout p19b pseudogenized. The salmonid p19 translations share moderate identities (23–30%) to zebrafish and mammalian p19 molecules, but their identity is supported by structural features, a conserved 4 exon/3 intron gene organization, and phylogenetic tree analysis.[185] Besides mammals and teleost fish, no p19 genes have been reported in other vertebrates to date.

The salmonid p19 genes are highly expressed in blood and gonad. Trout p19 gene expression is induced by bacterial and viral infection in vivo, by PAMPs (polyI:C and peptidoglycan), and by the proinflammatory cytokine IL-1β in primary HK macrophages.[185] Zebrafish p19 expression is also induced in vivo after infection with *Mycobacterium marinum* and in vitro by LPS.[213] These data may indicate functional roles of IL-23 in regulating the immune response in fish.

Since IL-23 is a heterodimer of a p40 subunit and a p19 subunit, and three p40 paralogs are present in fish, it is possible that teleost fish have up to three IL-23 isoforms in 3R teleost fish and up to six IL-23 isoforms in salmonids (Table 5.1). Since the trout IL-12 isoforms containing a single p35 paired with different p40 can have distinct bioactivity,[180] it is also possible that multiple IL-23 isoforms may be present in teleosts, with distinct functions to fine-tune a unique fish-Th17-like response with multiple IL-17A/F isoforms (see Section 6). The bioactivity of any fish IL-23 remains to be determined.

4.2.3 IL-27

IL-27 consists of the two subunits p28/IL-30 and EBI3 that signal via a receptor complex of gp130 and IL-27R (also known as WSX-1/TCCR). Being a heterodimeric cytokine that signals through gp130, IL-27 is either grouped into the IL-6 or the IL-12 family of cytokines. IL-27 is a multifaceted heterodimeric cytokine with pronounced pro- and antiinflammatory, as well as immunoregulatory, functions.[214]

The EBI3 gene was first identified in B lymphocytes as a gene induced by EBV infection.[215] It encodes a 34 kDa soluble type-1 cytokine receptor that is homologous to the p40 subunit of IL-12. EBI3 is able to associate with the p28 subunit to form IL-27,[216] or with the p35 subunit to form IL-35.[217,218] EBI3 genes are present in tetrapods, including mammals, birds, reptiles, amphibians, and coelacanth, as well as in cartilaginous and teleost fish.

Mammalian EBI3 is expressed in tonsil, spleen, and placental trophoblast, and is upregulated by activation of myeloid cells and regulatory T and B cells.[219] In half-smooth tongue sole (*Cynoglossus semilaevis*), EBI3 expression was high in immune organs (eg, blood, spleen, and HK) but less abundant in liver (Li et al., 2013). However, the constitutive expression of EBI3 in Atlantic salmon (and in rainbow trout, unpublished data) is low in immune organs (HK, spleen, blood, gills, and thymus), but is two orders higher in liver and one order higher in caudal kidney, compared to spleen.[8,185] The different expression patterns may suggest different roles of EBI3 in different species/lineages. Tongue sole rEBI3, at a nonphysiological concentration (10 μg/ml), induced the expression of proinflammatory cytokines (IL-1 and IL-8) and chemokines in PBL.[220]

Human and mouse p28 genes were also discovered by a computational approach.[216] Outside of mammals, p28 has only been characterized in fish. Two p28 paralogs (p28a and p28b) sharing 72% aa identity have been cloned in Atlantic salmon, and a single p28 gene has been found in other teleost fish.[184] A potential p28 gene also appears to exist in cartilaginous fish.[142] Mammalian p28 is expressed in cells of the myeloid lineage (mainly monocytes and activated dendritic cells) and plasmacytoid dendritic cells.[214] Both salmon p28 genes are highly expressed in immune relevant tissues, such as thymus, gills, spleen, and HK. This is in contrast to salmon EBI3 that is highly expressed in liver and caudal kidney. The expression of p28 is induced in HK cells by PAMPs and recombinant cytokines in vitro, and in spleen after injection of polyI:C in vivo.[184]

One IL-27 (p28/EBI3) isoform is present in mammals and potentially in 3R teleost fish. However, two IL-27 isoforms may exist in the 4R salmonids (Table 5.1). No bioactivity analysis has been reported for fish IL-27 to date.

4.2.4 IL-35

The broad presence of p35 and EBI3 from cartilaginous and teleost fish to coelacanth, amphibians, birds, reptiles, and mammals, described previously, suggests that IL-35 is likely present in all vertebrates. Due to the extra WGD, two IL-35 isoforms may exist in 3R teleost fish and three in 4R salmonids (Table 5.1).

The p35/EBI3 heterodimer was discovered in 1997 in mammals.[217] However, its function and physiological relevance were unknown until 2007, when the name IL-35 and function were given to this novel IL-12 family member.[218] IL-35 is produced mainly by regulatory T cells in contrast to other IL-12 family cytokines, which are mainly produced by antigen-presenting cells. It can also be produced by regulatory B cells and regulatory CD8+ T cells. IL-35 can signal via four receptor complexes: gp130/IL-12Rβ2, gp130/gp130, IL-12Rβ2/IL-12Rβ2, and IL-27Rα/IL-12Rβ2.[214] IL-35 exhibits its suppressive activities in a range of autoimmune diseases and cancer models by inhibition of proliferation, and induction of an IL-35-producing induced regulatory T-cell population, referred to as iTr35. No IL-35 bioactivity has been reported outside of mammals to date.

5 IL-10 FAMILY

The IL-10 family in mammals consists of IL-10, IL-19, IL-20, IL-22, IL-24, IL-26, and the interferons,[221] although IL-26 is absent in mice (see later in the chapter), showing that in particular species one or more of these genes may not be expressed. These genes are found at two loci: in humans on Chr 1q32 that contains IL-10, IL-19, IL-20, and IL-24, and on human Chr 12q15 that contains IL-22 and IL-26 (as well as IFN-γ). They have a common 5 exon/4 intron gene organization, suggesting that they have arisen by gene duplication from a common ancestor. The locus containing the IL-22 and IL-26 genes is well-conserved throughout gnathostome (jawed) vertebrate evolution, and these two genes have been reported in birds (eg, chicken[222,223]; turkey[224]), amphibians,[225] and bony fish.[226,227] However, in cartilaginous fish only IL-22 has been found at this locus.[160] Curiously, in mice it appears that the IL-22 and IL-26 genes have been duplicated locally, and whereas one of the IL-22 genes is still functional (IL-22α), the second IL-22 gene (IL-22β), and both IL-26 genes, are pseudogenes. However, it is not certain whether a full-length IL-26 gene paralog might exist in the genome of "wild" mice. Whereas the function of IL-22 has been investigated in some detail in different species, IL-26 is understudied.

5.1 IL-22

In fish, relatively high levels of IL-22 expression have been reported in mucosal tissues such as gills[226,228] and intestine.[226,229] Following pathogen challenge of immunized fish, a significantly increased expression is seen relative to control (unvaccinated) fish.[228] Increased expression of IL-22 is also seen in immune tissues, including gills of mullet, following challenge with *Streptococcus dysgalactiae*,[230] and in liver, spleen, and HK of turbot challenged with *A. salmonicida*.[229] Expression of IL-22 in whole larvae is also enhanced following exposure to *Yersinia ruckeri*, where it is thought to play a role in disease protection during early developmental stages.[231] In turbot, IL-22 expression is also highly induced by stimulation with PMA, as seen with HK, spleen, or intestinal cells.[229] In rag1-/- zebrafish, IL-22 expression is ~two-fold higher than in wild-type fish, with high expression in the HK, especially in macrophages.[232] In *Xenopus*, no constitutive expression is found, but IL-22 can be induced in spleen and intestine after LPS stimulation.[225] In chicken, constitutive expression was seen in thymus, spleen, and small intestine, but, curiously, LPS stimulation of lymphocytes decreased IL-22 expression.[223]

Only a few studies have looked at the bioactivity of IL-22 in nonmammalian species. In rainbow trout, rIL-22 enhanced the expression of antimicrobial peptides such as LEAP2, hepcidin, and β-defensins in splenocytes, showing that it promotes host innate immunity against microbes, as seen in mammals.[233] In turbot, rIL-22 induced the expression of hepcidin, IL-1β, IL-8, and TNF-α in HK cells, in a JAK/STAT-dependent manner,[232] and in zebrafish induced myeloperoxidase expression in enterocytes, as visualized in mpx:GFP/lysC:DsRED2 transgenic fish.[234] Fish injected with rIL-22 and infected with the bacterium *A. salmonicida* were found to have higher survival rates relative to control fish. The importance of IL-22 for disease resistance was also shown in zebrafish embryos, where knockdown of IL-22 with morpholinos decreased survival to infection with *A. hydrophila*, and even control fish given the morpholinos (ie, without infection) had a decreased survival.[232] In So-iny mullet, in vivo injection of rIL-22 increased the expression of β-defensin in liver, spleen, kidney, and gut tissue, and survival following infection with *Streptococcus dysgalactiae*.[230] Lastly, in chickens, rIL-22 had little effect on immune cells but increased expression of IL-8 and IL-10 in epithelial cells (chicken embryo kidney-cells), and at low doses (0.01 μg/ml) enhanced the stimulatory effect of LPS on expression of IL-1β, IL-6, IL-8, SAA and the antimicrobial peptide gallinacin-2 in these cells.[223] In addition, chicken rIL-22 enhanced IL-1β, IL-8, SAA, and LEAP2 expression in hepatocytes, which was further enhanced in the presence of LPS. rIL-22 can also induce IL-10 expression in chicken kidney cells.[235]

Modeling of the So-iny mullet IL-22 suggests that it has six alpha-helices, as seen in the human monomer, although helix A, C, and E are shorter, whereas the AB and DE loops are longer.[236] However, the cysteine residues do not form clear disulphide bonds. Recently, the crystal structure of zebrafish IL-22 has been determined.[234] The zebrafish molecule was most similar to the human IL-22 structure, with some differences located in the N-terminus, followed by human IL-20, then IL-19.

5.2 IL-26

Typically IL-26 shows either low or no constitutive expression in tissues. IL-26 was induced in intestine of fugu following polyI:C stimulation[226] and in spleen of *Xenopus* following polyI:C stimulation,[225] suggesting a possible role in antiviral defense.

5.3 IL-10

The IL-10 locus is also well-conserved, with IL-10 readily identifiable in all gnathostome vertebrates. However, the number of related genes and their homology to mammalian IL-10 family members varies. In the elephant shark, two additional IL-10 family genes are present next to IL-10, but show no clear homology to IL-19/20/24.[160] In bony fish, one additional gene is present that branches in phylogenetic tree analysis to the base of the IL-19/IL-20/IL-24 clades, suggesting that it is related to an ancestral gene that has subsequently duplicated in evolution.[237,234] Similarly, in *Xenopus*[238] and chicken,[235] a single additional IL-10 family gene is present next to IL-10 at this locus, referred to as IL-20 and IL-19, respectively.

In bony fish, IL-10 was first discovered in the fugu genome,[239] and has since been found in a wide range of fish species.[240–243] In trout two genes are present that differ in expression level and inducibility.[244] Constitutive expression is typically seen in immune tissues, as in carp/grass carp, where it is detectable in HK, gills, intestine, and spleen.[245] Expression can be upregulated in vitro by exposure to a variety of stimulants, such as LPS, PHA, or IL-21,[240,244–246] and in vivo by injection with (live or dead) bacteria.[244,247,248] Relatively few studies of IL-10 bioactivity have been performed in fish to date. In goldfish, rIL-10 pretreatment of monocytes can reduce the production of reactive oxygen species (ROS) in response to *A. salmonicida* or IFN-γ stimulation, and this is associated with phosphorylation and nuclear translocation of STAT3, and an increase of SOCS3 expression.[241] In carp, rIL-10 downregulated the production of ROS and nitrogen radicals (NOS) from neutrophils and macrophages, with the latter being more sensitive, and the expression of proinflammatory molecules such as IL-6, p35, and MHC class I/II in response to LPS stimulation,[249] again associated with STAT3 phosphorylation and induced SOCS3 expression. Effects on carp T and B cell responses were also apparent. rIL-10 increased the proliferation of a subset of memory T cells (primed by *Trypanoplasma borreli* infection in vivo) in response to antigen exposure (*T. borreli* lysate) in vitro, and increased the proliferation (whether from immunized or naive fish) and antibody secretion (total and antigen-specific) of immunoglobulin (Ig)M+ B cells.

In *Xenopus*, IL-10 has highest constitutive expression in spleen, kidney, and intestine, and was induced by LPS (ip) injection,[238] whereas in chicken, IL-10 is constitutively expressed in thymus, bursa of Fabricius, cecal tonsils, liver, and lung, and is induced in thymocytes by PHA stimulation and in macrophages by LPS stimulation.[250] Similar expression profiles are seen with turkey[251] and duck IL-10,[252] although in the latter case two splice variants are present: one lacking exon 5 and one with a spliced 3'UTR (with the last 400 nt from a downstream exon 6). IL-10 has also been shown to be induced by infection in birds, as seen with *Eimeria*-infected chickens,[250,253] where higher levels of IL-10 expression appear to correlate with disease susceptibility. Interestingly, intercrossing of different chicken lines has revealed an association between single nucleotide polymorphism (SNP) in the IL-10 (and MAPKAPK2) gene with *Salmonella enteritidis* burden, with potential for use in marker-assisted selection.[254] rIL-10 bioactivity has also been studied in these three species. Chicken and turkey rIL-10 has been shown to inhibit mitogen-induced IFN-γ synthesis in splenocytes,[250,251] whereas duck rIL-10 can inhibit mitogen-induced IL-2 expression in peripheral blood mononuclear-cells.[252]

In relation to the second gene found at the IL-10 locus in euteleostomi (bony fish and tetrapods), in trout the IL-20L gene is highly expressed following stimulation of RTS-11 cells (a trout macrophage cell line) with LPS, and following infection with the bacterial pathogen *Y. ruckeri*.[237] No studies on the expression of the IL-20 gene in *Xenopus* have yet been reported, but in chicken the IL-19 gene is highly expressed in spleen, heart, lung, and skin, and can be induced in the ileum by infection with *Ascaridia galli*[235] and by LPS stimulation of monocytes.[255] rIL-19 was able to induce the expression of IL-1β, IL-6, IL-8, and iNOS/nitric oxide, and to increase apoptosis in monocytes, whereas in splenocytes it increased IL-4, IL-13, and IFN-γ expression, and this effect was enhanced by preincubation with Con A.[255]

5.4 vIL-10

It should be noted that IL-10-like genes have been discovered in some viruses. Whereas they are well-known in mammalian viruses such as Herpesviridae and Poxviridae, more recently they have also been found in fish viruses (Alloherpesviridae).[256,257] The biological properties have yet to be studied in most cases, but in mammals they have broad immunosuppressive properties, despite the sequence identity usually being quite low relative to the host molecule. For example, the IL-10 molecule in eel (*Anguilla anguilla*) and the Anguillid herpesvirus-1 ORF25 have 33.6% identity, whereas the IL-10 molecule in carp with Cyprinid herpesvirus-3 (CyHV-3) ORF 134 have 26.9% identity. Injection of zebrafish with the CyHV-3 IL-10 mRNA increased the number of lysozyme-positive cells, as seen with zebrafish IL-10, and this effect could be inhibited by injection of a morpholino to one of the IL-10 receptor chains (IL-10R1). Although these transcripts are highly expressed during infection, in carp they do not appear to be essential for viral replication or virulence.[258]

6 IL-17 FAMILY

The first member of the IL-17 family of cytokines was discovered in rodents as CTLA-8 in 1993.[259] Since then it has become apparent that six isoforms are present in mammals, designated IL-17A-F. They share 20–50% identity, and, with the exception of IL-17A and IL-17F that are in tandem on Chr 6 (Fig. 5.3), they are found at different loci (eg, IL-17B on Chr 5, IL-17C on Chr 16, IL-17D on Chr 13, and IL-17E on Chr 14). Studies into the evolution of this cytokine family have unexpectedly found that they are an ancient lineage with homologs within the invertebrates. Multiple genes can be present within non-vertebrate species, as seen in Pacific oyster,[260] and they form a clade separate from the vertebrate molecules in phylogenetic tree analysis. Within vertebrates the most ancient isoform appears to be IL-17D, where agnathan species such as the Japanese lamprey *Lethenteron japonicum* possess a single isoform that clusters with IL-17D from other vertebrates.[46] It is constitutively expressed by most tissues, and is upregulated by LPS in cultured skin-cells. Interestingly, IL-17 has also been found to be produced by variable lymphocyte receptor (VLR) A+ lymphocytes in sea lamprey *Petromyzon marinus*, in response to the T-cell mitogen, PHA, in an analogous way to the response in T cells in gnathostome vertebrates.[261]

Within gnathostomes it seems likely that four genes were present in early species, equivalent to IL-17A/F, IL-17B, IL-17C, and IL-17D. In the case of

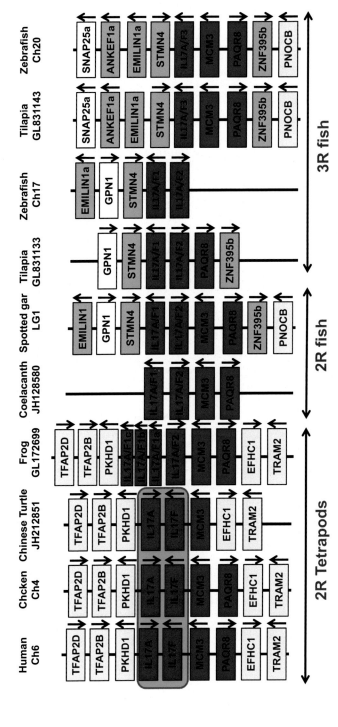

FIGURE 5.3   Synteny analysis of the IL-17A/F loci from 2R tetrapods, 2R and 3R teleost species. Schematic diagram shows the syntenically conserved genes in the IL-17A/F loci in 2R tetrapods (human chromosome Chr6, Chicken Chr4, Chinese turtle Chr JH212851, frog Chr GL172699); 2R fish (coelacanth Chr JH128580 and spotted gar Chr LG1), and 3R fish (tilapia Chr GL831133 and GL831143, and zebrafish Chr 11 and Chr20). An *arrow* indicates transcriptional direction. The synteny analysis was carried out using the Genomicus browser (http://www.genomicus.biologie.ens.fr/genomicus-74.01).

IL-17A/F, this molecule appears to have subsequently expanded in different lineages. Thus, the IL-17A/F genes have expanded to IL-17A/F1, -2, and -3 in teleost fish, or to IL-17A and IL-17F in reptiles, birds, and mammals. It should be noted that in the case of IL-17C, it is possible that this molecule subsequently diverged into IL-17C and IL-17E in early mammals, whereas in some teleost fish, two IL-17C genes are present.[262,264] This explanation of IL-17 evolution has yet to be verified, and in the case of IL-17A/F evolution in particular, other scenarios are possible, such as gene conversion (Fig. 5.4).

Thus, in cartilaginous fish, five IL-17-like genes were discovered in the elephant shark genome.[160] Two have homology to IL-17A and IL-17F, and are potentially two IL-17A/F genes. Two genes related to IL-17B and IL-17D are present that are potentially the true homologs of these molecules, and, lastly, one gene that is described as equivalent to IL-17C is present. Similarly, extensive

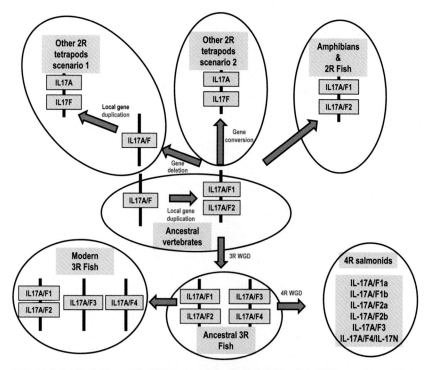

FIGURE 5.4   **Evolution of IL-17A/F genes in vertebrates.** Two IL-17A/F genes emerged via local gene duplication in the ancestral vertebrates. These two genes (IL-17A/F1 and IL-17A/F2) were preserved during the evolution of the 2R teleost fish and amphibians, but expanded by genome duplication in 3R fish that generated IL-17A/F1, 2, 3, and N; and in 4R salmonids that produced IL-17A/F1a, 1b, 2a, 2b, 3, and N. One of the two ancestral IL-17A/F genes might have been deleted, but the remaining gene was duplicated locally during evolution that produced the IL-17A and IL-17F genes in reptiles, birds, and mammals. Alternatively, the two ancestral IL-17A/F genes might have been converted to IL-17A and IL-17F in reptiles, birds, and mammals.

analysis of teleost fish genomes, initially in zebrafish, has revealed the presence of three IL-17A/F genes at two different loci (with IL-17A/F1 and IL-17A/F2 in tandem on chr 17), IL-17C, and IL-17D.[263] Subsequent analysis of the fugu genome revealed a second IL-17C locus, and the presence of what appeared to be a novel IL-17 family member that was termed IL-17N, giving seven IL-17 family members in this species.[264] In salmonids, the situation appears to be even more complex in that the 4R WGD that occurred in this lineage has given rise to further paralogs. Thus, rainbow trout and salmon possess two IL-17A/F1, two IL-17A/F2, and one IL-17A/F3, in addition to two IL-17C, one IL-17D, and one IL-17N, giving nine family members.[174] Most recently, it has become apparent that IL-17B is also present in at least some teleost fish groups, as seen in catfish[182] and eels (Wang, unpublished). With the additional IL-17A/F sequence information from further teleost species, it is now proposed that IL-17N is in fact an IL-17A/F, and it is likely that the IL-17A/F locus containing IL-17A/F1 and IL-17A/F2 was duplicated in teleosts to generate IL-17A/F3 (with high homology to IL-17A/F/1), and IL-17N (with homology to IL-17A/F2).[174]

Functional studies in teleost fish have shown complex patterns of expression that vary in a time-, tissue-, and paralog-dependent manner following infection or vaccination.[174,182,262,265] Interestingly, in carp infected with *Trypanosoma carassi,* induced p19 and p40(c) expression is seen, the necessary components of IL-23, and is correlated with IL-17A/F/2 expression, suggestive of a Th17-like response in this species.[266] In salmon, high levels of IL-17A/F2 (together with IL-17AR and TGF-β1) expression, but not IFN-γ or GATA3, correlate with the severity of side effects seen following injection with oil-adjuvanted vaccines,[267] also suggesting that Th17-type responses are involved. Lastly, in zebrafish overexpression of FoxP3 (a transcription factor involved in Treg differentiation) in developing embryos led to downregulation of IL-17A/F levels, whereas injection with a morpholino to FoxP3 enhanced IL-17A/F expression, hinting that IL-17 responses are tightly regulated at this level of phylogeny, potentially to prevent autoimmunity, as seen in mammals.[268]

Relatively few studies have reported the bioactivity of the IL-17 molecules in fish. In grass carp, rIL-17A/F1 can increase IL-1β, IL-6, IL-8, and TNF-α expression in HK leucocytes,[269] and in trout, rIL-17A/F/2a increases the expression of IL-6, IL-8, and an antimicrobial peptide (β-defensin 3) in splenocytes.[270] In the case of grass carp rIL-17D, it can also increase IL-1β, IL-8, and TNF-α expression in HK cells, but does not increase IL-6 expression,[269,271] hinting at subtle differences in the ability of different isoforms to induce proinflammatory genes.

No functional studies have been reported on the amphibian IL-17 family members, with IL-17B, IL-17C, and IL-17D all clearly present in *Xenopus,*[174,272] as well as genes likely equivalent to IL-17A/F1 and IL-17A/F2 (Fig. 5.3). In the case of *Xenopus,* in fact three IL-17A/F1 genes (a, b, c) can be found in tandem next to IL-17A/F2. However, in the amniotes, the IL-17A and IL-17F locus appears highly conserved, with both genes in the same orientation, suggesting that they are true orthologs of each other. Although no functional studies have been reported in reptiles, in chickens IL-17A and IL-17F are highly expressed in the gut, and the liver in the case of IL-17F, and in the CU205 (reticuloendotheliosis virus-transformed) chicken lymphoblast cell-line.[273,274] They can be induced in splenocytes by stimulation with ConA, LPS, and polyI:C, although with differences in kinetics and magnitude of induction. Similarly, duck IL-17A is induced by ConA stimulation of splenocytes.[275] Both chicken rIL-17A and rIL-17F have been shown to induce the expression of the proinflammatory cytokines IL-1β, IL-6, and IL-8 in chicken embryonic fibroblasts.[273,274] IL-17A has also been shown to play a role in the immunopathology caused by *Eimeria tenella* (intracellular apicomplexan parasite) infection, with rIL-17 administration increasing fecal oocyst shedding and cecal lesion score, but decreasing body weight, whereas anti-IL-17 treatment gave the converse effects.[276] However, comparative expression of IL-17A and IL-17F in intestinal tissue during *E. tenella* (cecum) or *E. maxima* (duodenum) infection has shown that IL-17F appears to be the main isoform upregulated.[273] Similarly, during experimental infection of chickens with the intracellular protozoal parasite *Cryptosporidium baileyi*, IL-17A expression was found increased in trachea and spleen, suggesting that it contributes to the inflammation seen during infection.[277] Curiously, both chicken and duck IL-17A have homology to ORF13 of *Herpesvirus saimiri* (HVS 13),[275,274] and perhaps this hints at the potential for immune evasion strategies targeting this pathway during herpesvirus infection in birds (as seen for IL-10 in other species).

7 TNF FAMILY

In mammals, the tumor necrosis factor superfamily (TNFSF) currently has 19 members[278] (Table 5.1), each of which had been identified under a different synonym until the current nomenclature assigned by the HUGO Gene Nomenclature Committee (HGNC[279]). Each member is a type II transmembrane molecule that contains a TNF homology domain and is thought to be active primarily in trimeric form, either on the cell surface or soluble after extracellular cleavage.[278] They are expressed predominately by activated immune cells, and elicit their biological effects by binding to type I transmembrane TNF superfamily receptors. They mediate a wide range of important functions, including embryogenesis, cell differentiation, homeostasis, immune system development, regulation of immune responses, inflammation, and anticancer defense.[278] With the increasing numbers of genomes available and the addition of transcriptomic data from a wide variety of species, a number of TNFSF members outside of mammals have now been identified, and it is possible to study how this family has evolved within a wide range of living organisms (Table 5.2).

7.1 Protostomian Invertebrates

The TNFSF is one of the few families in which ortholog genes from this group can be found within protostomian invertebrates. The initial discovery was

TABLE 5.2 Summary of the Currently Characterized TNFSF Members Within Vertebrates

	Other Synonyms	CD Number	Birds	Reptiles	Amphibians	Bony Fish	Cartilaginous Fish	Agnathans
TNFSF1	LT-a, TNF-b, TNFSF1B				✓	✓M	✓	
TNFSF2	TNF-a, DIF, Necrosin, Cytotoxin, TNFSF1A		✓P	✓M	✓	✓		
TNFSF3	LT-b, TNF-c				✓	✓		
TNFSF4	gp34, OX40L, CD134L, TXGP1	252	✓	✓	✓P		✓	
TNFSF5	CD40L, TRAP, Gp39, T-BAM	154	✓	✓	✓	✓	✓	
TNFSF6	FASL, APTL, APT1LG1, CD95L	178	✓	✓	✓	✓	✓P,M	
TNFSF7	CD27L	70						
TNFSF8	CD30L	153		✓	✓P			
TNFSF9	CD137L, 4-1BBL				✓			
TNFSF10	TRAIL, APO-2L	253	✓M	✓M	✓M	✓M	✓P,M	✓
TNFSF11	OPGL, RANKL, TRANCE, ODF, SOFA	254	✓	✓	✓M	✓		
TNFSF12	TWEAK, APO-3L, DR3L			✓	✓	✓		
TNFSF13	APRIL, TALL-2, TRDL-1	256						
TNFSF13B	BLyS, BAFF, TALL-1, THANK, TNFSF20, ZTNF4, TNFSF20	257	✓	✓	✓	✓M	✓M	
TNFSF14	LIGHT, HVEML	258	✓	✓	✓	✓		
TNFSF15	TL1, TL-1A, VEGI		✓	✓	✓	✓		
TNFSF18	GITRL, TL-6, AITRL		✓	✓P		✓	✓P	
TNFSF19	DEDD		✓	✓	✓	✓		

Squares colored yellow indicate where additional family members have recently been identified, using available genomes and sequence databases for analysis in this chapter. P, where a sequence has been predicted from the genome. M, where multiple sequences exist for this TNSF member.

within *Drosophila melanogaster*[280,281]; however, subsequent discoveries have been made within the molluscs *Haliotis discus discus*[282,283] and *Crassostrea gigas*,[157] and the crustacean *Marsupenaeus japonicus*[284] Investigations in *Drosophila* have shown Eiger to have highest homology with the TNF family member Ectodysplasin A (EDA) and shown to be involved in a variety of cellular and tissue processes, such as cell death, cell proliferation, tissue growth regulation, host defense, and pain sensitization.[281] A homolog to Eiger has also been identified in *M. japonicus*[284] where expression was highest in healthy tissues, such as the muscle, stomach, brain, and gill. Peptidoglycan (PG) or polyI:C stimulation of cells taken from the "lymphoid organ," that has been shown to be important in the elimination of microorganisms, increases the expression of this gene. All other TNFSF members identified within other invertebrates show varying homology to members of the mammalian TNFSF. The gene identified from *H. discus discus*[282] has a TNFSF homology domain and has been described as a homolog of TNFSF2. These investigations have shown that this gene can be upregulated in vivo, in response to lipopolysaccharide (LPS), pathogenic bacteria, or virus; moreover, by using in situ hybridization both tissue and circulating hemocytes can be stained positive for this gene. A more recent study has identified that it is possible for invertebrates to contain a number of TNFSF members, as 23 individual TNFSF genes can be found in the genome of *C. gigas*,[157] many of which have come from the duplication of genes. Functional diversity of each of these genes is predicted, due to differences in their expression in a variety of tissues. The role each of these TNFSF members have in the immune responses of these organisms remains unclear, and functional studies are required. In addition, caution should be taken in attempting to link sequences from invertebrates to homologs in vertebrates. Although it cannot be disputed that TNFSF members exist in invertebrates, any relation to a vertebrate gene may be purely coincidental, especially when the largest identity between the genes is mainly within the TNF homology domain, which is found in all TNFSF sequences.

7.2 Primitive Chordates and Basal Vertebrates: Cephalochordates, Urochordates, and Cyclostomata

Investigations have looked for the presence of TNFSF members within the most primitive chordates alive. Cephalochordates is a chordate subphylum that is represented by the Amphioxiformes (lancelets, also known as amphioxus), which are small, fish-like, filter-feeding animals found in shallow water, and are defined by the presence of a notochord that persists throughout their life. As described in more detail in chapter: Origin and Functions of Tunicate Hemocytes, urochordates are now considered the sister group of vertebrates. The Cyclostomata is a group of primitive vertebrates that comprises the jawless fishes, whose only living representatives are the lampreys and hagfishes. A draft amphioxus genome is available[285,286] and offers insights into vertebrate origins and the evolution of immune system components, as cephalochordates and vertebrates evolved from a common ancestor over 520 million years ago. In addition, a genome exists for the sea lamprey,[287] and a transcriptome has been created from leucocytes isolated from peripheral blood, collected from the inshore lamprey.[288] Using the amphioxus genome, the information on the tunicates *Ciona intestinalis*[289] and *Ciona savignyi*,[290] and the available lamprey transcriptome, a preliminary analysis of the immune gene repertoire has revealed that these groups contain members that belong to the TNFSF.[288–291] Two were identified within the lamprey, whereas amphioxus had around 24, many of which were clustered in one region of the genome. Of these, only five sequences were cloned from *Branchiostoma japonicum*, and expression analysis revealed differences in their expression patterns in a variety of tissues. Attempts were made to identify whether any of the amphioxus and agnathan TNFSF sequences were homologous to existing vertebrate TNFSF members. What can be concluded is that the amphioxus genes form three very separate groups, with one of these containing a large number that is thought to have some homology to vertebrate TNFSF10. Interestingly, genes from the artic lamprey and inshore hagfish do group well with other vertebrate TNFSF10 sequences.

7.3   Fish

Using available fish genomes and sequences that have been deposited into databases, a number of studies have already been carried out in an attempt to characterize the TNFSF members that exist in bony fish.[246,292] It is clear from these investigations that the diversification of the TNFSF occurred early in evolution, as fish have had an extensive number of homologs from this family identified. In addition, there may also be members of the TNFSF that are novel to this group of vertebrates.

7.3.1   TNFSF1-3

TNFSF2, also known as TNF-α, is a key cytokine in mammals that induces cell survival, apoptosis, and necrosis, and contributes to both physiological and pathological processes.[278] It plays an important role in systemic inflammation, and is one of the cytokines released during the acute-phase reaction (Locksley et al., 2001). This was one of the first cytokines characterized within teleosts, and had been initially isolated from Japanese flounder[293] and trout.[294] Since then, it has been identified in a wide range of bony fish, which includes zebrafish,[295] gilt-head seabream,[296] common carp,[297] channel catfish,[298] fugu,[299] tilapia,[300] Atlantic salmon,[37] mandarinfish,[301] sea bass,[302] ayu,[303] turbot,[304] goldfish,[305] large yellow croaker,[306] bluefin tuna,[307] striped trumpeter,[45] rock bream,[308] orange-spotted grouper,[309] grass carp,[310] and crucian carp.[311] Each of these sequences were shown to contain a transmembrane domain, a tumor necrosis factor-alpha converting enzyme (TACE) cut site, and the TNF ligand family signature, similar to their human homolog. In addition, expression has also been looked at, and is upregulated in HK or macrophage primary cell-cultures after treatment with immunostimulants such as LPS, ConA, or PMA, or is upregulated in various tissues such as HK, spleen, and blood from fish infected with bacterial or viral pathogens.

Of interest in teleosts is the presence of multiple isoforms of TNFSF2 that have been discovered within a variety of species. Two copies were initially found in rainbow trout[312] and four within the common carp,[297,313,314] which share high sequence identity, but was not unexpected, as both species are tetraploid.[315,316] Although the role of each of these genes was unclear, early investigations into their study patterns of expression showed that there were clear differences. However, with the discovery of at least two TNFSF2 genes within nontetraploid fish, such as bluefin tuna,[307] orange-spotted grouper,[309] zebrafish, and medaka,[317] along with an additional gene within rainbow trout,[318] it has become clear that teleosts have two very clear groups of TNFSF2 genes. Within the genomes of zebrafish and medaka,[317] it has been shown that members from group I and group II can be found on a different chromosome (Fig. 5.5), with conservation of similar genes around it, indicating that this was due to one of the duplication events that has occurred within bony fish.[315] Interestingly, in the bluefin tuna, zebrafish, and the trout there is a difference in expression of each group member in fish, or in cells stimulated with LPS. An analysis of sequences found within available fish genomes and databases shows that both groups of TNFSF2 molecules do exist in a variety of fish species. However, the role that each of these genes plays within the immune response of teleosts remains to be determined.

Some bioactivity studies have been carried out within selected species, with the early investigations using group I TNFSF2 proteins. A variety of activities were shown, including induction of proinflammatory factors in cells from immune tissues, recruitment of phagocytic cells, enhancement of phagocytic activity, enhancement of nitric oxide (NO) production, and regulation of nonspecific cytotoxic cells.[300,304,305,307,308,319,320] However, as more studies were carried out within different fish species, some inconsistencies with certain activities were seen, which were initially highlighted in common carp and sea bream,[323,324] especially with regard to the ability of TNFSF2 to activate phagocytes. These studies showed that TNFSF2 could act on phagocytes indirectly, by activating endothelial cells to produce stimulatory factors. To date, not all fish TNFSF2 molecules have been explored, and some of these differences could be attributed to the presence of multiple forms of this gene. Investigations have been carried out on the activities of members of the fish TNFSF2 group II. In bluefin tuna, similar activities were seen with regard to enhancement of phagocytic activity of peripheral blood leucocytes,[308] and, in trout, primary macrophages, induction of pro- and anti-inflammatory cytokines, antimicrobial peptides, and the macrophage growth factor, IL-34, were observed.[318] Apart from its role in the immune response

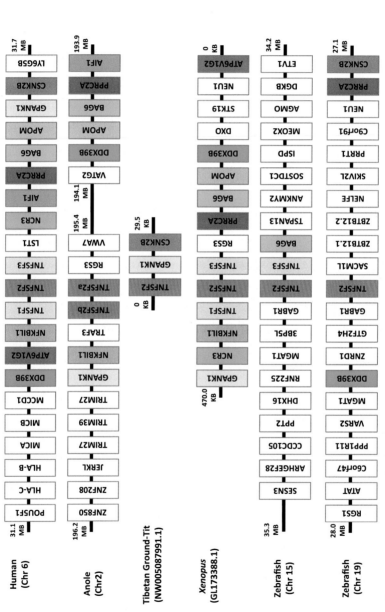

FIGURE 5.5   **Synteny analysis of the locus containing the TNFSF2 gene from human, reptile, bird, amphibian, and fish.** GeneID[321] and GENSCAN[322] were used to predict gene-coding regions of nonmammalian species to discover the gene order.

of fish, the activities of TNFSF2 in trout on other physiological pathways have also been investigated. A role within skeletal muscle metabolism was shown, where glucose uptake within trout muscle cells was stimulated,[325] and some involvement in ovarian function was found, having a stimulatory effect on oocyte maturation.[326]

To date, what still remains in question is the existence of fish homologs to TNFSF1 and TNFSF3, which in mammals are located, along with TNFSF2, next to each other on chromosome 6 in humans, within the major histo-compatibility complex (MHC) class III region.[327] TNFSF1, also known as TNF-β or LT-α, and TNFSF3, also known as LT-β, mediate a large variety of inflammatory and immunostimulatory responses, are involved in the formation of secondary lymphoid organs during development, and also play a role in apoptosis.[328] Initially in fugu and zebrafish,[299] a gene was discovered next to the already characterized TNFSF2, within the genomes of these species, which has been called TNF-new (TNF-n). Subsequent investigations identified homologs of this gene within medaka, zebrafish,[317] and trout,[329] where two genes were identified (TNF-n1 and TNF-n2). Although not functional evidence, phylogenetic analysis of these sequences with known vertebrate TNFSF1-3 sequences, has shown a closer relationship to TNFSF3 than to TNFSF1 and TNFSF2. This becomes clearer with the inclusion of *Xenopus* sequences, which are available for all three members[329] and is strengthened with the addition of a recently isolated sequence from the African lung-fish, where good identity to TNFSF3 is found.[330] Preliminary investigations have looked at the expression of TNF-n in the previously mentioned species. Constitutive expression of TNF-n is highest within the gill, liver, and intestine of zebrafish, and shows little change in HK cells stimulated with LPS.[331] In trout, it was shown that TNF-n1 had high constitutive expression in the gills and intestine, along with the spleen and HK, whereas there was little or no expression of TNF-n2 in any tissues.[329] However, no expression of either gene was found in unstimulated and stimulated macrophages, or in fibroblasts. The characterization of this gene from more fish species and functional studies are required, before its exact identity can be confirmed.

7.3.2 TNFSF13 and 13B

TNFSF13, also known as apoptosis-inducing ligand (APRIL), and TNFSF13B, also known as B-cell activating factor belonging to the TNF family (BAFF), are two related members of the TNF ligand superfamily that share receptors, however, their functions are not redundant.[332] TNFSF13B is a critical survival/maturation and proliferation factor for peripheral B cells, whereas APRIL appears to play a role in T-independent type II antigen responses and T-cell survival, but can also induce proliferation/survival of nonlymphoid cells,[333–336] To date, TNFSF13 has only been characterized in two cyprinid species, grass carp and zebrafish,[337,338] both of which contain a transmembrane domain, a TNF family signature, and a furin protease cleavage site. Searching the available sequence databases provides evidence to show that TNFSF13 can be found in a number of fish species, and is not restricted to this group of fish (Bird, unpublished). In grass carp, their expression was highest in the skin, spleen, and HK, and their involvement within the immune response was shown as expression was upregulated in these tissues as well as in gill and liver, in response to bacterial and viral pathogens. Functional activity of this molecule was observed in the zebrafish, with the recombinant protein shown to bind the surface of spleen lymphocytes and help prolong the survival of these lymphocytes.

TNFSF13B has been characterized in a larger number of fish species, which includes zebrafish,[339] mefugu,[340] Japanese sea perch,[341] grass carp,[342] yellow grouper,[343] miiuy croaker,[344] and tongue sole.[345] Similar to their human homolog, each of these sequences are shown to contain a transmembrane domain, a furin protease cleavage site, the TNF ligand family signature, and a conserved D-E loop (known as the "Flap"), which is unique to TNFSF13B and found in no other TNFSF. Comparison of the predicted 3D structure for the miiuy croaker and mefugu TNFSF13B with human revealed that they had a very similar folding pattern.[340,344] Where expression of this gene was studied in healthy tissues, it was consistently shown that it could be detected within immune-relevant tissues, where highest expression was in the spleen, followed by the HK. Exceptions to this were seen in the grass carp and miiuy croaker, where highest expression was in the skin, followed by the spleen and HK. Modulation of this expression was seen in response to bacterial and viral pathogens. In tongue sole, an increase in expression of TNFSF13B was seen in both the spleen and kidney, 6, 12, and 24 h after infection with *E. tarda*.[345] TNFSF13B expression was also significantly upregulated within the gill, liver, kidney, spleen, and skin of grass carp after *A. hydrophila* or *Aquareovirus* infection.[342] Recently highlighted, and similar to that found for TNFSF2 in fish, was the presence of more than one TNFSF13B gene in the miiuy croaker[344] and fugu,[346] which was termed TNFSF13B-like. An extensive search of the available fish genomes and sequences available within databases has revealed that many fish species have more than one TNFSF13B gene present, allowing two distinct groups to be observed. The relationship of each gene, with what is known in humans, has been investigated, and a prediction of the group II TNFSF13B gene 3D structure in the miiuy croaker shows that it has a very similar structure to the group I TNFSF13B.[344] In addition, mapping the position of each TNFSF13B gene in the genomes of selected fish species has shown that group I TNFSF13B genes are located in a region that shares conserved synteny with the human genome, whereas those in group II are located in a different region, where no synteny is observed.[346] However, this TNFSF13B-like gene is located next to another known TNF family member, ectodysplasin A (EDA). A preliminary investigation has looked at the role that these genes may have within the immune response of muiiy croaker, where the group I TNFSF13B is expressed at higher levels in the liver and kidney than the group II TNFSF13B during bacterial infection; however, this is reversed within the spleen. Limited functional studies have been carried out, however, group I TNFSF13B genes from selected fish species have been investigated using recombinant proteins. TNFSF13B has been shown to bind to the surface of lymphocytes[345] and to promote survival and proliferation of splenic B cells or lymphocytes in vitro.[339–341,343,345] In addition, overexpression of TNFSF13B in vivo enhanced macrophage activation and reduced bacterial infection, whereas knocking down the expression led to fish being more susceptible.[345]

As well as bony fish, TNFSF13B has also been characterized within a number of cartilaginous fish, such as the bamboo shark,[347] spiny dogfish,[348] and the small-spotted catshark.[349] All proteins were predicted to contain a transmembrane domain, TNF family signature, and furin protease cleavage site. Modeling of the protein structure in bamboo shark also revealed the presence of the long D-E loop that is specific to all other characterized TNFSF13B proteins. Expression in healthy tissues from all three species indicates expression is high in immune tissues, especially the spleen; however, in the spiny dogfish the pancreas also showed high constitutive expression. Stimulation of peripheral blood leucocytes with various mitogens showed that PWM, which is mitogenic for both T and B cells, had the greatest effect on TNFSF13 expression in the dogfish and catfish,[348,349] with polyI:C, LPS, ConA, PHA, and PMA having limited effects. In bamboo shark, functional activity of the protein was investigated and shown to stimulate the proliferation of mammalian B cells, however, its effects on cartilaginous fish cells remains to be seen. Interestingly, using sequences obtained from the available genomes and databases, it can be seen that, like bony fish, cartilaginous fish may also have two groups of TNFSF13B sequences, where the currently characterized bamboo shark belongs to group I and the dogfish and catshark belongs to group II, with sequences found in the elephant shark genome represented in both (Bird, unpublished).

7.3.3   Remaining TNFSF Members

Previous investigations using the available genomes and sequence databases has given good insight into which TNFSF members may exist in bony fish.[246,292] Along with the already characterized molecules mentioned previously, homologs for TNFSF5, TNFSF6, TNFSF10, TNFSF11, TNFSF12, TNFSF14, and TNFSF18 have been identified and have subsequently been characterized in a variety of fish species, where a transmembrane domain and a TNF homology domain was conserved in all cases. TNFSF5, also known as CD40 ligand (CD40L), is important in the promotion of v dependent B cell responses, where CD40L is expressed by activated T cells that engage CD40 expressed by B cells, inducing B cell proliferation, differentiation, Ig production, Ig isotype class-switching, and promotion of germinal center (GC) formation.[350] Initially this was identified within salmon,[351] but has also been discovered within *fugu*.[346] In *fugu*, highest constitutive expression was seen in the HK, liver, intestine, and heart, whereas in salmon it was observed in the HK, spleen, and gills, and was increased in HK leucocytes stimulated with PHA or ConA.[351] In addition, overexpression of CD40L in a salmon cell-line, which was cocultured with HK leucocytes, induced the rapid and long-lasting upregulation of key costimulatory molecules and cytokines that are important in T-helper cell responses.

TNFSF6, also known as Fas ligand (FasL), is predominantly expressed on activated T cells and natural killer-cells, and plays a crucial role in modulating immune responses by inducing cell-specific apoptosis.[352] Investigations in Japanese flounder[353] and *fugu*[346] have identified this family member. Both predicted amino-acid sequences were shown to contain a proline-rich N-terminal sequence, which is essential for protein expression on the cell surface, and FasL is the only member of the TNF family with this feature.[354] Constitutive expression was high in the *fugu* liver and heart,[346] whereas in flounder it was the kidney and thymus; moreover, cytotoxic activity of the recombinant flounder FasL protein was shown against a flounder cell-line.[353]

TNFSF10, also known as TNF-related apoptosis-inducing ligand (TRAIL), can induce apoptosis in various tumor cell-lines but not in normal cells, and administration in vivo can induce apoptosis in tumors with no cytotoxicity in normal organs or tissues.[355] TNFSF10 has been identified in a wide range of fish, including zebrafish,[295] grass carp,[356] mandarin fish,[357] and *fugu*.[346,358] A predicted 3D model using the *fugu* sequence showed that it was similar to the human and contained all of the important structural amino acids conserved in the same positions.[358] Constitutive mRNA expression was found in all tissues tested in each species, with the protein also widely expressed in the mandarin fish.[357] Functional activity has also been investigated, where overexpression of the protein in HeLa cells, or the effect of the recombinant protein on Jurkat or HeLa, induces apoptosis in these cell lines.[357,358] Interestingly in *fugu*, three genes have been identified with homology to TNFSF10, and multiple genes have also been shown to exist in other species, including *fugu*.[346] Despite their relatedness, each gene in *fugu* has a very different gene organization, however, their expression profiles are similar in healthy tissues and almost the same in HK cells stimulated with LPS or polyI:C. Phylogenetic analysis has shown that each of these TNFSF10 genes in fish forms distinct groups,[346] which is similar to our analysis showing that three very distinct groups of TNFSF10 can be seen (Bird, unpublished).

The remaining TNFSF members identified in fish have had limited investigations carried out. TNFSF12, also known as TNF-like weak inducer of apoptosis (TWEAK), has multiple biological activities, including stimulation of cell growth and angiogenesis, induction of inflammatory cytokines, and stimulation of apoptosis.[359] It has been characterized within the grass carp[338] and *fugu*,[346] where skin shows highest expression in both species, followed by spleen, HK, gill, and brain in the carp. In addition, bacterial and viral expression significantly upregulated TNFSF12 expression in carp spleen, HK, gill, and brain.[338] TNFSF14, also known as LT-related Inducible ligand that competes for Glycoprotein D binding to Herpesvirus entry mediator on T cells (LIGHT), functions as a costimulatory molecule for T cells and promotes the activation and expansion of T-cell populations.[360] Homologs of this gene have been investigated in zebrafish,[361] where highest constitutive expression was seen in the spleen, followed by HK, and in *fugu*[346] where expression was highest in the HK and liver. A recombinant protein was also shown to bind to the surface of zebrafish lymphocytes.[361] TNFSF18, also known as glucocorticoid-induced TNF receptor ligand (GITRL), participates in the immune response against tumors and infectious agents by influencing the activity of effector and regulatory T cells.[362] Only one functional study exists, where a homolog of this gene is found in the zebrafish.[363] Its activity has been looked at during development, where its knockdown results in disruption of embryogenesis. Lastly, within the databases, a sequence can be found within a number of bony fish with homology to TNFSF19 (also known as DEDD), which is a new member to the TNFSF. It is also a regulator and executor of the programmed cell-death pathway, with its overexpression shown to induce weak apoptosis.[364] This sequence groups well with TNFSF19 found within other vertebrate groups (Bird, unpublished).

Not much has been done to characterize these remaining TNFSF members in cartilaginous fish. Recently, a TNFSF5 homolog has been characterized in the small-spotted catshark.[349] In this study, expression was found to be highest within the gut, spleen, and gill, which correlated directly with a T-cell marker, TCRα, and its expression could be upregulated in PBLs, following stimulation with PHA, PMA, and PWM.[349] A search of the elephant shark genome and sequences available in databases has revealed that a number of other TNFSF members may exist. Phylogenetic analysis of these with representative sequences from each major vertebrate group shows that, along with TNFSF5, homologs to TNFSF6, TNFSF10, and TNFSF15 can also be identified, with multiple sequences available for TNFSF6 and TNFSF10. However, a number of sequences do exist in the elephant shark genome that belong to the TNFSF, but are difficult to assign to an existing homolog in humans.

7.4 Birds, Reptiles, and Amphibians

An interrogation of both the chicken and turkey genomes has allowed the identification of a number of TNFSF members that have been characterized within mammals.[221,223] However, TNFSF1, TNFSF2, TNFSF3, TNFSF7, TNFSF9, TNFSF12, TNFSF13, TNFSF14, and TNFSF19 remained unidentified within birds, and for some it was speculated that they may not be present within this vertebrate group. The absence of TNFSF1 and TNFSF3 was not unexpected, as these genes play an important role in lymph node development in mammals, which is lacking in birds.[328] Interestingly, the presence of TNFSF2 was expected, as TNF-α-like activity had been reported in chickens.[365] An examination of all available bird genomes has revealed a partial sequence with homology to TNFSF2 within the Tibetan ground-tit, *Pseudopodoces humilis*, on scaffold 880 (Accession no. NW_005087991.1). Using this sequence within a phylogenetic analysis does group it with other characterized TNFSF2 sequences, and prediction of genes on this scaffold does reveal that genes GPANK1 and CSNK2B can be determined, which are also found within regions of the human genome that contains TNFSF2, showing some conservation of synteny (Fig. 5.5). In addition to what has previously been characterized, an examination of all available bird sequence-data has also revealed the existence of a TNFSF14 and TNFSF19 homolog (Bird, unpublished).

Other than the discovery of gene sequences using bird genomes, limited information exists on the activity of these identified TNFSF genes in birds. The best characterized is TNFSF13B, where the gene has been isolated from chicken,[366,367] goose,[368] duck,[369] quail,[370] dove,[371] and ostrich.[372] In each of these studies, expression was highest within the spleen and bursa of fabricius, where lymphocyte concentrations are high, and the recombinant protein was shown to play an important role in the survival and proliferation of B cells in each species. The activity of recombinant chicken TNFSF5 has also been investigated, and shown to maintain proliferation of B cells in culture for up to 3 weeks and to maintain direct differentiation of cells toward a plasma-cell phenotype.[373] In addition, antigen-specific IgM and IgG was secreted by TNFSF5-activated B cells, taken from immunized birds. Lastly, TNFSF8, also known as CD30L, which plays an inhibitory role in modulating Ig class-switching in B cells,[374] along with TNFSF10 have also been loosely characterized in chicken. Both genes were shown to have high levels of expression in the spleen, in bursa of Fabricus, and in a chicken leukemia cell-line, IN24.[375]

Almost no studies have been carried out looking at the TNFSF members that are present within reptiles. One recent study exists that has isolated and characterized BAFF within the Yangtze alligator.[376] Real-time PCR indicated that the highest expression was within the spleen, and the recombinant protein was able to promote the survival of alligator spleen lymphocytes. In addition, this protein also showed some cross-reactivity in mammals, helping to promote the survival of mouse spleen cells in culture. To determine the other TNFSF members that exist within reptiles, a search of the green anole *Anolis carolinensis* genome[377] was carried out, along with the available reptile sequences within the databases. Many of the TNSF members that had been found in birds had a homolog within this vertebrate group (Table 5.2). Only TNFSF18 needed to be predicted from the genome, and was found on Scaffold chrUn0590 (Accession No. GL343782.1), along with a related sequence from the green sea turtle (Accession no. XP_007072858.1). The only main differences found were within *A. carolinensis*, where a homolog for TNFSF13 was identified (Accession no. XP_008120421.1), and a distinct region was discovered in the genome that contained a TNFSF2 homolog, which shared some synteny with the human and amphibian genomes (Fig. 5.5). Interestingly, two TNFSF2 genes are predicted within this region, with no sequence similarity to TNFSF1 and TNFSF3.

Amphibians have had some TNFSF members identified, which have been predicted using the *X. tropicalis* genome,[246,378] with a select few having been sequenced and functionally characterized. TNFSF2 was one of the first to be studied[379] in *Xenopus laevis*. In amphibians, it has been suggested that TNFSF2 may play an important role in tadpole metamorphosis, as TNFSF2 expression was prominent in the blood at prometamorphosis, and the recombinant protein found to suppress thyroid hormone induced apoptosis in a vascular endothelial cell-line.[379] More recently, homologs of *X. laevis* TNFSF10 and TNFSF13B have also been identified. Two homologs of TNFSF10 exist in *X. laevis*[380] and have been shown to play a role in erythroid maturation, which is similar to human studies.[381] TRAIL1 and TRAIL2 both show high expression within the liver and red blood cells during metamorphosis; in tadpoles, TRAIL1 was shown to accelerate hemoglobin switching and induce apoptosis in larval, but not adult, red blood cells. TNSF13B was isolated from *X. laevis*, and, similar to what was found in reptiles and birds, the expression was highest in the spleen, and the recombinant protein was able to promote survival and proliferation of lymphocytes from both *Xenopus* and mouse.[382] Lastly, using the *X. tropicalis* genome[378] and available databases, a search of the remaining TNFSF that had not yet been characterized was undertaken. This search revealed the presence of TNFSF4, TNFSF8, TNFSF9, TNFSF13, TNFSF14, TNFSF15, and TNFSF19 (Table 5.2). Of particular interest is the presence of TNFSF1 and TNFSF3, which have currently no homologs in reptiles or birds, and were first characterized in a study looking at a TNFSF member discovered within trout.[329] These two genes were identified due to the conservation of synteny that this species has with the human genome around the TNFSF2 gene. An analysis of Scaffold_752 (Accession no. GL173388.1) identified that TNFSF1, TNFSF2, and TNFSF3 were located next to each other, similar to what is found in the human genome, with conservation of other genes around them (Fig. 5.5).

REFERENCES

1. Bird S, Tafalla C. Teleost chemokines and their receptors. *Biology* 2015;**4**:756–84.
2. Chen J, Xu Q, Wang T, Collet B, Corripio-Miyar Y, Bird S, et al. Phylogenetic analysis of vertebrate CXC chemokines reveals novel lineage specific groups in teleost fish. *Dev Comp Immunol* 2013;**41**:137–52.
3. Nomiyama H, Osada N, Yoshie O. Systematic classification of vertebrate chemokines based on conserved synteny and evolutionary history. *Genes Cells* 2013;**18**:1–16.
4. Grimholt U, Hauge H, Hauge AG, Leong J, Koop BF. Chemokine receptors in Atlantic salmon. *Dev Comp Immunol* 2015;**49**:79–95.
5. Zou J, Redmond AK, Zhitao Q, Dooley H, Secombes CJ. The CXC chemokine receptors of fish: insights into CXCR evolution in the vertebrates. *Gen Comp Endocrinol* 2015;**215**:117–31.
6. Xu Q, Li R, Monte M, Jiang Y, Nie P, Holland JW, et al. Sequence and expression analysis of rainbow trout CXCR2, CXCR3a and CXCR3b aids interpretation of lineage-specific conversion, loss and expansion of these receptors during vertebrate evolution. *Dev Comp Immunol* 2014;**45**:201–13.
7. Wang T, Huang W, Costa MM, Secombes CJ. The gamma-chain cytokine/receptor system in fish: more ligands and receptors. *Fish Shellfish Immunol* 2011;**31**:673–87.
8. Secombes CJ, Wang T, Bird S. The interleukins of fish. *Dev Comp Immunol* 2011;**35**:1336–45.

9. Wang T, Secombes CJ. The cytokine networks of adaptive immunity in fish. *Fish Shellfish Immunol* 2013;**35**:1703–18.

10. Wang T, Secombes CJ. The evolution of IL-4 and IL-13 and their receptor subunits. *Cytokine* 2015;**75**:8–13.

11. Dinarello CA. IL-1: discoveries, controversies and future directions. *Eur J Immunol* 2010;**40**: 599–606.

12. Garlanda C, Dinarello CA, Mantovani A. The interleukin-1 family: back to the future. *Immunity* 2013;**39**:1003–18.

13. Dinarello CA. Biology of interleukin-1. *Faseb J* 1988;**2**:108–15.

14. Allan SM, Tyrrell PJ, Rothwell NJ. Interleukin-1 and neuronal injury. *Nat Rev Immunol* 2005;**5**:629–40.

15. Sigrist CJ, Cerutti L, de Castro E, Langendijk-Genevaux PS, Bulliard V, Bairoch A, Hulo N. PROSITE, a protein domain database for functional characterization and annotation. *Nucleic Acids Res* 2010;**38**:D161–6.

16. Dinarello CA. Interleukin-1. *Rev Infect Dis* 1984;**6**:51–95.

17. Oppenheim JJ, Kovacs EJ, Matsushima K, Durum SK. There is more than one interleukin-1. *Immunol Today* 1986;**7**:45–56.

18. Dinarello CA. Interleukin-1 and interleukin-1 antagonism. *Blood* 1991;**77**:1627–52.

19. Dinarello CA. The biological properties of interleukin-1. *Eur Cytokine Netw* 1994;**5**:517–31.

20. Dinarello CA. Biologic basis for interleukin-1 in disease. *Blood* 1996;**87**:2095–147.

21. Nakae S, Asano M, Horai R, Iwakura Y. Interleukin-1 beta, but not interleukin-1 alpha, is required for T-cell-dependent antibody production. *Immunology* 2001;**104**:402–9.

22. Nambu A, Nakae S, Iwakura Y. IL-1 beta, but not IL-1 alpha, is required for antigen-specific T cell activation and the induction of local inflammation in the delayed-type hypersensitivity responses. *Int Immunol* 2006;**18**:701–12.

23. Andersson J, Björk L, Dinarello CA, Towbin H, Andersson U. Lipopolysaccharide induces human interleukin-1 receptor antagonist and interleukin-1 production in the same cell. *Eur J Immunol* 1992;**22**:617–2623.

24. Kavita U, Mizel SB. Differential sensitivity of interleukin-1-alpha and interleukin-1-beta precursor proteins to cleavage by calpain, a calcium-dependent protease. *J Biol Chem* 1995;**270**:27758–65.

25. Dinarello CA. Immunological and inflammatory functions of the interleukin-1 family. *Annu Rev Immunol* 2009;**27**:519–50.

26. Weitzmann MN, Savage N. Nuclear internalization and DNA-binding activities of interleukin-1. Interleukin-1 receptor and interleukin-1 receptor complexes. *Biochem Biophys Res Commun* 1992;**187**:1166–71.

27. Burns K, Martinon F, Tschopp J. New insights into the mechanism of IL-1 beta maturation. *Cur Opin Immunol* 2003;**15**:26–30.

28. Miller DK, Calaycay JR, Chapman KT, Howard AD, Kostura MJ, Molineaux SM, Thornberry NA. The IL-1 beta converting enzyme as a therapeutic target. *Ann N Y Acad Sci* 1993;**696**:133–48.

29. Chin J, Kostura MJ. Dissociation of Il-1-Beta synthesis and secretion in human blood monocytes stimulated with bacterial-cell wall products. *J Immunol* 1993;**151**:5574–85.

30. Fantuzzi G, Ku G, Harding MW, Livingston DJ, Sipe JD, Kuida K, Flavell RA, Dinarello CA. Response to local inflammation of IL-1 beta-converting enzyme-deficient mice. *J Immunol* 1997;**158**:1818–24.

31. Schonbeck U, Mach F, Libby P. Generation of biologically active IL-1β by matrix metalloproteinases: a novel caspase-1 independent pathway of IL-1β processing. *J Immunol* 1998;**161**:3340–6.

32. Netea MG, Simon A, van de Veerdonk F, Kullberg BJ, Van der Meer JW, Joosten LA. IL-1 beta processing in host defense: beyond the inflammasomes. *PLoS Pathog* 2010;**6**: e1000661.

33. Weining K, Sick C, Kaspers B, Staeheli P. A chicken homolog of mammalian interleukin-1 beta: cDNA cloning and purification of active recombinant protein. *Eur J Biochem* 1998;**258**:994–1000.

34. Zhang Z, Chen B, Yuan L, Niu C. Acute cold stress improved the transcription of pro-inflammatory cytokines of Chinese soft-shelled turtle against *Aeromonas hydrophila*. *Dev Comp Immunol* 2015;**49**:127–37.

35. Zou J, Bird S, Minter R, Horton J, Cunningham C, Secombes C. Molecular cloning of the gene for interleukin-1β from *Xenopus laevis* and analysis of expression in vivo and in vitro. *Immunogenetics* 2000;**49**:332–8.

36. Zou J, Grabowski PS, Cunningham C, Secombes CJ. Molecular cloning of interleukin 1β from rainbow trout *Oncorhynchus mykiss* reveals no evidence of an ICE cut site. *Cytokine* 1999;**11**:552–60.

37. Ingerslev HC, Cunningham C, Wergeland HI. Cloning and expression of TNF-alpha IL-1 beta and COX-2 in an anadromous and landlocked strain of Atlantic salmon (*Salmo salar* L.) during the smolting period. *Fish Shellfish Immunol* 2006;**20**:450–61.

38. Fujiki K, Shin DH, Nakao M, Yano T. Molecular cloning and expression analysis of carp (*Cyprinus carpio*) interleukin-1 beta, high affinity immunoglobulin E Fc receptor gamma subunit and serum amyloid A. *Fish Shellfish Immunol* 2000;**10**:229–42.

39. Engelsma MY, Stet RJM, Saeij JP, Verburg-van Kemenade BM. Differential expression and haplotypic variation of two interleukin-1 beta genes in the common carp, *Cyprinus carpio* L. *Cytokine* 2003;**22**:21–32.

40. Bo YX, Song XH, Wu K, Hu B, Sun BY, Liu ZJ, Fu JG. Characterization of interleukin-1β as a proinflammatory cytokine in grass carp (*Ctenopharyngodon idella*). *Fish Shellfish Immunol* 2015;**46**:584–95.

41. Corripio-Miyar Y, Bird S, Tsamopoulos K, Secombes CJ. Cloning and expression analysis of two pro-inflammatory cytokines IL-1β and IL-8, in haddock (*Melanogrammus aeglefinus*). *Mol Immunol* 2007;**44**:1361–73.

42. Pelegrin P, Garcia-Castillo J, Mulero V, Meseguer J. Interleukin-1 beta isolated from a marine fish reveals up-regulated expression in macrophages following activation with lipopolysaccharide and lymphokines. *Cytokine* 2001;**16**:67–72.

43. Jiang S, Zhang D, Li J, Liu Z. Molecular characterization, recombinant expression and bioactivity analysis of the interleukin-1 beta from the yellowfin sea bream, *Acanthopagrus latus* (Houttuyn). *Fish Shellfish Immunol* 2008;**24**:323–36.

44. Lu DQ, Bei JX, Feng LN, Zhang Y, Liu XC, Wang L, Chen JL, Lin HR. Interleukin-1beta gene in orange-spotted grouper, *Epinephelus coioides*: molecular cloning, expression, biological activities and signal transduction. *Mol Immunol* 2008;**45**:857–67.

45. Covello JM, Bird S, Morrison RN, Battaglene SC, Secombes CJ, Nowak BF. Cloning and expression analysis of three striped trumpeter (*Latris lineata*) pro-inflammatory cytokines, TNF-alpha, IL-1beta and IL-8, in response to infection by the ectoparasitic, *Chondracanthus goldsmidi*. *Fish Shellfish Immunol* 2009;**26**:773–86.

46. Tsutsui S, Nakamura O, Watanabe T. Lamprey (*Lethenteron japonicum*) IL-17 upregulated by LPS-stimulation in the skin cells. *Immunogenetics* 2007;**59**:873–82.

47. Yu Y, Zhong Q, Li C, Jiang L, Sun Y, Wang X, Wang Z, Zhang Q. Molecular cloning and characterization of interleukin-1β in half-smooth tongue sole *Cynoglossus semilaevis*. *Vet Immunol Immunopathol* 2012;**146**:270–6.

48. Øvergård AC, Nepstad I, Nerland AH, Patel S. Characterisation and expression analysis of the Atlantic halibut (*Hippoglossus hippoglossus* L.) cytokines: IL-1β, IL-6, IL-11, IL-12β and IFNγ. *Mol Biol Rep* 2012;**39**:2201–13.

49. Lu XJ, Chen J, He YQ, Shi YH. Molecular characterization of an IL-1β gene from ayu (*Plecoglossus altivelis*). *Fish Shellfish Immunol* 2013;**34**:1253–9.

50. Lepen Pleić I, Secombes CJ, Bird S, Mladineo I. Characterization of three pro-inflammatory cytokines, TNFα1, TNFα2 and IL-1β, in cage-reared Atlantic bluefin tuna *Thunnus thynnus*. *Fish Shellfish Immunol* 2014;**36**:98–112.

51. Bird S, Wang T, Zou J, Cunningham C, Secombes CJ. The first cytokine sequence within cartilaginous fish: IL-1 beta in the small spotted catshark (*Scyliorhinus canicula*). *J Immunol* 2002;**168**:3329–40.

52. Bird S, Zou J, Wang T, Munday B, Cunningham C, Secombes CJ. Evolution of interleukin-1beta. *Cytokine Growth Factor Rev* 2002;**13**:483–502.

53. Cheng CS, Chen WT, Lee LH, Chen YW, Chang SY, Lyu PC, Yin HS. Structural and functional comparison of cytokine interleukin-1 beta from chicken and human. *Mol Immunol* 2011;**48**:947–55.

54. Koussounadis AI, Ritchie DW, Kemp GJ, Secombes CJ. Analysis of fish IL-1beta and derived peptide sequences indicates conserved structures with species-specific IL-1 receptor binding: implications for pharmacological design. *Curr Pharm Des* 2004;**10**:3857–71.

55. Scapigliati G, Costantini S, Colonna G, Facchiano A, Buonocore F, Bossù P, Cunningham C, Holland JW, Secombes CJ. Modelling of fish interleukin-1 and its receptor. *Dev Comp Immunol* 2004;**28**:429–41.

56. Costantini S, Facchiano AM, Randelli E, Casani D, Scapigliati G, Buonocore F. 3D modelling of three pro-inflammatory molecules in selected fish species. *Curr Pharm Des* 2010;**16**:4203–12.

57. Cheng CS, Lu WS, Tu IF, Lyu PC, Yin HS. Comparative analysis of receptor binding by chicken and human interleukin-1β. *J Mol Model* 2011;**17**:1283–94.

58. Michailidis G, Anastasiadou M, Guibert E, Froment P. Activation of innate immune system in response to lipopolysaccharide in chicken sertoli cells. *Reproduction* 2014;**148**:259–70.

59. Martini F, Fernández C, Segundo LS, Tarazona JV, Pablos MV. Assessment of potential immunotoxic effects caused by cypermethrin, fluoxetine, and thiabendazole using heat shock protein 70 and Interleukin-1β mRNA expression in the anuran *Xenopus laevis*. *Environ Toxicol Chem* 2010;**29**:2536–43.

60. Martini F, Fernández C, Tarazona JV, Pablos MV. Gene expression of heat shock protein 70, interleukin-1β and tumor necrosis factor α as tools to identify immunotoxic effects on *Xenopus laevis*: a dose-response study with benzo[a]pyrene and its degradation products. *Environ Pollut* 2012;**160**:28–33.

61. Zou J, Holland J, Pleguezuelos O, Cunningham C, Secombes CJ. Factors influencing the expression of interleukin-1 beta in cultured rainbow trout (*Oncorhynchus mykiss*) leucocytes. *Dev Comp Immunol* 2000;**24**:575–82.

62. Brubacher J, Secombes C, Zou J, Bols N. Constitutive and LPS induced gene expression in a macrophage like cell line from the rainbow trout (*Oncorhynchus mykiss*). *Dev Comp Immunol* 2000;**24**:565–74.

63. Engelsma M, Stet R, Schipper H, Verburg van Kemenade B. Regulation of interleukin-1 beta RNA expression in the common carp *Cyprinus carpio* L. *Dev Comp Immunol* 2001;**25**:195–203.

64. Øvergård AC, Nepstad I, Nerland AH, Patel S. Characterisation and expression analysis of the Atlantic halibut (*Hippoglossus hippoglossus* L.) cytokines: IL-1β, IL-6, IL-11 IL-12β and IFNγ. *Mol Biol Rep* 2012;**39**:2201–13.

65. Gonzalez SF, Buchmann K, Nielsen ME. Real-time gene expression analysis in carp (*Cyprinus carpio* L.) skin: inflammatory responses caused by the ectoparasite *Ichthyophthirius multifiliis. Fish Shellfish Immunol* 2007;**22**:641–50.

66. Orieux N, Douet DG, Le Hénaff M, Bourdineaud JP. Prevalence of *Flavobacterium psychrophilum* bacterial cells in farmed rainbow trout: characterization of metallothionein A and interleukin1-β genes as markers overexpressed in spleen and kidney of diseased fish. *Vet Microbiol* 2012;**162**:127–35.

67. Gonzalez SF, Huising MO, Stakauskas R, Forlenza M, Lidy Verburg-van Kemenade BM, Buchmann K, Nielsen ME, Wiegertjes GF. Real-time gene expression analysis in carp (*Cyprinus carpio* L.) skin: inflammatory responses to injury mimicking infection with ectoparasites. *Dev Comp Immunol* 2007;**31**:244–54.

68. Yoon Y, Yoon J, Jang MY, Na Y, Ko Y, Choi JH, Seok SH. High cholesterol diet induces IL-1β expression in adult but not larval zebrafish. *PLoS One* 2013;**8**:e66970.

69. Banerjee S, Leptin M. Systemic response to ultraviolet radiation involves induction of leukocytic IL-1β and inflammation in zebrafish. *J Immunol* 2014;**193**:1408–15.

70. Richard S, Prévot-D'Alvise N, Bunet R, Simide R, Couvray S, Coupé S, Grillasca JP. Effect of a glyphosate-based herbicide on gene expressions of the cytokines interleukin-1β and interleukin-10 and of heme oxygenase-1 in European sea bass (*Dicentrarchus labrax* L.). *Bull Environ Contam Toxicol* 2014;**92**:294–9.

71. Yan B, Han P, Pan L, Lu W, Xiong J, Zhang M, Zhang W, Li L, Wen Z. IL-1β and reactive oxygen species differentially regulate neutrophil directional migration and basal random motility in a zebrafish injury-induced inflammation model. *J Immunol* 2014;**192**: 5998–6008.

72. Scapigliati G, Buonocore F, Bird S, Zou J, Pelegrin P, Falasca C, Prugnoli D, Secombes C. Phylogeny of cytokines: molecular cloning and expression analysis of sea bass *Dicentrarchus labrax* interleukin-1 beta. *Fish Shellfish Immunol* 2001;**11**:711–26.

73. Jarrous N, Kaempfer R. Induction of human interleukin-1 gene expression by retinoic acid and its regulation at processing of precursor transcripts. *J Biol Chem* 1994;**269**:23141–9.

74. Pleguezuelos O, Zou J, Cunningham C, Secombes CJ. Cloning, sequencing, and analysis of expression of a second IL-1 beta gene in rainbow trout (*Oncorhynchus mykiss*). *Immunogenetics* 2000;**51**:1002–11.

75. Wang YP, Wang Q, Baoprasertkul P, Peatman E, Liu Z. Genomic organization, gene duplication, and expression analysis of interleukin-1 beta in channel catfish (*Ictalurus punctatus*). *Mol Immunol* 2006;**43**:1653–64.

76. Husain M, Bird S, van Zwieten R, Secombes CJ, Wang T. Cloning of the IL-1β3 gene and IL-1β4 pseudogene in salmonids uncovers a second type of IL-1β gene in teleost fish. *Dev Comp Immunol* 2012;**38**:431–46.

77. Taechavasonyoo A, Kondo H, Nozaki R, Suzuki Y, Hirono I. Identification of novel interleukin 1 beta family genes in Japanese flounder *Paralichthys olivaceus. Fish Shellfish Immunol* 2013;**34**:393–6.

78. Angosto D, Montero J, López-Muñoz A, Alcaraz-Pérez F, Bird S, Sarropoulou E, Abellán E, Meseguer J, Sepulcre MP, Mulero V. Identification and functional characterization of a new IL-1 family member IL-1Fm2 most evolutionarily advanced fish. *Innate Immun* 2014;**20**:487–500.

79. Meyer A, Van de Peer Y. From 2R to 3R: evidence for a fishspecific genome duplication (FSGD). *Bioessays* 2005;**27**:937–45.

80. Hong S, Zou J, Crampe M, Peddie S, Scapigliati G, Bols N, Cunningham C, Secombes CJ. The production and bioactivity of rainbow trout (*Oncorhynchus mykiss*) recombinant IL-1β. *Vet Immunol Immunopathol* 2001;**81**:1–14.

81. Hong S, Peddie S, Campos-Perez JJ, Zou J, Secombes CJ. The effect of intraperitoneally administered recombinant IL-1β on immune parameters and resistance to *Aeromonas salmonicida* in the rainbow trout (*Oncorhynchus mykiss*). *Dev Comp Immunol* 2003;**27**:801–12.

82. Emmadi D, Iwahori A, Hirono I, Aoki T. cDNA microarray analysis of interleukin-1 beta-induced Japanese flounder *Paralichthys olivaceus* kidney cells. *Fish Sci* 2005;**71**:519–30.

83. Benedetti S, Randelli E, Buonocore F, Zou J, Secombes CJ, Scapigliati G. Evolution of cytokine responses: IL-1 beta directly affects intracellular Ca2+ concentration of teleost fish leukocytes through a receptor-mediated mechanism. *Cytokine* 2006;**34**:9–16.

84. Taechavasonyoo A, Hirono I, Kondo H. The immune-adjuvant effect of Japanese flounder *Paralichthys olivaceus* IL-1β. *Dev Comp Immunol* 2013;**41**:564–8.

85. Yang X, Wei H, Qin L, Zhang S, Wang X, Zhang A, Du L, Zhou H. Reciprocal interaction between fish TGF-β1 and IL-1β is responsible for restraining IL-1β signaling activity in grass carp head kidney leukocytes. *Dev Comp Immunol* 2014;**47**:197–204.

86. Peddie S, Zou J, Secombes CJ. A biologically active IL-1β derived peptide stimulates phagocytosis and bactericidal activity in rainbow trout, *Oncorhynchus mykiss* (Walbaum), head kidney leucocytes in vitro. *J Fish Dis* 2002;**25**:351–60.

87. Hong S, Zou J, Collet B, Bols NC, Secombes CJ. Analysis and characterisation of IL-1 beta processing in trout, *Oncorhynchus mykiss*. *Fish Shellfish Immunol* 2004;**16**:453–9.

88. Pelegrin P, Chaves-Pozo E, Mulero V, Meseguer J. Production and mechanism of secretion of interleukin-1 beta from the marine fish gilthead seabream. *Dev Comp Immunol* 2004;**28**:229–37.

89. Nicholson DW, Thornberry NA. Caspases: killer proteases. *Trends Biochem Sci* 1997;**22**:299–306.

90. Reis MI, do Vale A, Pereira PJ, Azevedo JE, Dos Santos NM. Caspase-1 and IL-1β processing in a teleost fish. *PLoS One* 2012;**7**:e50450.

91. Vojtech LN, Scharping N, Woodson JC, Hansen JD. Roles of inflammatory caspases during processing of zebrafish interleukin-1β in *Francisella noatunensis* infection. *Infect Immun* 2012;**80**:2878–85.

92. Ogryzko NV, Hoggett EE, Solaymani-Kohal S, Tazzyman S, Chico TJ, Renshaw SA, Wilson HL. Zebrafish tissue injury causes upregulation of interleukin-1 and caspase-dependent amplification of the inflammatory response. *Dis Model Mech* 2014;**7**:259–64.

93. Irmler M, Hertig S, MacDonald H, Sadoul R, Bercherer J, Proudfoot A, Solari R, Tschopp J. Granzyme A is an interleukin-1beta converting enzyme. *J Exp Med* 1995;**181**:1917–22.

94. Black R, Kronheim S, Cantrell M, Deeley M, March C, Prickett K, et al. Generation of biologically active interleukin-1β by proteolytic cleavage of the inactive precursor. *J Biol Chem* 1998;**263**:9437–42.

95. Hazuda D, Strickler J, Kueppers F, Simon P, Young P. Processing of precursor interleukin-1 beta and inflammatory disease. *J Biol Chem* 1990;**265**:6318–22.

96. Mizutani H, Schechter N, Lazarus G, Black R, Kupper T. Rapid and specific conversion of precursor interleukin-1 beta (IL-1 beta) to an active IL-1 species by human mast cell chymase. *J Exp Med* 1991;**174**:821–5.

97. Okamura H, Tsutsui H, Komatsu T, Yutsudo M, Hakura A, Tanimoto T, Torigoe K, Okura T, Nukada Y, Hattori K, Akita K, Namba M, Tanabe F, Konishi K, Fukuda S, Kurimoto M. Cloning of a new cytokine that induces IFN-gamma production by T-cells. *Nature* 1995;**378**:88–91.

98. Ushio S, Namba M, Okura T, Hattori K, Nukada Y, Akita K, Tanabe F, Konishi K, Micallef M, Fujii M, Torigoe K, Tanimoto T, Fukuda S, Ikeda M, Okamura H, Kurimoto M. Cloning of the cDNA for human IFN-gamma Inducing factor, expression in *Escherichia coli*, and studies on the biologic activities of the protein. *J Immunol* 1996;**156**:4274–9.

99. Bazan J, Timans J, Kastelein R. A newly defined interleukin-1? *Nature* 1996;**379**:591.

100. Gu Y, Kuida K, Tsutsui H, Ku G, Hsiao K, Fleming M, Hayashi N, Higashino K, Okamura H, Nakanishi K, Kurimoto M, Tanimoto T, Flavell R, Sato V, Harding M, Livingston D, Su M. Activation of interferon-gamma inducing factor mediated by interleukin-1 beta converting enzyme. *Science* 1997;**275**:206–9.

101. Ghayur T, Banerjee S, Hugunin M, Butler D, Herzog L, Carter A, Quintal L, Sekut L, Talanian R, Paskind M, Wong W, Kamen R, Tracey D, Allen H. Caspase-1 processes IFN-gamma inducing factor and regulates LPS induced IFN-gamma production. *Nature* 1997;**386**:619–23.

102. Liu B, Novick D, Kim S, Rubinstein M. Production of a biologically active human interleukin-18 requires its prior synthesis as pro-IL-18. *Cytokine* 2000;**12**:1519–25.

103. Torigoe K, Ushio S, Okura T, Kobayashi S, Taniai M, Kunikata T, Murakami T, Sanou O, Kojima H, Fujii M, Ohta T, Ikeda M, Ikegami H, Kurimoto M. Purification and characterization of the human interleukin-18 receptor. *J Biol Chem* 1997;**272**:25737–42.

104. Puren A, Fantuzzi G, Dinarello C. Gene expression, synthesis, and secretion of interleukin-18 and interleukin-1 beta are differentially regulated in human blood mononuclear cells and mouse spleen cells. *Proc Natl Acad Sci USA* 1999;**96**:2256–61.

105. Akita K, Ohtsuki T, Nukada Y, Tanimoto T, Namba M, Okura T, Takakura-Yamamoto R, Torigoe K, Gu Y, Su M, Fujii M, Satoh-Itoh M, Yamamoto K, Kohno K, Ikeda M, Kurimoto M. Involvement of caspase-1 and caspase-3 in the production and processing of mature human interleukin-18 in monocytic THP 1 cells. *J Biol Chem* 1997;**272**:26595–603.

106. Tone M, Thompson S, Tone Y, Fairchild P, Waldmann H. Regulation of IL-18 (IFN-gamma inducing factor) gene expression. *J Immunol* 1997;**159**:6156–63.

107. Schneider K, Puehler F, Baeuerle D, Elvers S, Staeheli P, Kaspers B, Weining KC. cDNA cloning of biologically active chicken interleukin-18. *J Interferon Cytokine Res* 2000;**20**:879–83.

108. Kaiser P. Turkey and chicken interleukin-18 (IL18) share high sequence identity, but have different polyadenylation sites in their 3′ UTR. *Dev Comp Immunol* 2002;**26**:681–7.

109. Chen HY, Cui BA, Xia PA, Li XS, Hu GZ, Yang MF, Zhang HY, Wang XB, Cao SF, Zhang LX, Kang XT, Tu K. Cloning, in vitro expression and bioactivity of duck interleukin-18. *Vet Immunol Immunopathol* 2008;**123**:205–14.

110. Zou J, Bird S, Truckle J, Bols N, Horne M, Secombes C. Identification and expression analysis of an IL-18 homologue and its alternatively spliced form in rainbow trout (*Oncorhynchus mykiss*). *Eur J Biochem* 2004;**271**:1913–23.

111. Kato Z, Jee J, Shikano H, Mishima M, Ohki I, Ohnishi H, Li A, Hashimoto K, Matsukuma E, Omoya K, Yamamoto Y, Yoneda T, Hara T, Kondo N, Shirakawa M. The structure and binding mode of interleukin-18. *Nat Struct Biol* 2003;**10**:966–71.

112. Göbel TW, Schneider K, Schaerer B, Mejri I, Puehler F, Weigend S, Staeheli P, Kaspers B. IL-18 stimulates the proliferation and IFN-gamma release of CD4+ T cells in the chicken: conservation of a Th1-like system in a nonmammalian species. *J Immunol* 2003;**171**:1809–15.

113. Chen HY, Yang MF, Cui BA, Cui P, Sheng M, Chen G, Wang SJ, Geng JW. Construction and immunogenicity of a recombinant fowlpox vaccine coexpressing S1 glycoprotein of infectious bronchitis virus and chicken IL-18. *Vaccine* 2010;**28**:8112–9.

114. Chen HY, Zhao L, Wei ZY, Cui BA, Wang ZY, Li XS, Xia PA, Liu JP. Enhancement of the immunogenicity of an infectious laryngotracheitis virus DNA vaccine by a bicistronic plasmid encoding glycoprotein B and interleukin-18. *Antiviral Res* 2010;**87**:235–41.

115. Chen HY, Zhang HY, Li XS, Cui BA, Wang SJ, Geng JW, Li K. Interleukin-18-mediated enhancement of the protective effect of an infectious laryngotracheitis virus glycoprotein B plasmid DNA vaccine in chickens. *J Med Microbiol* 2011;**60**:110–6.

116. Mingxiao M, Ningyi J, Zhenguo W, Ruilin W, Dongliang F, Min Z, Gefen Y, Chang L, Leili J, Kuoshi J, Yingjiu Z. Construction and immunogenicity of recombinant fowlpox vaccines coexpressing HA of AIV H5N1 and chicken IL18. *Vaccine* 2006;**24**:4304–11.

117. Chen HY, Shang YH, Yao HX, Cui BA, Zhang HY, Wang ZX, Wang YD, Chao AJ, Duan TY. Immune responses of chickens inoculated with a recombinant fowlpox vaccine coexpressing HA of H9N2 avain influenza virus and chicken IL-18. *Antiviral Res* 2011;**91**:50–6.
118. Chen HY, Cui P, Cui BA, Li HP, Jiao XQ, Zheng LL, Cheng G, Chao AJ. Immune responses of chickens inoculated with a recombinant fowlpox vaccine coexpressing glycoprotein B of infectious laryngotracheitis virus and chicken IL-18. *FEMS Immunol Med Microbiol* 2011;**63**:289–95.
119. Li K, Gao H, Gao L, Qi X, Gao Y, Qin L, Wang Y, Wang X. Adjuvant effects of interleukin-18 in DNA vaccination against infectious bursal disease virus in chickens. *Vaccine* 2013;**31**:1799–805.
120. Rahman MM, Uyangaa E, Han YW, Kim SB, Kim JH, Choi JY, Eo SK. Enhancement of Th1-biased protective immunity against avian influenza H9N2 virus via oral co-administration of attenuated *Salmonella enterica* serovar *typhimurium* expressing chicken interferon-α and interleukin-18 along with an inactivated vaccine. *BMC Vet Res* 2012;**8**:105.
121. Lim KL, Jazayeri SD, Yeap SK, Mohamed Alitheen NB, Bejo MH, Ideris A, Omar AR. Antibody and T cell responses induced in chickens immunized with avian influenza virus N1 and NP DNA vaccine with chicken IL-15 and IL-18. *Res Vet Sci* 2013;**95**:1224–34.
122. Rahman MM, Uyangaa E, Han YW, Kim SB, Kim JH, Choi JY, Eo SK. Oral co-administration of live attenuated *Salmonella enterica* serovar *Typhimurium* expressing chicken interferon-α and interleukin-18 enhances the alleviation of clinical signs caused by respiratory infection with avian influenza virus H9N2. *Vet Microbiol* 2012;**157**:448–55.
123. Lim KL, Jazayeri SD, Yeap SK, Alitheen NB, Bejo MH, Ideris A, Omar AR. Co-administration of avian influenza virus H5 plasmid DNA with chicken IL-15 and IL-18 enhanced chickens immune responses. *BMC Vet Res* 2012;**8**:132.
124. Rahman MM1, Uyangaa E, Eo SK. Modulation of humoral and cell-mediated immunity against avian influenza and Newcastle disease vaccines by oral administration of *Salmonella enterica* serovar *typhimurium* expressing chicken interleukin-18. *Immune Netw* 2013;**13**:34–41.
125. Su BS, Shen PC, Hung LH, Huang JP, Yin HS, Lee LH. Potentiation of cell-mediated immune responses against recombinant HN protein of Newcastle disease virus by recombinant chicken IL-18. *Vet Immunol Immunopathol* 2011;**141**:283–92.
126. Wang C, Li X, Zhang C, Wu T, Li Y, Cheng X. A eukaryotic expression plasmid carrying chicken interleukin-18 enhances the response to newcastle disease virus vaccine. *Clin Vaccine Immunol* 2015;**22**:56–64.
127. Nakanishi K, Yoshimoto T, Tsutsui H, Okamura H. Interleukin-18 regulates both Th1 and Th2 responses. *Annu Rev Immunol* 2001;**19**:423–74.
128. Gibson MS, Fife M, Bird S, Salmon N, Kaiser P. Identification, cloning, and functional characterization of the IL-1 receptor antagonist in the chicken reveal important differences between the chicken and mammals. *J Immunol* 2012;**189**:539–50.
129. Gibson MS, Salmon N, Bird S, Kaiser P, Fife M. Identification, cloning and characterisation of interleukin-1F5 (IL-36RN) in the chicken. *Dev Comp Immunol* 2012;**8**:136–47.
130. Hannum CH, Wilcox CJ, Arend WP, Joslin FG, Dripps DJ, Heimdal PL, Armes LG, Sommer A, Eisenberg SP, Thompson RC. Interleukin-1 receptor antagonist activity of a human interleukin-1 inhibitor. *Nature* 1990;**343**:336–40.
131. Evans RJ, Bray J, Childs JD, Vigers GP, Brandhuber BJ, Skalicky JJ, Thompson RC, Eisenberg SP. Mapping receptor binding sites in interleukin (IL)-1 receptor antagonist and IL-1 beta by site-directed mutagenesis. Identification of a single site in IL-1ra and two sites in IL-1 beta. *J Biol Chem* 1995;**270**:11477–83.
132. Arend WP. Interleukin-1 receptor antagonist. *Adv Immunol* 1993;**54**:167–227.
133. Butcher C, Steinkasserer A, Tejura S, Lennard AC. Comparison of two promoters controlling expression of secreted or intracellular IL-1 receptor antagonist. *J Immunol* 1994;**153**:701–11.

134. Muzio M, Polentarutti N, Facchetti F, Peri G, Doni A, Sironi M, Transidico P, Salmona M, Introna M, Mantovani A. Characterization of type II intracellular IL-1 receptor antagonist (IL-1ra3): a depot IL-1ra. *Eur J Immunol* 1999;**29**:781–8.

135. Towne JE, Garka KE, Renshaw BR, Virca GD, Sims JE. Interleukin (IL)-1F6, IL-1F8, and IL-1F9 signal through IL-1Rrp2 and IL-1RAcP to activate the pathway leading to NF-kappaB and MAPKs. *J Biol Chem* 2004;**279**:13677–88.

136. Costelloe C, Watson M, Murphy A, McQuillan K, Loscher C, Armstrong ME, Garlanda C, Mantovani A, O'Neill LA, Mills KH, Lynch MA. IL-1F5 mediates anti-inflammatory activity in the brain through induction of IL-4 following interaction with SIGIRR/TIR8. *J Neurochem* 2008;**105**:1960–9.

137. Wang T, Bird S, Koussounadis A, Holland JW, Carrington A, Zou J, Secombes CJ. Identification of a novel IL-1 cytokine family member in teleost fish. *J Immunol* 2009;**183**:962–74.

138. Yao F, Yang Y, Wang X, Wei H, Zhang A, Zhou H. Molecular and functional characterization of an IL-β receptor antagonist in grass carp (*Ctenopharyngodon idella*). *Dev Comp Immunol* 2015;**49**:207–16.

139. Kaiser P, Mariani P. Promoter sequence exon:intron structure, and synteny of genetic location show that a chicken cytokine with T-cell proliferative activity is IL2 and not IL15. *Immunogenetics* 1999;**49**:26–35.

140. Díaz-Rosales P, Bird S, Wang TH, Fujiki K, Davidson WS, Zou J, Secombes CJ. Rainbow trout interleukin-2: cloning, expression and bioactivity analysis. *Fish Shellfish Immunol* 2009;**27**:414–22.

141. Bird S, Zou J, Kono T, Sakai M, Dijkstra JM, Secombes CJ. Characterisation and expression analysis of interleukin 2 (IL-2) and IL-21 homologues in the Japanese pufferfish, *Fugu rubripes*, following their discovery by synteny. *Immunogenetics* 2005;**56**:909–23.

142. Secombes CJ, Zou J, Bird S. Cytokines of cartilaginous fish. In: Smith SL, Sim RB, Flajnik MF, editors. *Immunobiology of the shark.* CRC Press: Boca Raton, FL; 2015. p. 123–42.

143. Liao W, Lin JX, Leonard WJ. Interleukin-2 at the crossroads of effector responses, tolerance, and immunotherapy. *Immunity* 2013;**38**:13–25.

144. Susta L, Diel DG, Courtney S, Cardenas-Garcia S, Sundick RS, Miller PJ, Brown CC, Afonso CL. Expression of chicken interleukin-2 by a highly virulent strain of Newcastle disease virus leads to decreased systemic viral load but does not significantly affect mortality in chickens. *Virol J* 2015;**12**:122.

145. Howard M, Farrar J, Hilfiker M, Johnson B, Takatsu K, Hamaoka T, Paul WE. Identification of a T cell-derived b cell growth factor distinct from interleukin 2. *J Exp Med* 1982;**155**:914–23.

146. Paul WE. History of interleukin 4. *Cytokine* 2015;**75**:3–7.

147. Brown KD, Zurawski SM, Mosmann TR, Zurawski G. A family of small inducible proteins secreted by leukocytes are members of a new superfamily that includes leukocyte and fibroblast-derived inflammatory agents, growth factors, and indicators of various activation processes. *J Immunol* 1989;**142**:679–87.

148. Avery S, Rothwell L, Degen WD, Schijns VE, Young J, Kaufman J, Kaiser P. Characterization of the first nonmammalian T2 cytokine gene cluster: the cluster contains functional single-copy genes for IL-3, IL-4, IL-13, and GM-CSF, a gene for IL-5 that appears to be a pseudogene, and a gene encoding another cytokine like transcript, KK34. *J Interferon Cytokine Res* 2004;**24**:600–10.

149. Sawant PM, Verma PC, Subudhi PK, Chaturvedi U, Singh M, Kumar R, Tiwari AK. Immunomodulation of bivalent Newcastle disease DNA vaccine induced immune response by co-delivery of chicken IFN-γ and IL-4 genes. *Vet Immunol Immunopathol* 2011;**144**:36–44.

150. Wang T, Huang W, Costa MM, Martin SA, Secombes CJ. Two copies of the genes encoding the subunits of putative interleukin (IL)-4/IL-13 receptors, IL-4Rα, IL-13Rα1 and IL-13Rα2, have been identified in rainbow trout (*Oncorhynchus mykiss*) and have complex patterns of expression and modulation. *Immunogenetics* 2011;**63**:235–53.

151. Li JH, Shao JZ, Xiang LX, Wen Y. Cloning, characterization and expression analysis of puffer-fish IL-4 cDNA: the first evidence of Th2-type cytokine in fish. *Mol Immunol* 2007;**44**:2078–86.

152. Bird S, Secombes CJ. *Danio rerio* partial mRNA for interleukin-4. GenBank Accession No. AM403245; 2006.

153. Ohtani M, Hayashi N, Hashimoto K, Nakanishi T, Dijkstra JM. Comprehensive clarification of two paralogous interleukin 4/13 loci in teleost fish. *Immunogenetics* 2008;**60**:383–97.

154. Dijkstra JM. T(H)2 and T-reg candidate genes in elephant shark. *Nature* 2014;**511**:E7–E10.

155. Wang T, Johansson P, Abós B, Holt A, Tafalla C, Jiang Y, Wang A, Xu Q, Qi Z, Huang W, Costa MM, Diaz-Rosales P, Holland JW, Secombes CJ. First in-depth analysis of the novel Th2-type cytokines in salmonid fish reveals distinct patterns of expression and modulation but overlapping bioactivities. *Oncotarget* 2016; doi: 10.18632/oncotarget.7295.

156. Lin AF, Xiang LX, Wang QL, Dong WR, Gong YF, Shao JZ. The DCSIGN of zebrafish: insights into the existence of a CD209 homologue in a lower vertebrate and its involvement in adaptive immunity. *J Immunol* 2009;**183**:7398–410.

157. Zhu L-Y, Pan P-P, Fang W, Shao J-Z, Xiang L-X. Essential role of IL-4 and IL-4Ra in interaction in adaptive immunity of zebrafish: insight into the origin of Th2-like regulatory mechanisms in ancient vertebrates. *J Immunol* 2012;**188**:5571–84.

158. Gao J, Zhao L, Wan YY, Zhu B. Mechanism of action of IL-7 and its potential applications and limitations in cancer immunotherapy. *Int J Mol Sci* 2015;**16**:10267–80.

159. Kono T, Bird S, Sonoda K, Savan R, Secombes CJ, Sakai M. Characterization and expression analysis of an interleukin-7 homologue in the Japanese pufferfish, *Takifugu rubripes*. *FEBS J* 2008;**275**:1213–26.

160. Venkatesh B, Lee AP, Ravi V, Maurya AK, Lian MM, Swann JB, et al. Elephant shark genome provides unique insights into gnathostome evolution. *Nature* 2014;**505**:174–9.

161. Farahani R, Sherkat R, Hakemi MG, Eskandari N, Yazdani R. Cytokines (interleukin-9, IL-17, IL-22 IL-25 and IL-33) and asthma. *Adv Biomed Res* 2014;**3**:127.

162. Kaplan MH, Hufford MM, Olson MR. The development and in vivo function of T helper 9 cells. *Nat Rev Immunol* 2015;**15**:295–307.

163. Choi KD, Lillehoj HS, Song KD, Han JY. Molecular and functional characterization of chicken IL-15. *Dev Comp Immunol* 1999;**23**:165–77.

164. Fang W, Xiang LX, Shao JZ, Wen Y, Chen SY. Identification and characterization of an interleukin-15 homologue from *Tetraodon nigroviridis*. *Comp Biochem Physiol B Biochem Mol Biol* 2006;**143**:335–43.

165. Wang T, Holland JW, Carrington A, Zou J, Secombes CJ. Molecular and functional characterization of IL-15 in rainbow trout *Oncorhynchus mykiss*: a potent inducer of IFN-gamma expression in spleen leukocytes. *J Immunol* 2007;**179**:1475–88.

166. Bae JS, Shim SH, Hwang SD, Kim JW, Park DW, Park CI. Molecular cloning and expression analysis of interleukin (IL)-15 and IL-15 receptor α from rock bream, *Oplegnathus fasciatus*. *Fish Shellfish Immunol* 2013;**35**:1209–15.

167. Bei JX, Suetake H, Araki K, Kikuchi K, Yoshiura Y, Lin HR, Suzuki Y. Two interleukin (IL)-15 homologues in fish from two distinct origins. *Mol Immunol* 2006;**43**:860–9.

168. Gunimaladevi I, Savan R, Sato K, Yamaguchi R, Sakai M. Characterization of an interleukin-15 like (IL-15L) gene from zebrafish (*Danio rerio*). *Fish Shellfish Immunol* 2007;**22**:351–62.

169. Dijkstra JM, Takizawa F, Fischer U, Friedrich M, Soto-Lampe V, Lefèvre C, Lenk M, Karger A, Matsui T, Hashimoto K. Identification of a gene for an ancient cytokine, interleukin 15-like, in mammals; interleukins 2 and 15 co-evolved with this third family member, all sharing binding motifs for IL-15Rα. *Immunogenetics* 2014;**66**:93–103.

170. Mishra A, Sullivan L, Caligiuri MA. Molecular pathways: interleukin-15 signaling in health and in cancer. *Clin Cancer Res* 2014;**20**:2044–50.

171. Wang T, Diaz-Rosales P, Costa MM, Campbell S, Snow M, Collet B, Martin SA, Secombes CJ. Functional characterization of a nonmammalian IL-21: rainbow trout *Oncorhynchus mykiss* IL-21 upregulates the expression of the Th cell signature cytokines IFN-gamma, IL-10, and IL-22. *J Immunol* 2011;**186**:708–21.

172. Wang HJ, Xiang LX, Shao JZ, Jia S. Molecular cloning, characterization and expression analysis of an IL-21 homologue from *Tetraodon nigroviridis*. *Cytokine* 2006;**35**:126–34.

173. Tangye SG. Advances in IL-21 biology—enhancing our understanding of human disease. *Curr Opin Immunol* 2015;**34**:107–15.

174. Rothwell L, Hu T, Wu Z, Kaiser P. Chicken interleukin-21 is costimulatory for T cells and blocks maturation of dendritic cells. *Dev Comp Immunol* 2012;**36**:475–82.

175. Wang T, Jiang Y, Wang A, Husain M, Xu Q, Secombes CJ. Identification of the salmonid IL-17A/F1a/b, IL-17A/F2b IL-17A/F3 and IL-17N genes and analysis of their expression following in vitro stimulation and infection. *Immunogenetics* 2015;**67**:395–412.

176. Janssens K, Slaets H, Hellings N. Immunomodulatory properties of the IL-6 cytokine family in multiple sclerosis. *Ann N Y Acad Sci* 2015;**1351**:52–60.

177. Dillon SR, Sprecher C, Hammond A, Bilsborough J, Rosenfeld-Franklin M, et al. Interleukin 31, a cytokine produced by activated T cells, induces dermatitis in mice. *Nat Immunol* 2004;**5**:752–60.

178. Cornelissen C, Lüscher-Firzlaff J, Baron JM, Lüscher B. Signaling by IL-31 and functional consequences. *Eur J Cell Biol* 2012;**91**:552–66.

179. Jones LL, Vignali DA. Molecular interactions within the IL-6/IL-12 cytokine/receptor superfamily. *Immunol Res* 2011;**51**:5–14.

180. Wang T, Husain M, Hong S, Holland JW. Differential expression, modulation, and bioactivity of distinct fish IL-12 isoforms: implication towards the evolution of Th1-like immune responses. *Eur J Immunol* 2014;**44**:1541–51.

181. Costa MM, Maehr T, Diaz-Rosales P, Secombes CJ, Wang T. Bioactivity studies of rainbow trout (*Oncorhynchus mykiss*) interleukin-6: effects on macrophage growth and antimicrobial peptide gene expression. *Mol Immunol* 2011;**48**:1903–16.

182. Schaper F, Rose-John S. Interleukin-6: biology, signaling and strategies of blockade. *Cytokine Growth Factor Rev* 2015;**26**:475–87.

183. Wang X, Li C, Thongda W, Luo Y, Beck B, Peatman E. Characterization and mucosal responses of interleukin 17 family ligand and receptor genes in channel catfish *Ictalurus punctatus*. *Fish Shellfish Immunol* 2014;**38**:47–55.

184. Husain M, Martin SA, Wang T. Identification and characterisation of the IL-27 p28 subunits in fish: cloning and comparative expression analysis of two p28 paralogues in Atlantic salmon *Salmo salar*. *Fish Shellfish Immunol* 2014;**41**:102–12.

185. Jiang Y, Husain M, Qi Z, Bird S, Wang T. Identification and expression analysis of two interleukin-23α (p19) isoforms, in rainbow trout *Oncorhynchus mykiss* and Atlantic salmon *Salmo salar*. *Mol Immunol* 2015;**66**:216–28.

186. Putoczki T, Ernst M. More than a sidekick: the IL-6 family cytokine IL-11 links inflammation to cancer. *J Leukoc Biol* 2010;**88**:1109–17.

187. Kaiser P, Rothwell L, Avery S, Balu S. Evolution of the interleukins. *Dev Comp Immunol* 2004;**28**:375–94.

188. Kaneda M, Odaka T, Suetake H, Tahara D, Miyadai T. Teleost IL-6 promotes antibody production through STAT3 signaling via IL-6R and gp130. *Dev Comp Immunol* 2012;**38**: 224–31.

189. Chen HH, Lin HT, Foung YF, Han-You Lin J. The bioactivity of teleost IL-6: IL-6 protein in orange-spotted grouper (*Epinephelus coioides*) induces Th2 cell differentiation pathway and antibody production. *Dev Comp Immunol* 2012;**38**:285–94.

190. Kawashima T, Hojyo S, Nishimichi N, Sato M, Aosasa M, Horiuchi H, Furusawa S, Matsuda H. Characterization and expression analysis of the chicken interleukin-11 receptor alpha chain. *Dev Comp Immunol* 2005;**29**:349–59.

191. Wang T, Holland JW, Bols N, Secombes CJ. Cloning and expression of the first nonmammalian interleukin-11 gene in rainbow trout *Oncorhynchus mykiss*. *FEBS J* 2005;**272**: 1136–47.

192. Huising MO, Kruiswijk CP, van Schijndel JE, Savelkoul HF, Flik G, Verburg-van Kemenade BM. Multiple and highly divergent IL-11 genes in teleost fish. *Immunogenetics* 2005;**57**:432–43.

193. Santos MD, Yasuike M, Kondo H, Hirono I, Aoki T. Teleostean IL11b exhibits complementing function to IL11a and expansive involvement in antibacterial and antiviral responses. *Mol Immunol* 2008;**45**:3494–501.

194. Nicola NA, Babon JJ. Leukemia inhibitory factor (LIF). *CytokineGrowth Factor Rev* 2015;**26**:533–44.

195. Fujiki K, Nakao M, Dixon B. Molecular cloning and characterisation of a carp (*Cyprinus carpio*) cytokine-like cDNA that shares sequence similarity with IL-6 subfamily cytokines CNTF, OSM, and LIF. *Dev Comp Immunol* 2003;**27**:127–36.

196. Abe T, Mikekado T, Haga S, Kisara Y, Watanabe K, Kurokawa T, Suzuki T. Identification, cDNA cloning, and mRNA localization of a zebrafish ortholog of leukemia inhibitory factor. *Comp Biochem Physiol B Biochem Mol Biol* 2007;**147**:38–44.

197. Wang T, Secombes CJ. Identification and expression analysis of two fish-specific IL-6 cytokine family members, the ciliary neurotrophic factor (CNTF)-like and M17 genes, in rainbow trout *Oncorhynchus mykiss*. *Mol Immunol* 2009;**46**:2290–8.

198. Ogai K, Kuwana A, Hisano S, Nagashima M, Koriyama Y, Sugitani K, Mawatari K, Nakashima H, Kato S. Upregulation of leukemia inhibitory factor (LIF) during the early stage of optic nerve regeneration in zebrafish. *PLoS One* 2014;**9**:e106010.

199. Hanington PC, Belosevic M. Interleukin-6 family cytokine M17 induces differentiation and nitric oxide response of goldfish (*Carassius auratus* L.) macrophages. *Dev Comp Immunol* 2007;**31**:817–29.

200. Pasquin S, Sharma M, Gauchat JF. Ciliary neurotrophic factor (CNTF): new facets of an old molecule for treating neurodegenerative and metabolic syndrome pathologies. *Cytokine Growth Factor Rev* 2015;**26**:507–15.

201. Maehiro S, Takeuchi A, Yamashita J, Hiraki T, Kawabata Y, Nakasone K, Hosono K, Usami T, Paul-Prasanth B, Nagahama Y, Oka Y, Okubo K. Sexually dimorphic expression of the sex chromosome-linked genes cntfa and pdlim3a in the medaka brain. *Biochem Biophys Res Commun* 2014;**445**:113–9.

202. Vlotides G, Zitzmann K, Stalla GK, Auernhammer CJ. Novel neurotrophin-1/B cell-stimulating factor-3 (NNT-1/BSF-3)/cardiotrophin-like cytokine (CLC)—a novel gp130 cytokine with pleiotropic functions. *Cytokine Growth Factor Rev* 2004;**15**:325–36.

203. Derouet D, Rousseau F, Alfonsi F, Froger J, Hermann J, et al. Neuropoietin, a new IL-6-related cytokine signalling through the ciliary neurotrophic factor receptor. *Proc Natl Acad Sci USA* 2004;**101**:4827–32.

204. Kobayashi M, Fitz L, Ryan M, Hewick RM, Clark SC, Chan S, Loudon R, Sherman F, Perussia B, Trinchieri G. Identification and purification of natural killer cell stimulatory factor (NKSF), a cytokine with multiple biologic effects on human lymphocytes. *J Exp Med* 1989;**170**:827–45.
205. Yoshiura Y, Kiryu I, Fujiwara A, Suetake H, Suzuki Y, Nakanishi T, Ototake M. Identification and characterization of *Fugu* orthologues of mammalian interleukin-12 subunits. *Immunogenetics* 2003;**55**:296–306.
206. Wang T, Husain M. The expanding repertoire of the IL-12 cytokine family in teleost fish: identification of three paralogues each of the p35 and p40 genes in salmonids, and comparative analysis of their expression and modulation in Atlantic salmon *Salmo salar*. *Dev Comp Immunol* 2014;**46**:194–207.
207. Huising MO, Kruiswijk CP, Flik G. Phylogeny and evolution of class-I helical cytokines. *J Endocrinol* 2006;**189**:1–25.
208. Nascimento DS, do Vale A, Tomás AM, Zou J, Secombes CJ, dos Santos NMS. Cloning, promoter analysis and expression in response to bacterial exposure of sea bass (*Dicentrarchus labrax* L.) interleukin-12 p40 and p35 subunits. *Mol Immunol* 2007;**44**:2277–91.
209. Tsai JL, Priya TA, Hu KY, Yan HY, Shen ST, Song YL. Grouper interleukin-12, linked by an ancient disulfide-bond architecture, exhibits cytokine and chemokine activities. *Fish Shellfish Immunol* 2014;**3**:27–37.
210. Zhang L, Zhang BC, Hu YH. Rock bream (*Oplegnathus fasciatus*) IL-12p40: identification, expression, and effect on bacterial infection. *Fish Shellfish Immunol* 2014;**39**:312–20.
211. Oppmann B, Lesley R, Blom B, Timans JC, Xu Y, et al. Novel p19 protein engages IL-12p40 to form a cytokine, IL-23, with biological activities similar as well as distinct from IL-12. *Immunity* 2000;**13**:715–25.
212. Floss DM, Schröder J, Franke M, Scheller J. Insights into IL-23 biology: from structure to function. *Cytokine Growth Factor Rev* 2015;**26**:569–78.
213. Holt A, Mitra S, van der Sar AM, Alnabulsi A, Secombes CJ, Bird S. Discovery of zebrafish (*Danio rerio*) Interleukin-23 alpha (IL-23α) chain, a subunit important for the formation of IL-23, a cytokine involved in the development of Th17 cells and inflammation. *Mol Immunol* 2011;**48**:981–91.
214. Aparicio-Siegmund S, Garbers C. The biology of interleukin-27 reveals unique pro- and anti-inflammatory functions in immunity. *Cytokine Growth Factor Rev* 2015;**26**:579–86.
215. Devergne O, Hummel M, Koeppen H, Le Beau MM, Nathanson EC, Kieff E, Birkenbach M. A novel interleukin-12 p40-related protein induced by latent Epstein-Barr virus infection in B lymphocytes. *J Virol* 1996;**70**:1143–53.
216. Pflanz S, Timans JC, Cheung J, Rosales R, Kanzler H, et al. IL-27, a heterodimeric cytokine composed of EBI3 and p28 protein, induces proliferation of naive CD4+ T cells. *Immunity* 2002;**16**:779–90.
217. Devergne O, Birkenbach M, Kieff E. Epstein-Barr virus-induced gene 3 and the p35 subunit of interleukin 12 form a novel heterodimeric hematopoietin. *Proc Natl Acad Sci USA* 1997;**94**:12041–6.
218. Collison LW, Workman CJ, Kuo TT, Boyd K, Wang Y, Vignali KM, Cross R, Sehy D, Blumberg RS, Vignali DA. The inhibitory cytokine IL-35 contributes to regulatory T-cell function. *Nature* 2007;**450**:566–9.
219. Sawant DV, Hamilton K, Vignali DA. Interleukin-35: expanding its job profile. *J Interferon Cytokine Res* 2015;**35**:499–512.
220. Li MF, Sun BG, Xiao ZZ, Sun L. First characterization of a teleost Epstein-Barr virus-induced gene 3 (EBI3) reveals a regulatory effect of EBI3 on the innate immune response of peripheral blood leukocytes. *Dev Comp Immunol* 2013;**41**:514–22.

221. Lutfalla G, Roest Crollius H, Stange-Thomann N, Jaillon O, Mogensen K, Monneron D. Comparative genomic analysis reveals independent expansion of a lineage-specific gene family in vertebrates: the class II cytokine receptors and their ligands in mammals and fish. *BMC Genomics* 2003;**4**:29.
222. Kaiser P, Poh TY, Rothwell L, Avery S, Balu S, Pathania US, et al. A genomic analysis of chicken cytokines and chemokines. *J Interferon Cytokine Res* 2005;**25**:467–84.
223. Kim S, Faris L, Cox CM, Sumners LH, Jenkins MC, Fetterer RH, Miska KB, Dalloul RA. Molecular characterization and immunological roles of avian IL-22 and its soluble receptor IL-22 binding protein. *Cytokine* 2012;**60**:815–27.
224. Dalloul RA, Long JA, Zimin AV, Aslam L, Beal K, Blomberg LA. Multi-platform next-generation sequencing of the domestic turkey (*Meleagris gallopavo*): genome assembly and analysis. *PLoS Biology* 2010;**8**:e1000475.
225. Qi ZT, Nie P. Comparative study and expression analysis of the interferon gamma gene locus cytokines in *Xenopus tropicalis*. *Immunogenetics* 2008;**60**:699–710.
226. Igawa D, Sakai M, Savan R. An unexpected discovery of two interferon gamma-like genes along with interleukin(IL)-22 and -26 from teleost: IL-22 and -26 genes have been described for the first time outside mammals. *Mol Immunol* 2006;**43**:999–1009.
227. Zou J, Yoshiura Y, Dijkstra JM, Sakai M, Ototake M, Secombes CJ. Identification of an interferon gamma homologue in Fugu, *Takifugu rubripes*. *Fish Shellfish Immunol* 2004;**17**:403–9.
228. Corripio-Miyar Y, Zou J, Richmond H, Secombes CJ. Identification of interleukin-22 in gadoids and examination of its expression level in vaccinated fish. *Mol Immunol* 2009;**46**:2098–106.
229. Costa MM, Pereiro P, Wang T, Secombes CJ, Figueras A, Novoa B. Characterization and gene expression analysis of the two main Th17 cytokines (IL-17A/F and IL-22) in turbot, *Scophthalmus maximus*. *Dev Comp Immunol* 2012;**38**:505–16.
230. Qi Z, Zhang Q, Wang Z, Zhao W, Chen S, Gao Q. Molecular cloning, expression analysis and functional characterization of interleukin-22 in So-iny mullet, *Liza haematocheila*. *Mol Immunol* 2015;**63**:245–52.
231. Chettri JK, Raida MK, Kania P, Buchmann K. Differential immune response of rainbow trout (*Oncorhynchus mykiss*) at early developmental stages (larvae and fry) against the bacterial pathogen *Yersinia ruckeri*. *Dev Comp Immunol* 2012;**36**:463–74.
232. Costa MM, Saraceni PR, Forn-Cuní G, Dios S, Romero A, Figueras A, Novoa B. IL-22 is a key player in the regulation of inflammation in fish and involves innate immune cells and PI3K signaling. *Dev Comp Immunol* 2013;**41**:746–55.
233. Monte M, Zou J, Wang T, Carrington A, Secombes CJ. Cloning, expression analysis and bioactivity studies of rainbow trout (*Oncorhynchus mykiss*) interleukin-22. *Cytokine* 2011;**55**:62–73.
234. Siupka P, Hamming OJ, Fretaud M, Luftalla G, Levraud J-P, Hartmann R. The crystal structure of zebrafish IL-22 reveals an evolutionary conserved structure highly similar to that of human IL-22. *Genes Immun* 2014;**15**:293–302.
235. Kaiser P. The avian immune genome—a glass half-full or half-empty? *Cytogenet Genome Res* 2007;**117**:221–30.
236. Qi Z, Shi R, Li S, Zang X, W ang Z. 3-D modelling and molecular dynamics simulation of interleukin-22 from the So-iny mullet, *Liza Haematocheila*. *Electron J Biotechnol* 2013;**16**:4.
237. Wang T, Díaz-Rosales P, Martin SAM, Secombes CJ. Cloning of a novel interleukin(IL)-20-like gene in rainbow trout *Oncorhynchus mykiss* gives an insight into the evolution of the IL-10 family. *Dev Comp Immunol* 2010;**34**:158–67.
238. Qi Z, Zhang Q, Wang Z, Zhao W, Gao Q. Cloning of interleukin-10 from African clawed frog (*Xenopus tropicalis*), with the finding of IL-19/20 homologue in the IL-10 locus. *J Immunol Res* 2015;**2015**:462138.

239. Zou J, Clark MS, Secombes CJ. Characterisation, expression and promoter analysis of an interleukin 10 homologue in the puffer fish, *Fugu rubripes*. *Immunogenetics* 2003;**55**:325–35.

240. Buonocore F, Randelli E, Bird S, Secombes CJ, Facchiano A, Costantini S, Scapigliati G. Interleukin-10 expression by real-time PCR and homology modelling analysis in the European sea bass (*Dicentrarchus labrax* L.). *Aquac Res* 2007;**270**:512–22.

241. Grayfer L, Hidgkinson JW, Hitchen SJ, Belosevic M. Characterization and functional analysis of goldfish (*Carassius auratus* L.) interleukin-10. *Mol Immunol* 2011;**48**:563–71.

242. Nam B-H, Moon J-Y, Park E-H, Kim Y-O, Kim D-G, Kong HJ, et al. Conserved gene structure and function of interleukin-10 in the teleost fish. *J Animal Vet Adv* 2014;**13**:774–82.

243. Karan S, Kaushik H, Saini N, Sahoo PK, Dixit A, Lalit CG. Genomic cloning and sequence analysis of interleukin-10 from *Labeo rohita*. *Bioinformation* 2014;**10**:623–9.

244. Harun NO, Costa MM, Secombes CJ, Wang T. Sequencing of a second interleukin-10 gene in rainbow trout *Oncorhynchus mykiss* and comparative investigation of the expression and modulation of the paralogues in vitro and in vivo. *Fish Shellfish Immunol* 2011;**31**:107–17.

245. Savan R, Igawa D, Sakai M. Cloning, characterization and expression analysis of interleukin-10 from the common carp, *Cyprinus carpio*. *Eur J Biochem* 2003;**270**:4647–54.

246. Glenney GW, Wiens GD. Early diversification of the TNF superfamily in teleosts: genomic characterization and expression analysis. *J Immunol* 2007;**178**:7955–73.

247. Pinto RD, Nascimento DS, Reis MIR, do Vale A, dos Santos NMS. Molecular characterization 3D modelling and expression analysis of sea bass (*Dicentrarchus labrax* L.) interleukin-10. *Mol Immunol* 2007;**44**:2056–65.

248. Swain B, Samanta M, Basu M, Panda P, Sahoo BR, Maiti NK, et al. Molecular characterization, inductive expression and mechanism of interleukin-10 gene induction in the Indian major carp (*Catla catla*). *Aquac Res* 2012;**43**:897–907.

249. Piazzon MC, Savelkoul HFJ, Pietretti D, Wiegertjes GF, Forlenza M. Carp Il10 has anti-inflammatory activities on phagocytes, promotes proliferation of memory T cells, and regulates B cell differentiation and antibody secretion. *J Immunol* 2015;**194**:187–99.

250. Rothwell L, Young JR, Zoorob R, Whittaker CA, Hesketh P, Archer A, et al. Cloning and characterization of chicken IL-10 and its role in the immune response to *Eimeria maxima*. *J Immunol* 2004;**173**:2675–82.

251. Powell F, Rothwell L, Clarkson M, Kaiser P. Development of reagents to study the turkey's immune response: cloning and characterization of two turkey cytokines, interleukin (IL)-10 and IL-13. *Vet Immunol Immunopathol* 2012;**147**:97–103.

252. Yao Q, Fischer KP, Tyrrell DL, Gutfreund KS. Genomic structure, molecular characterization and functional analysis of Pekin duck interleukin-10. *Dev Comp Immunol* 2012;**38**:30–43.

253. Haritova AM, Stanilova SA. Enhanced expression of IL-10 in contrast to IL-12B mRNA in poultry with experimental coccidiosis. *Exp Parasitol* 2012;**132**:378–82.

254. Ghebremicael SB, Hasenstein JR, Lamont SJ. Association of interleukin-10 cluster genes and *Salmonella* response in chicken. *Poultry Sci* 2008;**87**:22–6.

255. Kim S, Miska KB, McElroy AP, Jenkins MC, Fetterer RH, Cox CM, et al. Molecular cloning and functional characterization of avian interleukin-19. *Molec Immunol* 2009;**47**:476–84.

256. van Beurden SJ, Forlenza M, Westphal AH, Wiegertjes GF, Haenen OLM, Engelsma MY. The alloherpesviral components of interleukin-10 in European eel and common carp. *Fish Shellfish Immunol* 2011;**31**:1211–7.

257. Sunarto A, Liongue C, McColl KA, Adams MM, Bulach D, Crane M, Schat KA, et al. Koi herpesvirus encodes and expresses a functional interleukin-10. *J Virol* 2012;**86**:11512–20.

258. Ouyang P, Rakus K, Boutier M, Reschner A, Leroy B, Ronsmans M, et al. The IL-10 homologue encoded by cyprinid herpesvirus 3 is essential neither for viral replication in vitro nor for virulence in vitro. *Vet Res* 2013;**44**:53.

259. Rouvier E, Luciani MF, Mattei M-G, et al. CTLA-8, cloned from an activated T cell, bearing AU-rich messenger RNA instability sequences, and homologous to a herpesvirus saimiri gene. *J Immunol* 1993;**150**:5445–56.

260. Li J, Zhang Y, Zhang Y, Xiang Z, Tong Y, Qu F, Yu Z. Genomic characterization and expression analysis of five novel IL-17 genes in the Pacific oyster *Crassostrea gigas. Fish Shellfish Immunol* 2014;**40**:455–65.

261. Guo P, Hirano M, Herrin BR, Li J, Yu C, Sadlonova A, Cooper MD. Dual nature of the adaptive immune system in lampreys. *Nature* 2009;**459**:796–801.

262. Wang T, Martin SAM, Secombes CJ. Two interleukin-17C-like genes exist in rainbow trout *Oncorhynchus mykiss* that are differentially expressed and modulated. *Dev Comp Immunol* 2010;**34**:491–500.

263. Gunimaladevi I, Savan R, Sakai M. identification, cloning and characterization of interleukin-17 and its family from zebrafish. *Fish Shellfish Immunol* 2006;**21**:393–403.

264. Korenaga H, Kono T, Sakai M. Isolation of seven IL-17 family genes from the Japanese pufferfish *Takifugu rubripes. Fish Shellfish Immunol* 2010;**28**:809–18.

265. Zhang H, Shen B, Wu H, Gao L, Liu Q, Wang Q, et al. Th17-like immune response in fish mucosal tissues after administration of live attenuated *Vibrio anguillarum* via different vaccination routes. *Fish Shellfish Immunol* 2014;**37**:229–38.

266. Ribeiro CMS, Pontes MJSL, Bird S, Chadzinska M, Scheer M, Verburg-van Kemenade BML, Savelkoul HFJ, Wiegertjes GF. Trypanosomiasis-induced Th17-like immune responses in carp. *PLoS ONE* 2010;**5**:e13012.

267. Mutoloki S, Cooper GA, Marjara IS, Koop BF, Evensen O. High gene expression of inflammatory markers and IL-17A correlates with severity of injection site reactions of Atlantic salmon vaccinated with oil-adjuvanted vaccines. *BMC Genomics* 2010;**11**:336.

268. Quintana FJ, Iglesias AH, Farez MF, Caccamo M, Burns EJ, Kassam N, et al. Adaptive autoimmunity and foxp3-based immunoregulation in zebrafish. *PLoS ONE* 2010;**5**:e9478.

269. Du L, Feng S, Yin L, Wang X, Zhang A, Yang K, Zhou H. Identification and functional characterization of grass carp IL-17A/F1: an evaluation of the immunoregulatory role of teleost IL-17A/F1. *Dev Comp Immunol* 2015;**51**:202–11.

270. Monte M, Wang T, Holland JW, Zou J, Secombes CJ. Cloning and characterization of rainbow trout interleukin-17A/F2 (IL-17A/F2) and IL-17 receptor A: expression during infection and bioactivity of recombinant IL-17A/F2. *Infect Immun* 2013;**81**:340–53.

271. Du L, Qin L, Wang X, Zhang A, Wei H, Zhou H. Characterization of grass carp (*Ctenopharyngodon idella*) IL-17D: molecular cloning, functional implication and signal transduction. *Dev Comp Immunol* 2014;**42**:220–8.

272. Kumari J, Larsen AN, Bogwald J, Dalmo RA. Interleukin-17D in Atlantic salmon (*Salmo salar*): molecular characterization 3D modelling and promoter analysis. *Fish Shellfish Immunol* 2009;**27**:647–59.

273. Kim WH, Jeong J, Park AR, Yim D, Kim Y-H, Kim KD, et al. Chicken IL-17F: identification and comparative expression analysis in *Eimeria*-infected chickens. *Dev Comp Immunol* 2012;**38**:401–9.

274. Min W, Lillehoj HS. Isolation and characterization of chicken interleukin-17 cDNA. *J Interferon Cytokine Res* 2002;**22**:1123–8.

275. Yoo J, Jang SI, Kim S, Cho J-H, Lee H-J, Rhee MH, et al. Molecular characterization of duck interleukin-17. *Vet Immunol Immunopathol* 2009;**318**:318–22.

276. Zhang L, Liu R, Song M, Hu Y, Pan B, Cai J, Wang M. *Eimeria tenella*: interleukin-17 contributes to host immunopathology in the gut during experimental infection. *Exp Parasitol* 2013;**133**:121–30.

277. Zhao G-H, Cheng W-Y, Wang W, Jia Y-Q, Fang Y-Q, Du S-Z, Yu S-K. The expression dynamics of IL-17 and Th17 response relative cytokines in the trachea and spleen of chickens after infection with *Cryptosporidium baileyi*. *Parasites Vectors* 2014;**7**:212.

278. Aggarwal BB, Gupta SC, Kim JH. Historical perspectives on tumor necrosis factor and its superfamily: 25 years later, a golden journey. *Blood* 2012;**119**:651–65.

279. Gray KA, Daugherty LC, Gordon SM, Seal RL, Wright MW, Bruford EA. Genenames.org: the HGNC resources in 2013. *Nucleic Acids Res* 2013;**41**:D545–52 (Database issue).

280. Igaki T, Kanda H, Yamamoto-Goto Y, Kanuka H, Kuranaga E, Aigaki T, Miura M. Eiger, a TNF superfamily ligand that triggers the *Drosophila* JNK pathway. *EMBO J* 2002;**21**:3009–18.

281. Igaki T, Miura M. The Drosophila TNF ortholog Eiger: emerging physiological roles and evolution of the TNF system. *Semin Immunol* 2014;**26**:322–74.

282. De Zoysa M, Jung S, Lee J. First molluscan TNF-alpha homologue of the TNF superfamily in disk abalone: molecular characterization and expression analysis. *Fish Shellfish Immunol* 2009;**26**:625–31.

283. De Zoysa M, Nikapitiya C, Moon DO, Whang I, Kim GY, Lee J. A novel Fas ligand in mollusk abalone: molecular characterization, immune responses and biological activity of the recombinant protein. *Fish Shellfish Immunol* 2009;**27**:423–32.

284. Mekata T, Sudhakaran R, Okugawa S, Inada M, Kono T, Sakai M, Itami T. A novel gene of tumor necrosis factor ligand superfamily from kuruma shrimp *Marsupenaeus japonicus*. *Fish Shellfish Immunol* 2010;**28**:571–8.

285. Putnam NH, Butts T, Ferrier DE, Furlong RF, Hellsten U, Kawashima T, Robinson-Rechavi M, et al. The amphioxus genome and the evolution of the chordate karyotype. *Nature* 2008;**453**:1064–71.

286. Holland LZ, Albalat R, Azumi K, Benito-Gutiérrez E, Blow MJ, Bronner-Fraser M, Brunet F, et al. The amphioxus genome illuminates vertebrate origins and cephalochordate biology. *Genome Res* 2008;**18**:1100–11.

287. Smith JJ, Kuraku S, Holt C, Sauka-Spengler T, Jiang N, Campbell MS, Yandell MD, Manousaki T, et al. Sequencing of the sea lamprey (*Petromyzon marinus*) genome provides insights into vertebrate evolution. *Nat Genet* 2013;**45**:415–21.

288. Suzuki T, Kohara Shin-IT, Kasahara YM. Transcriptome analysis of hagfish leukocytes: a framework for understanding the immune system of jawless fishes. *Dev Comp Immunol* 2004;**28**:993–1003.

289. Parrinello N, Vizzini A, Arizza V, Salerno G, Parrinello D, Cammarata M, Giaramita FT, Vazzana M. Enhanced expression of a cloned and sequenced *Ciona intestinalis* TNFalpha-like (CiTNF alpha) gene during the LPS-induced inflammatory response. *Cell Tissue Res* 2008;**334**:305–17.

290. Zhang X, Luan W, Jin S, Xiang J. A novel tumor necrosis factor ligand superfamily member (CsTL) from *Ciona savignyi*: molecular identification and expression analysis. *Dev Comp Immunol* 2008;**32**:1362–73.

291. Huang S, Yuan S, Guo L, Yu Y, Li J, Wu T, Liu T, Yang M, Wu K, Liu H, Ge J, Yu Y, Huang H, Dong M, Yu C, Chen S, Xu A. Genomic analysis of the immune gene repertoire of amphioxus reveals extraordinary innate complexity and diversity. *Genome Res* 2008;**18**:1112–26.

292. Wiens GD, Glenney GW. Origin and evolution of TNF and TNF receptor superfamilies. *Dev Comp Immunol* 2011;**35**:1324–35.

293. Hirono I, Nam BH, Kurobe T, Aoki T. Molecular cloning, characterization, and expression of TNF cDNA and gene from Japanese flounder *Paralichthys olivaceus*. *J Immunol* 2000;**165**:4423–7.

294. Laing KJ, Wang T, Zou J, Holland J, Hong S, Bols N, Hirono I, Aoki T, Secombes CJ. Cloning and expression analysis of rainbow trout *Oncorhynchus mykiss* tumour necrosis factor-alpha. *Eur J Biochem* 2001;**268**:1315–22.

295. Bobe J, Goetz FW. Molecular cloning and expression of a TNF receptor and two TNF ligands in the fish ovary. *Comp Biochem Physiol B Biochem Mol Biol* 2001;**129**:475–81.

296. García-Castillo J, Pelegrín P, Mulero V, Meseguer J. Molecular cloning and expression analysis of tumor necrosis factor alpha from a marine fish reveal its constitutive expression and ubiquitous nature. *Immunogenetics* 2002;**54**:200–7.

297. Saeij JP, Stet RJ, de Vries BJ, van Muiswinkel WB, Wiegertjes GF. Molecular and functional characterization of carp TNF: a link between TNF polymorphism and trypanotolerance? *Dev Comp Immunol* 2003;**27**:29–41.

298. Zou J, Secombes CJ, Long S, Miller N, Clem LW, Chinchar VG. Molecular identification and expression analysis of tumor necrosis factor in channel catfish (*Ictalurus punctatus*). *Dev Comp Immunol* 2003;**27**:845–58.

299. Savan R, Kono T, Igawa D, Sakai M. A novel tumor necrosis factor (TNF) gene present in tandem with the TNF-alpha gene on the same chromosome in teleosts. *Immunogenetics* 2005;**57**:140–50.

300. Praveen K, Evans DL, Jaso-Friedmann L. Constitutive expression of tumor necrosis factor-alpha in cytotoxic cells of teleosts and its role in regulation of cell-mediated cytotoxicity. *Mol Immunol* 2006;**43**:279–91.

301. Xiao J, Zhou ZC, Chen C, Huo WL, Yin ZX, Weng SP, Chan SM, Yu XQ, He JG. Tumor necrosis factor-alpha gene from mandarin fish, *Siniperca chuatsi*: molecular cloning, cytotoxicity analysis and expression profile. *Mol Immunol* 2007;**44**:3615–22.

302. Nascimento DS, Pereira PJ, Reis MI, do Vale A, Zou J, Silva MT, Secombes CJ, dos Santos NM. Molecular cloning and expression analysis of sea bass (*Dicentrarchus labrax* L.) tumor necrosis factor-alpha (TNF-alpha). *Fish Shellfish Immunol* 2007;**23**:701–10.

303. Uenobe M, Kohchi C, Yoshioka N, Yuasa A, Inagawa H, Morii K, Nishizawa T, Takahashi Y, Soma G. Cloning and characterization of a TNF-like protein of *Plecoglossus altivelis* (ayu fish). *Mol Immunol* 2007;**44**:1115–22.

304. Ordás MC, Costa MM, Roca FJ, López-Castejón G, Mulero V, Meseguer J, Figueras A, Novoa B. Turbot TNFalpha gene: molecular characterization and biological activity of the recombinant protein. *Mol Immunol* 2007;**44**:389–400.

305. Grayfer L, Walsh JG, Belosevic M. Characterization and functional analysis of goldfish (*Carassius auratus* L.) tumor necrosis factor-alpha. *Dev Comp Immunol* 2008;**32**:532–43.

306. Xie FJ, Zhang ZP, Lin P, Wang SH, Zou ZH, Wang YL. Cloning and infection response of tumour-necrosis factor alpha in large yellow croaker *Pseudosciaena crocea* (Richardson). *J Fish Biol* 2008;**73**:1149–60.

307. Kadowaki T, Harada H, Sawada Y, Kohchi C, Soma G, Takahashi Y, Inagawa H. Two types of tumor necrosis factor-alpha in bluefin tuna (*Thunnus orientalis*) genes: molecular cloning and expression profile in response to several immunological stimulants. *Fish Shellfish Immunol* 2009;**27**:585–94.

308. Kim MS, Hwang YJ, Yoon KJ, Zenke K, Nam YK, Kim SK, Kim KH. Molecular cloning of rock bream (*Oplegnathus fasciatus*) tumor necrosis factor-alpha and its effect on the respiratory burst activity of phagocytes. *Fish Shellfish Immunol* 2009;**27**:618–24.

309. Lam FW, Wu SY, Lin SJ, Lin CC, Chen YM, Wang HC, Chen TY, Lin HT, Lin JH. The expression of two novel orange-spotted grouper (*Epinephelus coioides*) TNF genes

in peripheral blood leukocytes, various organs, and fish larvae. *Fish Shellfish Immunol* 2011;**30**:618–29.

310. Zhang A, Chen D, Wei H, Du L, Zhao T, Wang X, Zhou H. Functional characterization of TNF-α in grass carp head kidney leukocytes: induction and involvement in the regulation of NF-κB signaling. *Fish Shellfish Immunol* 2012;**33**:1123–32.

311. Kajungiro RA, Xue L, Aynealem M. Molecular cloning and expression patterns of two tumor necrosis factor al pha genes in Crucian carp (*Carassius carassius*). *Mol Biol (Mosk)* 2015;**49**:138–48.

312. Zou J, Wang T, Hirono I, Aoki T, Inagawa H, Honda T, Soma GI, Ototake M, Nakanishi T, Ellis AE, Secombes CJ. Differential expression of two tumor necrosis factor genes in rainbow trout *Oncorhynchus mykiss*. *Dev Comp Immunol* 2002;**26**:161–72.

313. Savan R, Sakai M. Presence of multiple isoforms of TNF alpha in carp (*Cyprinus carpio* L.): genomic and expression analysis. *Fish Shellfish Immunol* 2004;**17**:87–94.

314. Zhao X, Duan D, Feng X, Chen Y, Sun Z, Jia S, He J, Wang B, Li W, Zhang J, Wang W, Yang Z, Lu Q. Molecular cloning and expression analysis of common carp *Cyprinus carpio* tumor necrosis factor-α. *Fisheries Sci* 2012;**78**:1229–36.

315. Berthelot C, Brunet F, Chalopin D, Juanchich A, Bernard M, Noël B, Bento P, Da Silva C, Labadie K, et al. The rainbow trout genome provides novel insights into evolution after whole-genome duplication in vertebrates. *Nat Commun* 2014;**5**:3657.

316. Xu P, Zhang X, Wang X, Li J, Liu G, Kuang Y, Xu J, Zheng X, Ren L, Wang G, Zhang Y, Huo L, Zhao Z, et al. Genome sequence and genetic diversity of the common carp, *Cyprinus carpio*. *Nat Genet* 2014;**46**:1212–9.

317. Kinoshita S, Biswas G, Kono T, Hikima J, Sakai M. Presence of two tumor necrosis factor (tnf)-α homologs on different chromosomes of zebrafish (*Danio rerio*) and medaka (*Oryzias latipes*). *Mar Genomics* 2014;**13**:1–9.

318. Hong S, Li R, Xu Q, Secombes CJ, Wang T. Two types of TNF-α exist in teleost fish: phylogeny, expression, and bioactivity analysis of type-II TNF-α3 in rainbow trout *Oncorhynchus mykiss*. *J Immunol* 2013;**191**:5959–72.

319. García-Castillo J, Chaves-Pozo E, Olivares P, Pelegrín P, Meseguer J, Mulero V. The tumor necrosis factor alpha of the bony fish seabream exhibits the in vivo proinflammatory and proliferative activities of its mammalian counterparts, yet it functions in a species-specific manner. *Cell Mol Life Sci* 2004;**61**:1331–40.

320. Zou J, Peddie S, Scapigliati G, Zhang Y, Bols NC, Ellis AE, Secombes CJ. Functional characterisation of the recombinant tumor necrosis factors in rainbow trout, *Oncorhynchus mykiss*. *Dev Comp Immunol* 2003;**27**:813–22.

321. Blanco E, Abril JF. Computational gene annotation in new genome assemblies using GeneID. *Methods Mol Biol* 2009;**537**:243–61.

322. Burge CB, Karlin S. Finding the genes in genomic DNA. *Curr Opin Struct Biol* 1998;**8**: 346–54.

323. Roca FJ, Mulero I, López-Muñoz A, Sepulcre MP, Renshaw SA, Meseguer J, Mulero V. Evolution of the inflammatory response in vertebrates: fish TNF-alpha is a powerful activator of endothelial cells but hardly activates phagocytes. *J Immunol* 2008;**181**:5071–81.

324. Forlenza M, Magez S, Scharsack JP, Westphal A, Savelkoul HF, Wiegertjes GF. Receptor-mediated and lectin-like activities of carp (*Cyprinus carpio*) TNF-alpha. *J Immunol* 2009;**183**:5319–32.

325. Vraskou Y, Roher N, Díaz M, Antonescu CN, MacKenzie SA, Planas JV. Direct involvement of tumor necrosis factor-alpha; in the regulation of glucose uptake in rainbow trout muscle cells. *Am J Physiol Regul Integr Comp Physiol* 2011;**300**:R716–23.

326. Crespo D, Mañanós EL, Roher N, MacKenzie SA, Planas JV. Tumor necrosis factor alpha may act as an intraovarian mediator of luteinizing hormone-induced oocyte maturation in trout. *Biol Reprod* 2012;**86**:1–12.

327. Li DH, Havell EA, Brown CL, Cullen JM. Woodchuck lymphotoxin-alpha, -beta and tumor necrosis factor genes: structure, characterization and biological activity. *Gene* 2000;**242**:295–305.

328. Ruddle NH. Lymphoid neo-organogenesis: lymphotoxin's role in inflammation and development. *Immunol Res* 1999;**19**:119–25.

329. Kono T, Zou J, Bird S, Savan R, Sakai M, Secombes CJ. Identification and expression analysis of lymphotoxin-beta like homologues in rainbow trout *Oncorhynchus mykiss*. *Mol Immunol* 2006;**43**:1390–401.

330. Tacchi L, Larragoite ET, Muñoz P, Amemiya CT, Salinas I. African lungfish reveal the evolutionary origins of organized mucosal lymphoid tissue in vertebrates. *Curr Biol* 2015;**25**:2417–24.

331. Kinoshita S, Biswas G, Kono T, Hikima J, Sakai M. Presence of two tumor necrosis factor (tnf)-α homologs on different chromosomes of zebrafish (*Danio rerio*) and medaka (*Oryzias latipes*). *Mar Genomics* 2014;**13**:1–9.

332. Schneider P. The role of APRIL and BAFF in lymphocyte activation. *Curr Opin Immunol* 2005;**17**:282–9.

333. Stein JV, López-Fraga M, Elustondo FA, Carvalho-Pinto CE, Rodríguez D, Gómez-Caro R, De Jong J, Martínez-A C, Medema JP, Hahne M. APRIL modulates B and T cell immunity. *J Clin Invest* 2002;**109**:1587–98.

334. Mackay F, Schneider P, Rennert P, Browning J. BAFF AND APRIL: a tutorial on B cell survival. *Annu Rev Immunol* 2003;**21**:231–64.

335. Mackay F, Leung H. The role of the BAFF/APRIL system on T cell function. *Semin Immunol* 2006;**18**:284–9.

336. Rolink AG, Melchers F. BAFFled B cells survive and thrive: roles of BAFF in B-cell development. *Curr Opin Immunol* 2002;**14**:266–75.

337. Min C, Liang Z, Cui X, Wang Q, Chen Y, Zhang S. Molecular cloning and partial functional characterization of a proliferation inducing ligand (APRIL) in zebrafish (*Danio rerio*). *Dev Comp Immunol* 2012;**37**:202–6.

338. Pandit NP, Shen YB, Chen Y, Wang WJ, Li JL. Molecular characterization, expression, and immunological response analysis of the TWEAK and APRIL genes in grass carp, *Ctenopharyngodon idella*. *Genet Mol Res* 2014;**13**:10105–20.

339. Liang Z, Kong Y, Luo C, Shen Y, Zhang S. Molecular cloning, functional characterization and phylogenetic analysis of B-cell activating factor in zebrafish (*Danio rerio*). *Fish Shellfish Immunol* 2010;**29**:233–40.

340. Ai H, Shen Y, Min C, Pang S, Zhang J, Zhang S, Zhao Z. Molecular structure, expression and bioactivity characterization of TNF13B (BAFF) gene in mefugu, *Takifugu obscures*. *Fish Shellfish Immunol* 2011;**30**:1265–74.

341. Cui XW, Li JF, Xiao W, Xuan Y, Tian AY, Xu XZ, Zhang SQ. Molecular cloning, expression and functional analysis of TNF13b (BAFF) in Japanese sea perch, *Lateolabrax japonicas*. *Int Immunopharmacol* 2012;**12**:34–41.

342. Pandit NP, Shen Y, Wang W, Chen Y, Li J. Identification of TNF13b (BAFF) gene from grass carp (*Ctenopharyngodon idella*) and its immune response to bacteria and virus. *Dev Comp Immunol* 2013;**39**:460–4.

343. Xiao W, Long W, Liu GY, Sui CL, Guo XR, Tian A, Ji CB, Cui XW, Zhang SQ. Molecular cloning, expression and functional analysis of B-cell activating factor (BAFF) in yellow grouper, *Epinephelus awoara*. *Mol Immunol* 2014;**59**:64–70.

344. Meng F, Sun Y, Xu T. Comparative genomic of the BAFF and BAFF-like genes and immune response to bacteria of miiuy croaker (*Miichthys miiuy*). *Fish Shellfish Immunol* 2015;**43**: 191–9.

345. Sun Y, Sun L. CsBAFF, a teleost B cell activating factor promotes pathogen-induced innate immunity and vaccine-induced adaptive immunity. *PLoS One* 2015;**10**:e0136015.

346. Biswas G, Kinoshita S, Kono T, Hikima J, Sakai M. Evolutionary evidence of tumor necrosis factor super family members in the Japanese pufferfish (*Takifugu rubripes*): comprehensive genomic identification and expression analysis. *Mar Genomics* 2015;**22**:25–36.

347. Ren W, Pang S, You F, Zhou L, Zhang S. The first BAFF gene cloned from the cartilaginous fish. *Fish Shellfish Immunol* 2011;**31**:1088–96.

348. Li R, Dooley H, Wang T, Secombes CJ, Bird S. Characterisation and expression analysis of B-cell activating factor (BAFF) in spiny dogfish (*Squalus acanthias*): cartilaginous fish BAFF has a unique extra exon that may impact receptor binding. *Dev Comp Immunol* 2012;**36**: 707–17.

349. Li R, Redmond AK, Wang T, Bird S, Dooley H, Secombes CJ. Characterisation of the TNF superfamily members CD40L and BAFF in the small-spotted catshark (*Scyliorhinus canicula*). *Fish Shellfish Immunol* 2015;**47**:381–9.

350. Elgueta R, Benson MJ, de Vries VC, Wasiuk A, Guo Y, Noelle RJ. Molecular mechanism and function of CD40/CD40L engagement in the immune system. *Immunol Rev* 2009;**229**: 152–72.

351. Lagos LX, Iliev DB, Helland R, Rosemblatt M, Jørgensen JB. CD40L—a costimulatory molecule involved in the maturation of antigen presenting cells in Atlantic salmon (*Salmo salar*). *Dev Comp Immunol* 2012;**38**:416–30.

352. Hughes PD, Belz GT, Fortner KA, Budd RC, Strasser A, Bouillet P. Apoptosis regulators Fas and Bim cooperate in shutdown of chronic immune responses and prevention of autoimmunity. *Immunity* 2008;**28**:197–205.

353. Kurobe T, Hirono I, Kondo H, Saito-Taki T, Aoki T. Molecular cloning, characterization, expression and functional analysis of Japanese flounder *Paralichthys olivaceus* Fas ligand. *Dev Comp Immunol* 2007;**31**:687–95.

354. Blott EJ, Bossi G, Clark R, Zvelebil M, Griffiths GM. Fas ligand is targeted to secretory lysosomes via a prolinerich domain in its cytoplasmic tail. *J Cell Sci* 2001;**114**:2405–16.

355. MacFarlane M. TRAIL-induced signalling and apoptosis. *Toxicol Lett* 2003;**139**:89–97.

356. Chang MX, Nie P, Xie HX, Wang GL, Gao Y. Characterization and expression analysis of TNF-related apoptosis inducing ligand (TRAIL) in grass carp *Ctenopharyngodon idella*. *Vet Immunol Immunopathol* 2006;**110**:51–63.

357. Gao Y, Chang MX, Sun BJ, Nie P. TRAIL in the mandarin fish *Siniperca chuatsi*: gene and its apoptotic effect in HeLa cells. *Fish Shellfish Immunol* 2007;**24**:55–66.

358. Li JF, Ai HX, Zhang J, Du MX, Zhang Z, Zhang JX, Zhang SQ. Molecular cloning, functional characterization and phylogenetic analysis of TRAIL in Japanese pufferfish *Takifugu rubripes*. *J Fish Biol* 2011;**79**:747–60.

359. Wiley SR, Winkles JA. TWEAK, a member of the TNF superfamily, is a multifunctional cytokine that binds the TweakR/Fn14 receptor. *Cytokine Growth Factor Rev* 2003;**14**: 241–9.

360. Wang J, Fu YX. The role of LIGHT in T cell-mediated immunity. *Immunol Res* 2004;**30**: 201–14.

361. Tian AY, Yang HJ, Zhu SC, Zhang YS, Jiang ZA, Song JY, Liu HZ, Zhang SQ. Isolation and characterization of LIGHT (TNFSF14) gene homologue in zebrafish (*Danio rerio*). *Int Immunopharmacol* 2012;**14**:629–34.

362. Nocentini G, Ronchetti S, Cuzzocrea S, Riccardi C. GITR/GITRL: more than an effector T cell co-stimulatory system. *Eur J Immunol* 2007;**37**:1165–9.

363. Poulton LD, Nolan KF, Anastasaki C, Waldmann H, Patton EE. A novel role for glucocorticoid-induced TNF receptor ligand (Gitrl) in early embryonic zebrafish development. *Int J Dev Biol* 2010;**54**:815–25.

364. Valmiki MG, Ramos JW. Death effector domain-containing proteins. *Cell Mol Life Sci* 2009;**66**:814–30.

365. Rautenschlein S, Subramanian A, Sharma JM. Bioactivities of a tumour necrosis-like factor released by chicken macrophages. *Dev Comp Immunol* 1999;**23**:629–40.

366. Koskela K, Nieminen P, Kohonen P, Salminen H, Lassila O. Chicken B-cell-activating factor: regulator of B-cell survival in the bursa of fabricius. *Scand J Immunol* 2004;**59**:449–57.

367. Schneider K, Kothlow S, Schneider P, Tardivel A, Göbel T, Kaspers B, Staeheli P. Chicken BAFF-a highly conserved cytokine that mediates B cell survival. *Int Immunol* 2004;**16**:139–48.

368. Dan WB, Guan ZB, Zhang C, Li BC, Zhang J, Zhang SQ. Molecular cloning, in vitro expression and bioactivity of goose B-cell activating factor. *Vet Immunol Immunopathol* 2007;**118**:113–20.

369. Guan ZB, Ye JL, Dan WB, Yao WJ, Zhang SQ. Cloning, expression and bioactivity of duck BAFF. *Mol Immunol* 2007;**44**:1471–6.

370. Chen CM, Ren WH, Yang G, Zhang CS, Zhang SQ. Molecular cloning, in vitro expression and bioactivity of quail BAFF. *Vet Immunol Immunopathol* 2009;**130**:125–30.

371. Lu W, Cao P, Cai X, Yu J, Hu C, Cao M, Zhang S. Molecular cloning, expression, and bioactivity of dove B lymphocyte stimulator (doBAFF). *Vet Immunol Immunopathol* 2009;**128**:374–80.

372. Yang K, Xiao K, Huang H, Lu S, Zhong J, Ansari AR, Khaliq H, Song H, Liu H, Peng K. Molecular cloning, expression and bioactivity of B cell activating factor (BAFF) in African ostrich. *Int Immunopharmacol* 2015;**28**:686–94.

373. Kothlow S, Morgenroth I, Tregaskes CA, Kaspers B, Young JR. CD40 ligand supports the long-term maintenance and differentiation of chicken B cells in culture. *Dev Comp Immunol* 2008;**32**:1015–26.

374. Cerutti A, Schaffer A, Goodwin RG, Shah S, Zan H, Ely S, Casali P. Engagement of CD153 (CD30 ligand) by CD30-positive T cells inhibits class switch DNA recombination and antibody production in human IgD-positive IgM-positive B cells. *J Immunol* 2000;**165**:786–94.

375. Abdalla SA, Horiuchi H, Furusawa S, Matsuda H. Molecular cloning and characterization of chicken tumor necrosis factor (TNF)-superfamily ligands, CD30L and TNF-related apoptosis inducing ligand (TRAIL). *J Vet Med Sci* 2004;**66**:643–50.

376. Zhang JX, Song R, Sang M, Sun SQ, Ma L, Zhang J, Zhang SQ. Molecular and functional characterization of BAFF from the Yangtze alligator (*Alligator sinensis*, Alligatoridae). *Zoology* 2015;**118**:325–33.

377. Alföldi J, Di Palma F, Grabherr M, Williams C, Kong L, Mauceli E, Russell P, Lowe CB, Glor RE, et al. The genome of the green anole lizard and a comparative analysis with birds and mammals. *Nature* 2011;**477**:587–91.

378. Hellsten U, Harland RM, Gilchrist MJ, Hendrix D, Jurka J, Kapitonov V, Ovcharenko I, Putnam NH, et al. The genome of the Western clawed frog *Xenopus tropicalis*. *Science* 2010;**328**:633–6.

379. Mawaribuchi S, Tamura K, Okano S, Takayama S, Yaoita Y, Shiba T, Takamatsu N, Ito M. Tumor necrosis factor-alpha attenuates thyroid hormone-induced apoptosis in vascular endothelial cell line XLgoo established from Xenopus tadpole tails. *Endocrinology* 2008;**149**:3379–89.

380. Tamura K, Mawaribuchi S, Yoshimoto S, Shiba T, Takamatsu N, Ito M. Tumor necrosis factor-related apoptosis-inducing ligand 1 (TRAIL1) enhances the transition of red blood cells from the larval to adult type during metamorphosis in *Xenopus*. *Blood* 2010;**115**:850–9.

381. Secchiero P, Melloni E, Heikinheimo M, Mannisto S, Di Pietro R, Iacone A, Zauli G. TRAIL regulates normal erythroid maturation through an ERK-dependent pathway. *Blood* 2004;**103**:517–22.

382. Yang L, Zhou L, Zong X, Cao X, Ji X, Gu W, Zhang S. Characterization of the molecular structure, expression and bioactivity of the TNFSF13B (BAFF) gene of the South African clawed frog, *Xenopus laevis*. *Int Immunopharmacol* 2013;**15**:478–87.

Chapter 6

The Evolution of Complement System Functions and Pathways in Vertebrates

Miki Nakao, Tomonori Somamoto

Department of Bioscience and Biotechnology, Faculty of Agriculture,
Kyushu University, Hakozaki, Fukuoka, Japan

1 INTRODUCTION

The complement is a major humoral system of innate immunity. The mammalian system, the best characterized to date, is composed of more than 30 distinct plasma proteins and membrane-bound proteins, and mediates various immune effector functions, including elimination of invading pathogens, promotion of inflammatory responses, and clearance of apoptotic cell and necrotic cell debris, as well as modulation of humoral and cellular responses of adaptive immunity.[1,2]

The mammalian system is equipped with three well-defined activation pathways—the classical, alternative, and lectin pathways—to proteolytically convert C3, the central complement component, into its activated fragments C3a and C3b, followed by activation of the terminal lytic pathway, which damages the target-cell membrane. (Fig. 6.1)

The classical activation pathway is triggered upon recognition of an antigen-bound antibody by C1, followed by the proteolytic cascade involving C4 and C2, which form a C4bC2a complex or the C3-convertase. The lectin pathway is activated by various microbial carbohydrates, defined as the pathogen-associated molecular patterns (PAMPs). PAMPs are recognized by two distinct serum lectins, mannose-binding lectin (MBL) and ficolin (FCN), which are oligomeric proteins coupling with the MBL-associated serine proteases (MASPs) for the proteolytic activation of C4 and C2, as in the classical activation pathway.[3] Since C1 and MBL/FCN-MASPs require Ca^{2+} ion to maintain their quaternary structure, and C2 needs Mg^{2+} ion for its proper conformation, these two pathways proceed in the presence of both Ca^{2+} and Mg^{2+} at a millimolar level.[4] The initiation of the third activation pathway, the alternative pathway, does not rely on any clear recognition molecules. Instead, certain exogenous activators such

The Evolution of the Immune System. http://dx.doi.org/10.1016/B978-0-12-801975-7.00006-2

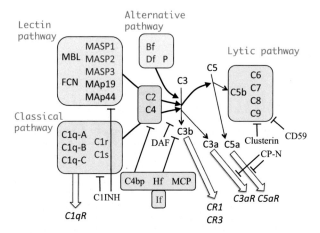

FIGURE 6.1 Activation pathways, receptors, and regulators of mammalian complement system. Complement components for activation are in gothic letters, receptors are in italic, and negative regulators are in roman fonts. Components with proteolytic activity are shown in red. Abbreviations: MBL, mannose-binding lectin; FCN, ficolin; MASP, MBL-associated serine protease; P, properdin; C1INH, C1-inhibitor; CR, complement receptor; C4bp, C4-binding protein; DAF, decay-accelerating factor; MCP, membrane-cofactor protein; If, factor I; CP-N, carboxypeptidase N. Thick arrows indicate proteolytic actions and block arrows mean receptor-ligand recognitions.

as bacterial lipopolysaccharide and fungal β-glucans lead to spontaneous C3 activation or C3-tickover, thanks to the formation of a C3-convertase, C3bBb, involving C3, factor B, and factor D. In this case, the normal suppression operated by various regulators of complement activation is overcome.[1]

Upon proteolytic activation by the C3-convertases, the nascent C3b can bind covalently to target-cell surface using its intrachain thioester bond, allowing further formation of surface-bound C3bBb; thus the alternative pathway can amplify C3-activation on the target surface.[1] At the same time, C3b can bind to C4bC2a or C3bBb to form trimolecular complexes, C4bC2aC3b, or C3bBbC3b, respectively, which can cleave C5 into its activated fragments C5a and C5b. The latter initiates molecular gathering of the terminal components C6 through C9 to form the membrane-attack complex (MAC) in the lytic pathway.[1]

In addition to the cytotoxicity against the target cell, the activated fragments of C3 and C5 mediate various innate immune-effector functions, including opsonization of target cells and promotion of inflammatory responses.[2] Namely, C3b and its further degradation product iC3b are recognized by complement receptors type 1 and type 3 (CR1 and CR3), respectively, expressed on phagocytes. On the other hand, C3a and C5a stimulate various leukocytes through interaction with their specific receptors C3aR and C5aR, respectively, inducing degranulation and chemotaxis.[5]

The potent physiological activities of the complement are tightly controlled at various steps of the activation cascades to prevent excess or misdirected activation, which may damage host tissues in a proximity of the complement activation sites. C1-inihibitor (C1INH) inactivates MASPs, C1r, and C1s; C4-binding protein and factor H enhance degradation of C4b and C3b by factor I protease (If); membrane-cofactor protein (MCP) and decay-accelerating factor (DAF) disturb the C3-convertase formation in an If-dependent and independent manner, respectively; serum carboxypeptidase N attenuates anaphylatoxic activities of C3a and C5a by removing their C-terminal Arg; CD59 inhibits the MAC formation on the host cell.[5]

Taxonomically, vertebrate is a subphylum of the Chordata phylum, composed of two superclasses, Agnatha (jawless cyclostome species), such as hagfish and lamprey, and Gnathostomata (jawed species), which includes cartilaginous and bony fishes, amphibians, reptiles, birds, and mammals.[6] As an evolution mechanism of vertebrates, the 2R hypothesis was proposed by Ohno (1970)[7] and is now well-accepted by a number of phylogenetic and genomic evidence.[8] According to the 2R hypothesis, a vertebrate ancestor (?) should have undergone two rounds of whole-genome duplication (WGD), which was probably tetraploidization of chromosomes. The first round of WGD is considered to occur prior to the appearance of the first jawless vertebrates, and the second before the emergence of the jawed vertebrates. In the immune system, this whole genome duplication is believed to have contributed to creation of the adaptive immunity made up of immunoglobulins (Igs), T-cell receptors (TCRs), and the major histocompatibility complex (MHC). Interestingly, a large (and the most common) bony fish group, teleost, has experienced an additional WGD (designated 3R) at a stem stage of the lineage, and this further large-scale gene duplication is believed to have impacted a teleost-specific diversification both in morphology and physiology.[9]

2 INVERTEBRATE COMPLEMENT SYSTEM REPRESENTING AN ANCESTRAL ARCHITECTURE OF VERTEBRATE SYSTEM

Comprehensive searches of complement-related components by molecular cloning, as well as genomic and transcriptomic database surveys from a number of invertebrate animal phyla, including Cnidaria,[10] Arthropoda,[11] and Mollusca,[12] have illustrated an original architecture of the ancestral complement system. The ancestral complement was probably an opsonic system composed of C3, Bf, and MASP. In this system, MASP could be activated upon sensing of PAMPs by some pattern-recognition molecule, resulting in activation of Bf, which in turn proteolytically activates C3 into C3a and C3b fragments to mediate inflammatory and phagocytic cellular responses, respectively.[13]

Although the complement system had lost in some protostome invertebrate lineages such as nematodes and insects, the basic architecture as an opsonic system has been well-maintained in deuterostome invertebrate phyla such as the Echinodermata and the Chordata subphyla Cephalochordata and Urochordata.[13] In chapter: Origin and Functions of Tunicate Hemocytes, Cima et al.

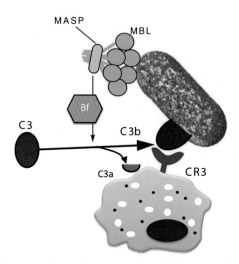

FIGURE 6.2   Architecture of the opsonic-only complement system of invertebrate chordates as a prototype that evolved into vertebrate systems. Mannose-binding lectin-like collectin complexed with its associated serine protease (MASP) recognizes PAMPs and triggers proteolytic C3-activation directly or through factor B-like protease. C3b, an activated C3 fragment, tags the target and enhances its phagocytosis mediated by CR3-like complement receptors.

briefly describe the complement elements discovered in Urochordates. The architecture of a prototypic complement system in the chordates seems to be a combination of the lectin and the alternative pathways, composed of MBL-like lectin as a PAMPs sensor, Bf as a C3-activating enzyme, C3 as an opsonin, and C3b-receptors on phagocytes (Fig. 6.2).

In the chapter, we deal with phylogeny of the complement pathways, complement receptors, and regulatory factors in vertebrates, from the molecular and functional points of view, with a reference to the contribution of the WGD, postulated by the 2R hypothesis. Evolutionary impact of additional WGD occurring in a stem lineage of teleost on the complement system will also be discussed.

3   PHYLOGENY OF COMPLEMENT PATHWAYS

Genomic and transcriptomic approaches in recent years have accelerated identification of homologues of the mammalian complement components in lower vertebrates and invertebrates. Table 6.1 is an update of the phylogenetic distribution of components, pathways, and physiological activities of a complement system, focusing more on the vertebrate system, modified from the preceding information in the literature.[14]

3.1   Lectin Pathway

In mammals, pattern-recognition molecules of the lectin pathway are two collectins, MBL and CL-K1, and three ficolins, namely FCN1, FCN2, and FCN3.[3,15]

TABLE 6.1 Complement Components, Receptors, and Regulatory Factors Identified in Representative Vertebrate Classes[a]

	Invertebrate	Vertebrate					
		Agnatha	Gnathostome				
			Fish		Amphibia	Tetrapods	
	Cephalo-chordate/urochordate	Jawless cyclostome	Cartilaginous fish	Bony fish (teleost)		Birds	Mammals
MBL		o		o		o	o
FCN	o	o		x	o	o	o
MASP1		o		x	o	x	o
MASP2				o	o	o	o
MSAP3	o	o	o	o	o	o	o
MAp19							o
MAp44				o		o	o
C1q		o		o	o		o
C1r				o	o	o	o
C1s				o	o	o	o
C3	o	o	o	o	o	o	o
C4			o	o	o	o	o
C5			o	o	o	o	o
Bf	o	o	o	o	o	o	o

(Continued)

TABLE 6.1 Complement Components, Receptors, and Regulatory Factors Identified in Representative Vertebrate Classes[a] (cont.)

	Invertebrate	Vertebrate						
		Agnatha	Gnathostome					
			Fish			Tetrapods		
	Cephalo-chordate/ urochordate	Jawless cyclostome	Cartilaginous fish	Bony fish (teleost)	Amphibia	Birds	Mammals
C2			o?	o?	o		o
Df				o			o
C6			o	o	o		o
C7				o	o		o
C8α			o	o	o		o
C8β			o	o			o
C8γ				o			o
C9	o		o	o	o		o
Hf		o		o	o		o
DAF					o		o
MCP				o			o
CR1							o
CR2							o

Factor						
C4bp						o
If	o	o			o	o
C1INH			o	o		o
P			o			o
CR3			o			o
C1qR				o		o
C3aR				o		o
C5aR						o
CPaseN				o		o
CD59	o		o		o	o

The marks "o" and "x" indicate the presence and the absence, respectively, of the factor supported by evidence in the literature or database.

While MBL and FCN partly share binding specificity toward monosaccharide ligands such as GlcNAc, these two lectins recognize distinct PAMPs such as bacterial peptidoglycans and fungal β-1,3-glucans, respectively.[16] In nonmammalian vertebrates, genes encoding MBL, CL-K1 (COLLEC11), and an FCN have been identified in chickens; those encoding three FCN homologues have been reported for *Xenopus*; three types of collectins—MBL, GalBL, and CL-K1—have been found in teleost species, and an MBL homologue has been isolated from lamprey.[15,17–19]

Interestingly, teleosts probably lack any homologue of FCN defined as a collagenous lectin with a C-terminal fibrinogen-like domain, but possess GalBL, an MBL-like collectin with galactose-directed binding specificity.[19,20] Therefore GalBL may be a functional homologue of FCN in teleost, but this hypothesis needs verification by functional assay at the protein level.

Another interesting point in evolution of vertebrate collectins is a conservation of MBL and CL-K1 from teleosts up to mammals. These two collectins are classified into two distant groups, designated "classical" collectins, including MBL, SP-A, and SP-D, and "novel" collectins, including CL-K1, CL-P1, and CL-L1, although they all share the same domain organization, namely N-terminal Cys-rich region, collagenous stalk, neck region, and C-terminal C-type lectin domain. The existence of the classical and novel collectins in teleosts, chickens, and mammals suggest their ancient evolutionary origin and functional importance in the recognition of pathogen and other danger-associated molecular patterns.[15]

A group of homologous protease, termed MBL-associated serine proteases (MASPs), are complexed with the collectins and FCNs, and play an essential role in triggering a proteolytic cascade for C3- and C4-activation.[21] In human, five MASP-like proteins with and without proteolytic activity are produced from two distinct genes, MASP1/3 gene and MASP2 gene. The MASP1/3 gene produces two proenzymes, MASP1 and MASP3, and a truncated form without catalytic domain, MAp44 or MAP-1, through alternative polyadenylation and splicing of mRNA. On the other hand, the MASP2 gene produces a proenzyme MASP2 and a noncatalytic truncated form, MAp19 (sMAP), as splicing variants.[22]

In the mammalian system, MASP2 is responsible for proteolytic activation of C4 and C2, leading to a formation of the C3-convertase, C4bC2a.[21] MASP1 can cleave proenzymes MASP2 and MASP3 into its active form and also profactor D into active factor D, in addition to many other noncomplement substrates, such as coagulation factor XIII, prothrombin, and kininogen.[23,24] Natural substrate of MASP3 has long remained unclear, but a recent report demonstrated that MASP3, as well as MASP1, converts pro-factor D into active factor D, implying its crucial role in triggering the alternative pathway activation.[23] Roles of MAp19 and MAp44 are still to be analyzed, though negative regulatory effects on lectin pathway activation by competing with MASP1, MASP2, and MASP3 have been speculated.[22,25]

An origin of the MASP1/3 gene can be traced back to an ancestral invertebrate chordate based on identification in cephalochordates, urochordates, agnathan (lamprey), and jawed vertebrates (shark, teleost, and frog).[26] On the other hand, the MASP2 gene seems to have occurred after emergence of agnathans, but before that of teleosts, and to have been retained in all the jawed vertebrates.[18]

It is intriguing that MASP1 gene encoding a protein with MASP1-specific serine protease domain is probably missing in teleosts and chickens, even after a comprehensive survey of genomic-sequence data.[27] Mammalian MASP1 is believed to play various roles in not only the complement lectin pathway, but also in coagulation and inflammation.[24] Thus, the absence of an MASP1 gene raises an interesting issue on the evolution of MASP1-mediated functional linkage between innate immunity and other physiological pathways.

It should also be noted that MAp44 also has an ancient origin. It was first described in a teleost species, the common carp, as a truncated isoform of MASP3, designated MRP, with domain organization of CUB1-EGF-CUB2-SCR1.[28] After identification of its mammalian homolog, named MAp44, generated by exactly the same splicing patterns as those of carp, a similar homologue has been found in urochordates, in which MAp44 is encoded by a distinct gene, but not as a splicing variant. Based on such strong conservation, MAp44 may be an important regulator of lectin pathway activation, rather than MAp19, which only appears in mammals.[22]

3.2   Alternative Pathway

The basic architecture of the alternative pathway, composed of C3 and factor B, seems to be tightly conserved in any group of vertebrates, as supported by identification of the two core components from all the vertebrate classes.[14] This pathway is believed to be important to amplify the generation of C3a and C3b, which are responsible for most of the complement-mediated defense and inflammatory functions.[1,2]

There is a divergence in the polypeptide structure in C3 between lampreys and the more recent jawed species. Namely, whereas C3 of jawed species has a two-chain structure composed of α- and β-chains linked by a disulfide bond, lamprey C3 has a mammalian C4-like three-chain structure (α-, β-, and γ-chains), caused by insertion of a posttranslational processing site to cleave into α- and γ-chains.[29,30] It is interesting that C3 of hagfish, another jawless species, keeps the two-chain protein in spite of the presence of a similar processing site.[31]

There is also a slight but significant structural difference in Bf between jawless and jawed vertebrates. While the serine protease domain shows a trypsin-like substrate specificity cleaving at C-terminal Arg residue corresponding to C-terminus of C3a region, an Asp residue that defines the specificity is located at different positions in their primary structures. In lamprey, as in invertebrate species, the Asp is six residues N-terminal from the active Ser. Conversely, the Asp is found at 39–42 residues C-terminal side of the active Ser in all the jawed vertebrate species analyzed so far. Thus, it is suggested that a structural specialization of the Bf serine protease domain has occurred in a common ancestor of Gnathostomes.[32]

Another intriguing issue on phylogeny of the alternative pathway is the occurrence of factor D. To date, a serine protease clearly identified as factor D has been found only in jawed vertebrates, except for cartilaginous fish.[14] Since proteolytic conversion of Bf, a proenzyme, into an active Bb fragment seems essential for the alternative pathway activation, it is very interesting to identify a protease responsible for the Bf cleavage. So far, even comprehensive transcriptomic approaches have not detected any Df-like molecule in jawless species.[33]

3.3 Classical Pathway

The classical pathway, as detected by antibody-dependent and Ca^{2+}- and Mg^{2+}-dependent hemolytic activity, has long been demonstrated in the jawed vertebrate species, including sharks, teleosts, and tetrapods.[34,35] This antibody dependency is attributable to a C1q subcomponent of C1, which recognizes immunoglobulins complexed with an antigen. The divalent cation-requirement reflects that C1 is a Ca^{2+}-dependent complex of C1q, C1r, and C1s, and that C2 needs coordination of Mg^{2+} for its normal conformation, as does Bf.[5]

C1q, a member of the C1q family, is composed of many proteins with an N-terminal collagenous region and a C-terminal C1q-like globular domain. In mammals, C1q is a hetero 18-mer, made up with six chains each of C1q-A, C1q-B, and C1q-C polypeptides.[5] As a subcomponent of C1, C1q is responsible for recognition of antigen-bound Ig Fc-region and other natural ligands. In the serum, C1q is complexed with two molecules each of C1r and C1s, which are serine proteases responsible of C4 activation.[5] In human chromosome 1, C1q-A, C1q-C, and C1q-B genes are located in tandem in this order. Conservation of the heterooligomeric composition of C1q, with the A, B, and C-chains, and their tandem gene arrangement has been reported in zebrafish.[36] Since C1q binds to a range of nonantibody ligands such as LPS and pentraxins, the classical pathway may be triggered by various PAMPs in an antibody-independent manner in vivo.[37]

Complement C1q-like molecules have also been identified as a N-acetylglucosamine (GlcNAc)-binding serum protein from two agnathan species, lamprey and hagfish.[38,39] Lamprey C1q is a homo-oligomer coupled with MASP-A, which is a MASP orthologue that activates C3. It was recently reported that lamprey C1q recognizes the variable lymphocyte receptor B (VLRB), a functional alternative of immunoglobulins, bound to target antigen cells, and may possibly lead to its cytolysis.[40] Hagfish GlcNAc-binding C1q showed an affinity to agarobiose and recognized a wide spectrum of PAMPs and microbes.[39]

C4, a C3 homologue composed of three disulfide-linked polypeptides, α-, β-, and γ-chains, covalently binds to the target surface through the thioester site, and provides a platform for binding of C2 to construct the classical pathway C3-convertase. Thus, emergence of C4 would have played a key role for establishment of the classical pathway. C4-encoding cDNAs or C4 proteins have been isolated from all the jawed vertebrates as low as cartilaginous and bony fish, but not from jawless species.[41,42]

In the mammalian classical pathway, C2 plays a role homologous to that of Bf in the alternative pathway, providing a catalytic subunit of the C3-convertase, C4bC2a, for proteolytic C3 activation.[5] From a jawless species, lamprey, two Bf/C2-like sequences have been cloned and identified as ancestral components yet to diverge into Bf and C2, functioning in the alternative pathway C3-convertase.[33] In cartilaginous and bony fish, two Bf/C2-like sequences as divergent as that between mammalian Bf and C2 have been cloned from a single species. Phylogenetic analyses of these Bf/C2-like molecules, however, did not show clear assignment to either Bf or C2, making it unclear whether cartilaginous and bony fish have functional C2.[42] More data on their functions, such as ability of C3-convertase formation with C4b or C3b, are still needed to answer this question. Interestingly, it has been reported that depletion of a Bf-like protein from trout serum resulted in total loss of its hemolytic activity through both the alternative and classical pathway, suggesting that teleost Bf also functions as C2 in the classical activation cascade.[43] Thus, presence or absence of a functional C2 molecule in fish is a key issue to better understand evolution of the classical pathway, from a functional point of view, in the lower vertebrates. The C2 molecule clearly identified as a classical pathway component seems to have evolved before the divergence of Amphibia from the tetrapod lineage, as evidenced by phylogenetic sequence analysis and functional assay.[14]

3.4   Lytic Pathway

Lytic activity clearly attributable to the complement system has been described only in jawed vertebrates, in which a group of terminal components, including C6, C7, C8, and C9 have been identified at both DNA and protein levels.[42,44–47] On the other hand, a natural hemolytic activity of lamprey serum is caused by a single 25-kDa protein and shows no relation to the lamprey complement system, which is only opsonic.[29] Agreeing well, comprehensive genomic and transcriptomic searches have found no sequences similar to C6, C7, C8, or C9 from lamprey or hagfish databases.[33]

In a recent publication, Nonaka classified the terminal complement components into two subgroups, the C6-like (C6 and C7) and the C9-like (C8α, C8β, and C9), based on the presence and absence of C-terminal FIMAC domains.[13] This classification is functionally relevant because the C6-like components interact with C5b through the FIMAC domains to start MAC formation, whereas C9-like components show no direct binding to C5b due to the lack of FIMAC domains.[48] Although C9-like molecules have been found in cephalochordates and urochordates, it seems unlikely that they are functionally connected, with their opsonic-complement cascade even lacking C5, according to the structure–function relationship of the terminal components.[18] Nevertheless, that invertebrate C9-like molecule might represent an ancestor of the terminal components seen in the jawed vertebrates.

Among the terminal components, C8 has a novel quaternary structure in that it is composed of three polypeptides, which are C8α and C8β, homologous to each other, and C8γ, belonging to a remote protein family, lipocalin.[49] C8γ has been cloned from teleost and mammals, and the mammalian C8-like three-chain structure has also been confirmed at the protein level in teleosts.[35,49,50] In cartilaginous fish, the presence of C8γ remains to be proven.

In the functional point of view, C9 play a key role to complete the formation of a barrel-shaped membrane–attack complex, but is optional for lysis of particular target cells, as reported for hemolysis of rabbit erythrocytes, which can be lysed without C9.[51] Although molecular mechanisms of the complement-mediated cytolysis without C9 are still to be clarified, it should be noted that the C9-independent rabbit-cell lysis has also been described in the bony fish complement, suggesting tight conservation of the membrane-attack mechanism by the terminal components.[52,53]

4 PHYLOGENY OF COMPLEMENT RECEPTORS

Complement receptors play crucial roles in mediating biodefense responses of the complement system by sensing various active fragments of complement components. Mammalian complement receptors include opsonic receptors such as C1q-receptor, CR1, CR3, and CR4, anaphylatoxin receptors such as C3a-receptor and C5a receptor, and immunomodulating receptors such as CR2.[1,2,5]

Opsonic function of the complement system has been described in bony fish and higher vertebrates, in which C3b and iC3b are candidates of opsonic complement ligand.[5,54,55] At the molecular level, CR3 subunits, or integrin CD18 and CD11, have been cloned from bony fish and mammals.[42] Although none of the CR3 subunits have been found in the jawless species, CD18/CD11 homologues have been shown to mediate opsonic function of the complement in a urochordate species.[56] Therefore, CR3-mediated opsonization is considered to be a well-conserved mechanism for pathogen elimination in all the vertebrate species. Other opsonic receptors homologous to C1q-receptor and CR1 are not clearly recognized outside of mammals.

Complement fragments corresponding to mammalian C3a, C4a, and C5a have been described in bony fish.[42] Similarly, jawless fish C3 can also release a corresponding C3a fragment, although its function is yet to be analyzed. C3a- and C5a-receptors have been identified also in bony fish, and chemotactic and anaphylatoxic response induced by C3a and C5a have been described in cartilaginous and bony fish and higher vertebrates.[42,57] In jawless species, chemotactic response of leukocytes seemingly attributable to complement anaphylatoxins have been reported in hagfish, but the ligand and receptors that mediated the chemotaxis have not been identified, yet.[58]

Mammalian CR2 expressed on B cells modulates antibody response by recognizing C3d, a terminal activation fragment of C3, bound to a foreign antigen.[59] While generation of C3d-like fragments is evident in bony fish, no direct CR2 homologue has been found in this group.[60] It would be particularly interesting if the bony fish complement has such immunomodulatory connection to the adaptive immunity, not only from an evolutionary aspect, but also from a practical point of view. This would indeed represent the basis for the development of a molecular adjuvant utilizing fish C3d fragments for disease prevention in aquaculture.

5   PHYLOGENY OF THE REGULATORY MECHANISM OF COMPLEMENT ACTIVATION

Although potent physiological activities of the complement system are crucial for effective pathogen elimination, they can potentially damage host cells in case of excessive or misdirected activation, resulting in an allergic or auto-immune pathology. Therefore, a complement system must be equipped with appropriate regulators to prevent such side effects. Controlling excessive complement activation on nonself targets and complement attack misdirected to the host cell needs both soluble and membrane-bound regulators of complement activation. In mammals, as soluble regulators, C1-inhibitor (C1INH) inactivates C1r/C1s and MASPs, C4-binding protein (C4bp) and factor H (Hf) promote proteolytic degradation of C4b and C3b, respectively, and clusterin interferes with fluid-phase formation of the membrane-attack complex.[1,5] Mammalian membrane-bound regulators are membrane-cofactor protein (MCP or CD46), CR1 (CD35), and decay-accelerating factor (DAF or CD55), which attenuate C3-convertase formation, and CD59, which inhibits MAC formation.[1,5]

Recent phylogenetic analysis of C1INH has depicted that the presence of C1INH in bony fish, reptiles, birds, and mammals, but absence in lamprey and amphibians, based on genomic database survey, suggests that C1INH has occurred in a common ancestor of jawed vertebrates.[61]

C4bp, Hf, MCP, and CR1 act as cofactors of factor I protease (If) that catalyze degradation of C4b and C3b fragments into their inactive forms, whereas DAF enhances dissociation of the C3-convertases, C3bBb and C4bC2a.[5] Factor I and its potential cofactors homologous to Hf have been identified from both jawed and jawless vertebrates.[42,33,62] Therefore, proteolytic C3b-degradation dependent on Hf-like and If-like regulators seems to be an ancestral regulatory mechanism of C3 activation. Membrane-bound cofactors of If, which are CD46-like, have been identified from bony fish, amphibians, and mammals,[5,63–65] suggesting its ancient origin, whereas the membrane-bound RCA from jawless species is yet to be identified. On the other hand, any RCA protein with DAF-like activity has not been found in the lower vertebrates, probably due to the lack of a functional assay method to evaluate the decay-acceleration of the C3-convertase complex.

In mammalian genomes, genes encoding RCA proteins are located in two tight clusters present in the same chromosome, group 1 cluster contains several factor H-like soluble proteins (Hf and Hf-related proteins), and group 2 cluster contains C4bp, DAF, CR2, CR1, and MCP-like soluble and membrane-bound proteins. Similar gene clusters have been reported from chickens, Xenopus, and zebrafish, indicating that the gene clustering has been well-conserved while varying the number of the members in the clusters.[63–67]

It is interesting that zebrafish possess a group 1 RCA gene cluster with a comparable number of the Hf-like genes to that of humans, but with much fewer members of group 2 genes,[64,67] despite a high degree of isotypic diversity of C3 and C4, which would be recognized by these RCA molecules.

CD59 has been cloned from bony fish, hagfish, and even some invertebrate parasites such as *Schistosoma mansoni*, suggesting its "prevertebrate" ancient origin.[68–70] However, the parasite CD59 showed no complement inhibition,[70] and the hagfish complement even lacks lytic activity. There is also no direct evidence for CD59 to inhibit MAC formation in bony fish, which do possess the lytic pathway. A recent study reported that recombinant CD59 from zebrafish-bound bacteria, and their PAMPs such as LPS and LTA, showed a slight antibacterial activity.[71] It is interesting data, but could be evaluated if such activities are immune-relevant in vivo.

6 EVOLUTIONARY SIGNIFICANCE OF MULTIPLE ISOFORMS IN TELEOST COMPLEMENT COMPONENTS

Bony fish is divided into two classes, Actinopteryii, or the ray-finned fishes, and Sarcopterygii, or the lobe-finned fishes, such as coelacanth. Teleost is a major infraclass of Actinopteryii, believed to have arisen in the Triassic period, and contains a very diverse extant species more than 26,000.[72] An important phylogenetic feature of teleost is that a whole-genome duplication occurred in its stem lineage, as evidence by a number of researches.[9] This duplication is believed to have provided genetic raw materials for further diversification, as seen in their morphology, physiology, and behavior.

A striking feature of the teleost complement system is an isotypic diversity of several components.[42,73] Since multiple isoforms of rainbow trout C3 have been first described at the protein level,[74] a number of studies, including protein isolation and molecular cloning, have uncovered the presence of multiple isoforms of complement components, receptors, and regulatory factors.[42]

Whereas several isotypes are limited to pseudotetraploid species such as carp and trout, indicating that they arose from the lineage-specific tetraploidization, some duplicates such as those of C3, C4, and C7 are commonly seen in various species, regardless of the chromosome ploidy. Thus, the whole-genome duplication probably played a crucial role to increase the number of isoforms of these complement components, although it is difficult to trace the exact gene-duplication scenario to generate the isotypes.

From a functional point of view, diversity of C3 and C4 has drawn our best attention because the sequence divergence between the isotypes includes a functionally important amino acid substitution at the position that determines binding specificity of these components. In most species other than teleost, C3 is encoded by a single-copy gene and has a His residue at about 100 residues C-terminal from the thioester site.[73] Thus, we designate it His-type C3. This His residue plays a catalytic role in cleavage and covalent binding of the thioester, enabling nascent His-type

C3b to bind to hydroxyl-groups by transacylation on the target surface or to surrounding water.[75] In vitro mutagenesis studies revealed that substitution of this catalytic His with other less nucleophilic residues, such as Ser and Asp, dramatically changes the binding specificity of the thioester toward amino-groups, which can directly cleave the thioester.[75] Very interestingly, teleost species analyzed so far, such as trout, carp, zebrafish, and medaka fish, possess both the His-type C3 and C3 carrying a Ser, Gln, Asp, or Ala at the catalytic position, designated non-His type C3, suggesting that the two C3 types show different functions, such as binding specificities against targets. At the protein level, C3 isoforms purified from trout and sea bream have been reported to show different binding specificities to various complement-activating model targets, such as sheep and rabbit erythrocytes, bacteria, and the yeast cell-wall.[76] We have tried to correlate the binding specificity of the thioester to hydroxyl- or amino-groups with binding spectra of His- and non-His-types of C3 against natural complement-activating targets, using monoclonal antibodies specific to His-type (C3-H1) and non-His-types (C3-S) of carp complement. The results showed that C3-S showed a wider range of binding spectrum than that of C3-H1, suggesting that non-His-type C3 unique to teleost play more prominent roles in complement activation and pathogen elimination (Table 6.2).

TABLE 6.2 Distinct Binding Spectra of His-Type and Non-His-Type C3 Isotypes of Carp Complement Determined by ELISA or Flow Cytometer

Targets	Assay	Binding	
		C3-H1 (His-type)	C3-S (non-His-type)
Poly-L-lysine	ELISA[a]	−	+
Glycogen (oyster)	ELISA	+	+
LPS (*E. coli* o44:B5)[b]	ELISA	+	+
LTA (*S. aureus*)[c]	ELISA	−	+
IC[d]	ELISA	+	+
Erythrocyte (rabbit)	FCM[e]	+	+
Erythrocyte (sheep)	FCM	−	+
Baker's yeast	FCM	+	+
Staphylococcus aureus	FCM	−	+
Escherichia coli DH5α	FCM	+	+
Aeromonas hydrophila	FCM	+	+
Aeromonas salmonicida	FCM	−	+
Edawardsiella tarda	FCM	−	+

[a]*Enzyme-linked immunoadsorbent assay.*
[b]*Lipopolysaccharide.*
[c]*Lipoteichoic acid.*
[d]*Immune complex of hen egg lysozyme and antilysozyme carp IgM.*
[e]*Flow cytometry.*

However, their target-binding specificities do not clearly correlate with the preference of hydroxyl- or amino-group by carp C3-H1 and C3-S, respectively.[77]

Other complement proteins also likely show some different functional activities between the isoforms, based on their amino-acid sequence diversity, especially at functionally important sites.[42,73] More functional analyses are needed, to gain comprehensive and convincing conclusions on the biological impacts of diversification of complement-component isoforms and their significance to the evolution of a complement system.

7   CONCLUDING REMARKS

It is reasonable to hypothesize that a prototype of the vertebrate complement system is well-represented by the system of cephalochordate and urochordate, that is, the invertebrate species of the chordate phylum, where MBL-like collectin, MASP, Bf, and C3 constitute an opsonic system with

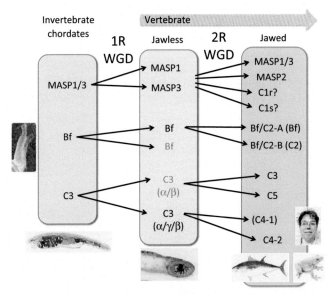

FIGURE 6.3   Hypothetical diversifications of MASP/C1r/C1s, Bf/C2, and C3/C4/C5 families driven by two rounds (1R and 2R) of WGD. Invertebrate chordates include urochordates (ascidian) and cephalochordates (amphioxus), and jawless vertebrates contain lamprey and hagfish. Genes in gray color are postulated to be lost in the extant species, but might be retained in a possible lineage ancestral to the derived class. C3 (α/β) and C3 (α/γ/β) represent C3 composed of α- and β-chains and C3 having C4-like α-, γ-, and β-chain structure, respectively. Evolutionary correspondences between MASP1/MASP2 genes of jawless species and MASP1/3, MASP2, and C1r/C1s of jawed vertebrates are unclear. Bf/C2-A and Bf/C2-B identified in cartilaginous and bony fish may correspond to Bf and C2, respectively, of higher vertebrates, but the assignments are not convincing enough on phylogenetic analyses based on the sequence data available so far. C4-1 lineage is found only in some cartilaginous and bony fish species, and might be lost in the descendent classes, whereas C4-2 seems to be maintained in all the lineages of jawed vertebrates.

a pattern-recognition ability.[13] An evolutionary scenario of the complement system, starting from the prototype to the system observed in jawed vertebrates, can be summarized as follows: (1) The complement system of jawless species remains opsonic with no cytolytic activity. An important development is recruitment of C1q, in addition to MBL, as a pattern-recognition molecule to activate C3. C1q may possibly connect VLR-dependent antigen recognition and the complement system in an analogous way to the classical pathway in jawed vertebrates.

(2) The classical and lytic pathways emerged, seemingly together, in a common ancestor of jawed vertebrates. C4, C2, and C1r/C1s in the classical pathway were most likely generated by gene duplication from C3, Bf, and MASP, respectively. For the establishment of the lytic pathway, more gene duplication events should have been needed, such as generations of C5 from C3, and that of C6, C7, C8, and C9 from their C9-like common ancestor, which is missing in the extant jawless vertebrates. Here, we attempt to fit this scenario to the 2R hypothesis of vertebrate evolution by postulating that some of the duplicated gene has been lost in the extant jawless species after the first round GWD, while they kept in a lineage directly ancestral to the jawed vertebrates until the second round GWD happened, as shown in Fig. 6.3. Overall, the 2R hypothesis reasonably explains the genomic mechanism to acquire the classical and lytic pathways in the vertebrate complement system.

ACKNOWLEDGMENTS

This work was supported in part by a grant in aid from Ministry of Education, Science, Culture and Sports, Japan (25292127 to MN).

REFERENCES

1. Walport MJ. Complement. First of two parts. *N Engl J Med* 2001;**344**(14):1058–66.
2. Le Friec Gl, Kemper C. Complement: coming full circle. *Arch Immunol Ther Exp (Warsz)* 2009;**57**(6):393–407.
3. Endo Y, Takahashi M, Fujita T. Lectin complement system and pattern recognition. *Immunobiology* 2006;**211**(4):283–93.
4. Herpers BL, de Jong BA, Dekker B, Aerts PC, van Dijk H, Rijkers GT, van Velzen-Blad H. Hemolytic assay for the measurement of functional human mannose-binding lectin: a modification to avoid interference from classical pathway activation. *J Immunol Methods* 2009;**343**(1):61–3.
5. Law SKA, Reid KBM. *Complement*. 2nd ed. Oxford: IRL Press; 1995.
6. Vertebrate. From wikipedia, the free encyclopedia. http://en.wikipedia.org/wiki/vertebrate; 2015
7. Ohno S. *Evolution by gene duplication*. New York: Springer-Verlag; 1970.
8. Kasahara M. The 2R hypothesis: an update. *Curr Opin Immunol* 2007;**19**(5):547–52.
9. Sato Y, Nishida M. Teleost fish with specific genome duplication as unique models of vertebrate evolution. *Env Biol Fish* 2010;**88**(2):169–88.
10. Kimura A, Sakaguchi E, Nonaka M. Multi-component complement system of cnidaria: C3, Bf, and MASP genes expressed in the endodermal tissues of a sea anemone *Nematostella vectensis*. *Immunobiology* 2009;**214**(3):165–78.

11. Sekiguchi R, Nonaka M. Evolution of the complement system in protostomes revealed by de novo transcriptome analysis of six species of arthropoda. *Dev Comp Immunol* 2015;**50**(1):58–67.

12. Prado-Alvarez M, Rotllant J, Gestal C, Novoa B, Figueras A. Characterization of a C3 and a factor B-like in the carpet-shell clam *Ruditapes decussatus*. *Fish Shellfish Immunol* 2009;**26**(2):305–15.

13. Nonaka M. Evolution of the complement system. *Subcell Biochem* 2014;**80**:31–43.

14. Dodds AW, Matsushita M. The phylogeny of the complement system and the origins of the classical pathway. *Immunobiology* 2007;**212**(4–5):233–43.

15. Ohtani K, Suzuki Y, Wakamiya N. Biological functions of the novel collectins CL-L1, CL-K1, and CL-P1. *J Biomed Biotechnol* 2012;**2012**:493945.

16. Ma YG, Cho MY, Zhao M, Park JW, Matsushita M, Fujita T, et al. Human mannose-binding lectin and L-ficolin function as specific pattern recognition proteins in the lectin activation pathway of complement. *J Biol Chem* 2004;**279**(24):25307–12 11.

17. Kakinuma Y, Endo Y, Takahashi M, Nakata M, Matsushita M, Takenoshita S, Fujita T. Molecular cloning and characterization of novel ficolins from *Xenopus laevis*. *Immunogenetics* 2003;**55**(1):29–37.

18. Nakao M, Kajiya T, Sato Y, Somamoto T, Kato-Unoki Y, Matsushita M, et al. Lectin pathway of bony fish complement: identification of two homologs of the mannose-binding lectin associated with MASP2 in the common carp (*Cyprinus carpio*). *J Immunol* 2006;**177**(8):5471–9.

19. Takahashi M, Iwaki D, Matsushita A, Nakata M, Matsushita M, Endo Y, Fujita T. Cloning and characterization of mannose-binding lectin from lamprey (Agnathans). *J Immunol* 2006;**176**(8):4861–8.

20. Niu D, Peatman E, Liu H, Lu J, Kucuktas H, Liu S, et al. Microfibrillar-associated protein 4 (MFAP4) genes in catfish play a novel role in innate immune responses. *Dev Comp Immunol* 2011;**35**(5):568–79.

21. Matsushita M, Endo Y, Fujita T. Structural and functional overview of the lectin complement pathway: its molecular basis and physiological implication. *Arch Immunol Ther Exp (Warsz)* 2013;**61**(4):273–83.

22. Yongqing T, Drentin N, Duncan RC, Wijeyewickrema LC, Pike RN. Mannose-binding lectin serine proteases and associated proteins of the lectin pathway of complement: two genes, five proteins and many functions? *Biochim Biophys Acta* 2012;**1824**(1):253–62.

23. Sekine H, Takahashi M, Iwaki D, Fujita T. The role of MASP-1/3 in complement activation. *Adv Exp Med Biol* 2013;**735**:41–53.

24. Dobó J, Schroeder V, Jenny L, Cervenak L, Závodszky P, Gál P. Multiple roles of complement MASP-1 at the interface of innate immune response and coagulation. *Mol Immunol* 2014;**61**(2):69–78.

25. Degn SE, Hansen AG, Steffensen R, Jacobsen C, Jensenius JC, Thiel S. MAp44, a human protein associated with pattern recognition molecules of the complement system and regulating the lectin pathway of complement activation. *J Immunol* 2009;**183**(11):7371–8.

26. Endo Y, Nonaka M, Saiga H, Kakinuma Y, Matsushita A, Takahashi M, et al. Origin of mannose-binding lectin-associated serine protease (MASP)-1 and MASP-3 involved in the lectin complement pathway traced back to the invertebrate, amphioxus. *J Immunol* 2003;**170**(9):4701–7.

27. Lynch NJ, Khan SU, Stover CM, Sandrini SM, Marston D, Presanis JS, et al. Composition of the lectin pathway of complement in *Gallus gallus*: absence of mannan-binding lectin-associated serine protease-1 in birds. *J Immunol* 2005;**174**(8):4998–5006.

28. Nagai T, Mutsuro J, Kimura M, Kato Y, Fujiki K, Yano T, et al. A novel truncated isoform of the mannose-binding lectin-associated serine protease (MASP) from the common carp (*Cyprinus carpio*). *Immunogenetics* 2000;**51**(3):193–200.

29. Nonaka M, Fujii T, Kaidoh T, Natsuume-Sakai S, Nonaka M, Yamaguchi N, et al. Purification of a lamprey complement protein homologous to the third component of the mammalian complement system. *J Immunol* 1984;**133**(6):3242–9.

30. Nonaka M, Takahashi M. Complete complementary DNA sequence of the third component of complement of lamprey Implication for the evolution of thioester containing proteins. *J Immunol* 1992;**148**(10):3290–5.

31. Fujii T, Nakamura T, Tomonaga S. Component C3 of hagfish complement has a unique structure: identification of native C3 and its degradation products. *Mol Immunol* 1995;**32**(9):633–42.

32. Terado T, Smith SL, Nakanishi T, Nonaka MI, Kimura H, Nonaka M. Occurrence of structural specialization of the serine protease domain of complement factor B at the emergence of jawed vertebrates and adaptive immunity. *Immunogenetics* 2001;**53**(3):250–4.

33. Kimura A, Ikeo K, Nonaka M. Evolutionary origin of the vertebrate blood complement and coagulation systems inferred from liver EST analysis of lamprey. *Dev Comp Immunol* 2009;**33**(1):77–87.

34. Nonaka M, Smith SL. Complement system of bony and cartilaginous fish. *Fish Shellfish Immunol* 2000;**10**(3):215–28.

35. Nakao M, Yano T. Structural and functional identification of complement components of the bony fish, carp (*Cyprinus carpio*). *Immunol Rev* 1998;**166**:27–38.

36. Hu YL, Pan XM, Xiang LX, Shao JZ. Characterization of C1q in teleosts: insight into the molecular and functional evolution of C1q family and classical pathway. *J Biol Chem* 2010;**285**(37):28777–86.

37. Nayak A, Pednekar L, Reid KB, Kishore U. Complement and non-complement activating functions of C1q: a prototypical innate immune molecule. *Innate Immun* 2012;**18**(2):350–63.

38. Matsushita M, Matsushita A, Endo Y, Nakata M, Kojima N, Mizuochi T, et al. Origin of the classical complement pathway: lamprey orthologue of mammalian C1q acts as a lectin. *Proc Natl Acad Sci U S A*. 2004;**101**(27):10127–31.

39. Yamaguchi T, Takamune K, Kondo M, Takahashi Y, Kato-Unoki Y, Nakao M, et al. Hagfish C1q: its unique binding property. *Dev Comp Immunol* 2014;**43**(1):47–53.

40. Wu F, Chen L, Liu X, Wang H, Su P, Han Y, et al. Lamprey variable lymphocyte receptors mediate complement-dependent cytotoxicity. *J Immunol* 2013;**190**(3):922–30.

41. Terado T, Okamura K, Ohta Y, Shin DH, Smith SL, Hashimoto K, Takemoto T, et al. Molecular cloning of C4 gene and identification of the class III complement region in the shark MHC. *J Immunol* 2003;**171**(5):2461–6.

42. Nakao M, Tsujikura M, Ichiki S, Vo TK, Somamoto T. The complement system in teleost fish: progress of post-homolog-hunting researches. *Dev Comp Immunol* 2011;**35**(12):1296–308.

43. Sunyer JO, Zarkadis I, Sarrias MR, Hansen JD, Lambris JD. Cloning, structure, and function of two rainbow trout Bf molecules. *J Immunol* 1998;**161**(8):4106–14.

44. Wang Y, Zhang M, Wang C, Ye B, Hua Z. Molecular cloning of the alpha subunit of complement component C8 (CpC8α) of whitespotted bamboo shark (*Chiloscyllium plagiosum*). *Fish Shellfish Immunol* 2013;**35**(6):1993–2000.

45. Wang Y, Xu S, Su Y, Ye B, Hua Z. Molecular characterization and expression analysis of complement component C9 gene in the whitespotted bambooshark *Chiloscyllium plagiosum*. *Fish Shellfish Immunol* 2013;**35**(2):599–606.

46. Kimura A, Nonaka M. Molecular cloning of the terminal complement components C6 and C8beta of cartilaginous fish. *Fish Shellfish Immunol* 2009;**27**(6):768–72.

47. Aybar L, Shin DH, Smith SL. Molecular characterization of the alpha subunit of complement component C8 (GcC8alpha) in the nurse shark (*Ginglymostoma cirratum*). *Fish Shellfish Immunol* 2009;**27**(3):397–406.

48. Thai CT, Ogata RT. Complement components C5 and C7: recombinant factor I modules of C7 bind to the C345C domain of C5. *J Immunol* 2004;**173**(7):4547–52.

49. Kaufman KM, Sodetz JM. Genomic structure of the human complement protein C8γ: homology to the lipocalin gene family. *Biochemistry* 1994;**33**(17):5162–6.

50. Papanastasiou AD, Zarkadis IK. The gamma subunit of the eighth complement component (C8) in rainbow trout. *Dev Comp Immunol* 2006;**30**(5):485–91.

51. Müller-Eberhard HJ. The membrane attack complex. In: Müller-Eberhard HJ, Miescher PA, editors. *Complement*. New York: Springer-Verlag; 1985. p. 227–75.

52. Uemura T, Yano T, Shiraishi H, Nakao M. Purification and characterization of the eighth and ninth components of carp complement. *Mol Immunol* 1996;**33**(11–12):925–32.

53. Nakao M, Uemura T, Yano T. Terminal components of carp complement constituting a membrane attack complex. *Mol Immunol* 1996;**33**(11–12):933–7.

54. Boshra H, Li J, Sunyer JO. Recent advances on the complement system of teleost fish. *Fish Shellfish Immunol* 2006;**20**(2):239–62.

55. Nakao M, Fujiki K, Kondo M, Yano T. Detection of complement receptors on head kidney phagocytes of the common carp *Cyprinus carpio*. *Fish Sci* 2003;**69**(5):929–35.

56. Miyazawa S, Nonaka M. Characterization of novel ascidian beta integrins as primitive complement receptor subunits. *Immunogenetics* 2004;**55**(12):836–44.

57. Smith SL. Shark complement: an assessment. *Immunol Rev* 1998;**166**:67–78.

58. Newton RA, Raftos DA, Raison RL, Geczy CL. Chemotactic responses of hagfish (Vertebrata Agnatha) leucocytes. *Dev Comp Immunol* 1994;**18**(4):295–303.

59. Carroll MC, Isenman DE. Regulation of humoral immunity by complement. *Immunity* 2012;**37**(2):199–207.

60. Nakao M, Miura C, Itoh S, Nakahara M, Okumura K, Mutsuro J, et al. A complement C3 fragment equivalent to mammalian C3d from the common carp (*Cyprinus carpio*): generation in serum after activation of the alternative pathway and detection of its receptor on the lymphocyte surface. *Fish Shellfish Immunol* 2004;**16**(2):139–49.

61. Kumar A, Bhandari A, Sarde SJ, Goswami C. Molecular phylogeny of C1 inhibitor depicts two immunoglobulin-like domains fusion in fishes and ray-finned fishes specific intron insertion after separation from zebrafish. *Biochem Biophys Res Commun* 2014;**450**(1):219–26.

62. Kimura Y, Inoue N, Fukui A, Oshiumi H, Matsumoto M, Nonaka M, et al. A short consensus repeat-containing complement regulatory protein of lamprey that participates in cleavage of lamprey complement 3. *J Immunol* 2004;**173**(2):1118–28.

63. Tsujikura M, Nagasawa T, Ichiki S, Nakamura R, Somamoto T, Nakao M. A CD46-like molecule functional in teleost fish represents an ancestral form of membrane-bound regulators of complement activation. *J Immunol* 2015;**194**(1):262–72.

64. Wu J, Li H, Zhang S. Regulator of complement activation (RCA) group 2 gene cluster in zebrafish: identification, expression, and evolution. *Funct Integr Genomics* 2012;**12**(2):367–77.

65. Oshiumi H, Suzuki Y, Matsumoto M, Seya T. Regulator of complement activation (RCA) gene cluster in *Xenopus tropicalis*. *Immunogenetics* 2009;**61**(5):371–84.

66. Oshiumi H, Shida K, Goitsuka R, Kimura Y, Katoh J, Ohba S, et al. Regulator of complement activation (RCA) locus in chicken: identification of chicken RCA gene cluster and functional RCA proteins. *J Immunol* 2005;**175**(3):1724–34.

67. Sun G, Li H, Wang Y, Zhang B, Zhang S. Zebrafish complement factor H and its related genes: identification, evolution, and expression. *Funct Integr Genomics* 2010;**10**(4):577–87.

68. Papanastasiou AD, Georgaka E, Zarkadis IK. Cloning of a CD59-like gene in rainbow trout expression and phylogenetic analysis of two isoforms. *Mol Immunol* 2007;**44**(6):1300–6.

69. dos Remedios NJ, Ramsland PA, Hook JW, Raison RL. Identification of a homologue of CD59 in a cyclostome: implications for the evolutionary development of the complement system. *Dev Comp Immunol* 1999;**23**(1):1–14.

70. Farias LP, Krautz-Peterson G, Tararam CA, Araujo-Montoya BO, Fraga TR, Rofatto HK, et al. On the three-finger protein domain fold and CD59-like proteins in *Schistosoma mansoni*. *PLOS Negl Trop Dis* 2013;**7**(10):e2482.

71. Sun C, Wu J, Liu S, Li H, Zhang S. Zebrafish CD59 has both bacterial-binding and inhibiting activities. *Dev Comp Immunol* 2013;**41**(2):178–88.

72. Teleostei. from wikipedia, the free encylopedia.http://en.wikipedia.org/wiki/teleostei; 2015

73. Nakao M, Mutsuro J, Nakahara M, Kato Y, Yano T. Expansion of genes encoding complement components in bony fish: biological implications of the complement diversity. *Dev Comp Immunol* 2003;**27**(9):749–62.

74. Nonaka M, Nonaka M, Irie M, Tanabe K, Kaidoh T, Natsuume-Sakai S, et al. Identification and characterization of a variant of the third component of complement (C3) in rainbow trout (*Salmo gairdneri*) serum. *J Biol Chem* 1985;**260**(2):809–15.

75. Gadjeva M, Dodds AW, Taniguchi-Sidle A, Willis AC, Isenman DE, Law SK. The covalent binding reaction of complement component C3. *J Immunol* 1998;**161**(2):985–90.

76. Sunyer JO, Zarkadis IK, Lambris JD. Complement diversity: a mechanism for generating immune diversity? *Immunol today* 1998;**19**(11):519–23.

77. Ichiki S, Kato-Unoki Y, Somamoto T, Nakao M. The binding spectra of carp C3 isotypes against natural targets independent of the binding specificity of their thioester. *Dev Comp Immunol* 2012;**38**(1):10–6.

Chapter 7

Antiviral Immunity: Origin and Evolution in Vertebrates

Jun Zou*, Rosario Castro**, Carolina Tafalla[†]

*Scottish Fish Immunology Research Centre, University of Aberdeen, Zoology Building, Aberdeen, United Kingdom; **Animal Health Research Center (CISA-INIA), Carretera de Algete a El Casar, Valdeolmos (Madrid), Spain; [†]Animal Health Research Center (CISA-INIA), Carretera de Algete a El Casar, Valdeolmos (Madrid), Spain

1 INTRODUCTION

Viruses are infectious agents of ancestral origin with particular characteristics that place them at the edge of living forms. They are intracellular pathogens that lack a cellular structure and need the host cellular resources for their replication. Despite the fact that viruses have no complete autonomy to exist, they can reproduce themselves through self-assembly and are subjected to natural selection. These pathogens can infect all types of cells throughout the living kingdoms, although most of them have a limited range of hosts and are species-specific. Consequently, cellular mechanisms aimed at blocking viral entry and replication have evolved in both unicellular organisms and complex multicellular species. The innate arm of the immune system is an ancient form of host defense against pathogens, with evolutionary conserved mechanisms in both invertebrate and vertebrate lineages. These mechanisms are triggered through a diversified system of receptors called pattern recognition receptors (PRRs) that recognize particular conserved microbial structures, including proteins, lipids, lipoproteins, glycans, and nucleic acids of viruses, bacteria, fungi, or parasites (pathogenic or nonpathogenic), generally referred to as pathogen-associated molecular patterns (PAMPs). PRRs, which are germline encoded, include large gene families consisting of closely related but polymorphic members, and in vertebrates include membrane-bound receptors such as Toll-like receptors (TLRs), and cytosolic sensors such as retinoic acid-inducible gene-I (RIG-I)-like receptors (RLRs) and nucleotide-binding oligomerisation domain (NOD)-like receptors (NLRs).[1,2] Due to their critical role and their efficiency, these innate defense tools have been largely conserved through evolution, even if there is a significant degree of polymorphism and diversity intra- and inter-species, likely due to evolutionary pressures to match rapidly evolving ligands (pathogens). Viral nucleic acids,

The Evolution of the Immune System. http://dx.doi.org/10.1016/B978-0-12-801975-7.00007-4

including single stranded RNA (ssRNA), double stranded RNA (dsRNA), or DNA, are one of the common viral features suitable for innate immune recognition by PRRs.[3] Upon PAMP recognition, PRRs activate a signaling cascade that leads to an upregulation of cytokine genes as messengers of an inflammatory response that mediates the recruitment of cells to the site of intrusion, activates antimicrobial effector systems, and stimulates adaptive immunity (in vertebrates), all of them ultimately focused on the clearance of the intruder.[4,5] The interferon (IFN) system is the key cytokine network released after viral sensing. In fact, the name "interferon" was given by Isaacs and Lindenmann,[6] based on the ability of these molecules to "interfere" with viral progression. IFNs are pleiotropic cytokines that function as key regulators of the antiviral response. Three groups of IFNs have been described in mammals, based on their biological and structural properties, including type I, type II, and type III IFN. Type I and type III IFNs are directly induced by virus infection, promoting the transcription of antiviral genes through a single pathway. The type II IFN, on the other hand, functions as a regulatory cytokine of innate and adaptive immunity through a slightly different pathway.[7] Since type III IFN has only been recently identified in mammals and there is almost no information available in other vertebrate groups, in this review we will focus on type I IFN. Once an infected cell has secreted type I IFN in response to viral stimuli, this IFN signals in the producer and neighboring cells through type I IFN receptors that are present on nearly every nucleated cell. This signaling ultimately leads to the induction of IFN stimulated genes (ISGs) with different roles in a large number of immune pathways, many of which are capable of blocking intracellular viral replication at different levels.

In the current chapter, we provide an overview of IFN-mediated antiviral immunity in vertebrates, from early viral recognition to the antiviral activity of ISGs. The purpose of the chapter is to provide a general overview of this complex system, focusing on the most relevant functions and molecules, and specifically highlighting commonalities and unique features among vertebrate groups to provide an evolutionary perspective.

2 VIRUS-SENSING PATTERN RECOGNITION RECEPTORS

Virus detection can be accomplished either at the extracellular surface of cells or intracellularly, for viruses that have either been internalized by membrane-enclosed structures (ie, derived from phagocytosis of microbes or infected apoptotic cells) or for viruses that actively enter the cytoplasm. In general, the induction of antiviral immunity initiates with the recognition of viral nucleic acids by TLRs, RLRs, and NLRs, and/or recognition of viral glycoproteins by TLRs[8] (Fig. 7.1). Signaling through these receptors leads to the activation of immune effector molecules, mainly the induction of the IFN system that mediates the primary early response. Although all nucleated cells express some kind of PRRs, innate immune cells such as dendritic cells, macrophages, and lymphocytes are specially equipped to sense pathogens and initiate an immune response.[1]

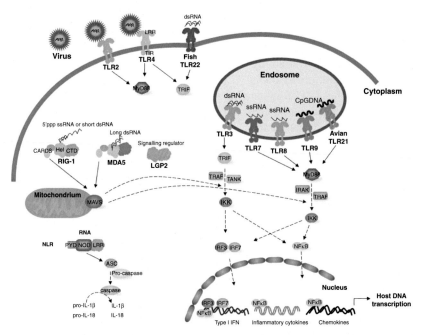

FIGURE 7.1   Schematic representation of viral-sensing pathways by PRRs in vertebrates.
TLRs. Viral glycoproteins (mammalian TLR2, TLR4), RNA (TLR3, TLR7, TLR8, fish TLR22), or
DNA (TLR9, avian TLR21) induce TLR activation and downstream signaling via MyD88 (TLR2,
TLR4, TLR7, TLR8, TLR9, avian TLR21) or via TRIF (TLR3, TLR4, fish TLR22) adaptors. Activation of MyD88 and TRIF leads to interaction with IRAK, TRAF, TANK, and IKK proteins to
activate IF-κB and IRF3/7 transcription factors that translocate to the nucleus and bind to cytokine
gene promoters, starting DNA transcription.[18,19,222] *RLRs.* Once activated by viral RNA, RIG-I and
MDA5 bind the mitochondrial adaptor MAVS through homotypic CAR—CAR interactions, leading to activation of IF-κB and IRF3/7 transcription factors. LGP2 receptors are proposed as regulators of RIG-I and MDA5 activities, but also recognize RNA in their own right.[2] *NLRs.* NLRs that
sense viral RNA induce the catalytic activity of caspases via the ASC adaptor, triggering the cleavage of pro-IL-1β and pro-IL-18 to their mature forms.[1,54]

2.1   Toll-Like Receptor Family

The first identified and best characterized PRR family is that of the membrane-
bound TLRs. TLRs were first described in the fruit fly *Drosophila melanogaster*
as receptors with a developmental function. They were later identified in humans and other species, and the nature of their immune-related function was
subsequently revealed in both vertebrates and invertebrates.[9–11] Similar structures are also found in bacteria and plants, revealing the ancient origin of these
receptors. TLRs are type I transmembrane proteins that form homo- or heterodimers. Each TLR molecule consists of an N-terminal domain, responsible for the
detection of PAMPs, containing numerous variable leucine-rich repeat (LRR)
facing toward the extracellular space or the endosomal lumen; a transmembrane

domain; and a cytosolic Toll-interleukin 1 (IL-1) receptor (TIR) domain that is involved in downstream signal transduction and the recruitment of adaptor molecules with TIR domains through homotypic TIR/TIR interactions.[5,12] In contrast to the high variability in the LRR motifs, the cytoplasmic TIR domain is highly conserved among TLRs and across species.[13] In both agnathans and gnathostomes, a TLR system has been characterized at the molecular level, and phylogenetic studies suggest a true orthology of this system among vertebrates.[14,15] The TLR2 subfamily, TLR3, TLR5, TLR7/8, as well as the fish-type TLR21/22, are essentially conserved in the lamprey (*Lethenteron japonicum*) and teleosts, suggesting that lampreys and jawed vertebrates share the same ancestral TLR repertoire composed of hybrid mammalian- and fish-type TLRs, which may represent the origin of the TLR repertoire in vertebrates.[16,17] Because an extensive review of the evolution of the TLR system can be found in chapter: The Evolution of Toll-like receptor system in Teleosts, in this chapter we will focus exclusively on viral sensing TLRs.

In mammals, viral nucleic acid recognition is achieved by the endosomal TLRs, namely TLR3, 7, 8, and 9, whereas in fish extracellular TLR22[18] or avian endosomal TLR21[19] are also involved in viral recognition. Endosomal TLR3 is the only mammalian TLR that signals solely via the TIR domain-containing adaptor, inducing IFN-β (TRIF), whereas the other TLRs, including endosomal TLR7, 8, and 9, depend on myeloid differentiation factor-88 (MyD88) for signaling. Fish TLR22 recruits TRIF for signaling, whereas avian TLR21 signals via the MyD88 adaptor. Both signaling adaptors, TRIF or MyD88, subsequently activate two main pathways. One is the activation of the IκB kinase (IKK) complex that leads to nuclear translocation of the transcription factor nuclear factor (NF)-κB to upregulate the expression of inflammatory cytokines and chemokines. Additionally, TLRs also activate the IFN regulatory factor (IRF) transcription factors 3/7 pathways that are crucial for the induction of type I IFNs[2,20,21] (Fig. 7.1). Although TLR families show distinct features among vertebrates, several components of the downstream TLR signaling pathways have been identified across vertebrates and are structurally and functionally well-conserved.[22,23] TLR3 specifically recognizes dsRNAs, such as the genomes of dsRNA viruses or dsRNAs generated as intermediate products during the replication of ssRNA viruses, or DNA viruses such as herpesviruses, as a by-product of symmetrical transcription.[3] TLR7 and TLR8 are known to sense guanosine/uridine (GU)-rich ssRNA of RNA viruses. Endosomal TLR9 is a DNA-sensing TLR and specifically binds unmethylated cytosine-guanosine (CpG)-containing oligodeoxynucleotides (CpG-ODN) present in bacteria and DNA viruses, which are rare in the vertebrate genome.[3]

True orthologues of mammalian TLR3 exist in lower vertebrates, and there is structural and functional evidence of a similar involvement in virus detection. For example, the organization of the exon/intron boundaries is highly conserved between the fish and human *tlr3* gene, and fish TLR3 conserves all key residues for binding to dsRNA.[24–26] Reports on the transcriptional upregulation of *tlr3* in response to different viral stimuli have provided indirect evidence of a conserved role for fish *tlr3*. These include evidence for an upregulation of *tlr3* after poly I:C stimulation in lamprey[17] or after exposure to the dsRNA virus in species such as grass carp (*Ctenopharyngo donidella*) and rare minnow (*Gobio cyprisrarus*)[27] or to the ssRNA virus in species such as zebrafish (*Danio rerio*)[28] and rainbow trout (*Oncorhynchus mykiss*).[29,30] More direct evidence of an equivalent antiviral role includes the increased IFN response of a trout fibroblastic cell-line transfected with *tlr3* following stimulation with poly I:C.[18] A role of avian TLR3 in ssRNA virus-recognition has also been described during infection with a highly pathogenic avian influenza virus (HPAIV).[19] All of these findings indicate that the common ancestor of mammals, teleosts, and agnathans likely contained a dsRNA recognition system involving TLR3 capable of detecting diverse viral families.

While TLR3 is an endosomal dsRNA receptor, fish TLR22 is a TLR3 analogue, sensing the presence of dsRNA outside the cells. TLR22 is widely conserved among teleosts and amphibians, but it is likely absent in avian or mammalian genomes, and it has been proposed as a TLR required for aquatic vertebrates[16] that evolves under positive selection.[31] Thus, teleosts possess two dsRNA-sensing TLRs, TLR3 at the endosomal compartment and TLR22 at the cell surface, with a functional difference regarding location and dsRNA discrimination by length. TLR3 recognizes preferentially short dsRNAs (<1 kbp), whereas TLR22 recognizes longer fragments (>1 kbp).[18,26]

TLR7, 8, and 9 form an evolutionary cluster, present in both mammals and teleosts, all localized in intracellular vesicles such as endosomes and the endoplasmic reticulum (ER). TLR7 and 8 are present in lamprey and were mapped to the TLR7/8 cluster of jawed vertebrates.[17] TLR7 and 8 sense viral-derived ssRNA, whereas TLR9 senses DNA CpG-ODN motifs. Interestingly, although a *tlr7* ortholog has been found in chickens, chicken *tlr8* is a pseudogene disrupted by several introns, and *tlr9* seems to have been deleted from avian genomes over evolutionary time.[19,32] Although the chicken genome does not contain *tlr9*, avian TLR21 has an immune function similar to mammalian TLR9 as a CpG-ODN receptor. This nonmammalian receptor is an endosomal TLR and is also present in *Xenopus tropicalis*, teleost fish, and lamprey.[16,19] Phylogenetic analysis indicates that TLR21 is a member of the TLR11 subfamily, together with mouse TLR12 and 13 and teleost TLR20. Although avian TLR21 is known to be involved in CpG-ODN sensing, the functionality of fish TLR21 remains to be determined. Furthermore, a number of fish TLR genes may have experienced insertion of additional introns after the divergence from tetrapods.[14,33] Among these, *tlr9* genes have different numbers of exons in fish species than in mammals.[34]

Mammalian TLR2 and TLR4, present on the cellular plasma membrane, have also been shown to recognize viral components, including envelope proteins and surface hemagglutinin proteins, such as the hemagglutinin of varicella virus, herpes simplex virus-1, human cytomegalovirus, and mouse mammary tumor virus.[35] Little information is available today on the recognition of viral pathogens by TLR2 or TLR4 in other vertebrates. TLR4 is thought to be absent in several fish, as in the salmonids, but has been identified in cyprinid species and catfish (*Ictalurus punctatus*).[15] An induction of *tlr4* has been reported after viral infection in cyprinids,[15,27] but the fact that the two coreceptors needed by mammalian TLR4 to recognize viral structures, namely myeloid differentiation protein-2 (MD-2) and CD14, are absent from the fish genomes means that the function of fish TLR4 signaling is still to be characterized. On the other hand, the G proteins of novirhabdoviruses are known to trigger the synthesis of IFN in rainbow-trout cells, suggesting that the fish immune system conserves the capacity to recognize viral glycoproteins.[36,37]

2.2 RIG-Like Receptor Family

The other main group of PRRs acting in viral RNA detection are the RLRs, which are Asp-Glu-x-Asp/His (DExD/H)-box helicases. RLRs are mobilized to sense viral RNA species in the cytosol during intracellular viral invasion and replication, leading to a potent induction of type I IFNs in most cell types (in contrast to the more immune cell-restricted expression pattern of TLRs). The RLR family is expressed ubiquitously in the cytoplasm and belongs to the IFN-stimulated gene (ISG) family, and, consequently, is subject to positive feedback regulation by IFN.[38] It consists of three members: RIG-I, melanoma differentiation-associated gene 5 (MDA5), and laboratory of genetics and physiology 2 (LGP2).

RIG-I and MDA5 share a similar domain structure, composed of two N-terminal caspase activation and recruitment domains (CARDs) required for downstream signaling; a central DExD/H-box RNA helicase domain with the capacity to hydrolyze ATP; and a C-terminal domain (CTD). Once activated, RIG-I and MDA5 are subsequently recruited to the mitochondrial antiviral signaling (MAVS) adaptor, followed by homotypic CARD-CARD interaction with the adaptor and initiation of downstream signaling via MAVS oligomerization, leading to mobilization of NF-kB and IRFs for cytokine gene-induction (IFN and pro-inflammatory cytokines) (Fig. 7.1). In contrast to TLRs that are restricted to the endosomal compartment, RLRs are in close contact with host RNAs in the cytoplasm, thus suggesting the existence of a precise mechanism for the discrimination of self versus nonself. Indeed, RIG-I is activated by short, uncapped 5′-triphosphate (5′ppp) ssRNA motifs juxtaposed to a short region of dsRNA, generated by viral RNA polymerases. In contrast, eukaryotic cells do not produce dsRNA, and mRNA transcripts are blocked at their 5′-ends by a 7-methyl-guanosine group.[39,40] Interestingly, several viruses have evolved a mechanism to remove their own 5′ppp groups to avoid detection by RIG-I.[41,42] Although both RIG-I and MDA5 are able to sense dsRNA, RIG-I recognizes short dsRNA, whereas MDA5 discriminates long dsRNA, generated during the course of virus infection.[43] Consequently, MDA5, but not RIG-I, responds to poly I:C stimulation, leading to IFN production. Furthermore, RIG-I can also detect DNA from either bacteria or DNA viruses through the DNA-dependent RNA polymerase III.[44]

The third member of the RIG-like receptor family, LGP2, lacks the signaling CARDs. Since embryonic fibroblasts from mice, with a targeted deletion of LGP2, produce increased amounts of IFN-β and active NF-κB in response to transfected poly-I:C relative to wild-type cells, LGP2 has been proposed as a negative regulator of RIG-I signaling.[45] However, more recent studies have demonstrated that LGP2 is a positive upstream regulator of RIG-I and MDA5 signaling, facilitating viral RNA recognition by RIG-I and MDA5 through its ATPase domain.[46]

Using a combination of gene modeling, phylogenetics, structural analysis, population genetics, and molecular-functional characterization of ancestral and extant RLRs, Mukherjee and coworkers found that the RLR-based system had arisen with the emergence of multicellularity.[47] Early functional differentiation of RLRs occurred in metazoan evolution through a series of gene duplication events followed by modifications of the RNA-binding domain, suggesting a course of multiple adaptive changes in sensitivity and specificity of these receptors throughout metazoan evolution, in parallel with viral evolution.[47] MDA5 and LGP2 appear to be common to all fish genomes, whereas RIG-I had been lost from some fish species that belong to the Acanthopterygii class.[48] To date, RIG-I orthologs have been found in primitive fish species such as those in the classes Ostariophysi, Protacanthopterygii, and Paracanthopterygii, as well as in Agnatha (lamprey) and in the Sarcopterygii (coelacanth), suggesting that RIG-I could have been lost after divergence of the Acanthopterygii from the Paracanthopterygii.[14,48,49] Similarly, the chicken genome, unlike that of ducks, geese, and finches, also lacks *rig-I* but contains *mda5* and *lgp2*, which functionally compensate for the absence of RIG-I. For example, while duck RIG-I is the cytosolic recognition element for HPAIV, chicken cells sense the virus through MDA5.[19]

Several studies have reported the induction of RLR mRNA expression in different fish tissues after viral infection, IFN treatment, or poly I:C treatment, as observed in mammals.[14,50] Concerning specific antiviral effects, overexpression of trout MDA5 and LGP2 resulted in a significant accumulation of Myxovirus (Mx)-resistance transcripts, which correlated with an enhancement of protection against viral infection.[14,50] Likewise, a recent study performed in Japanese flounder also revealed that MDA5 knockdown reduced the antiviral and immune effects of poly I:C.[51]

2.3 NOD-Like Receptor Family

TLRs and RLRs are important for the production of type I IFNs and several other cytokines, whereas NLRs play a major role in the regulation of IL-1β (Fig. 7.1). NLRs primarily recognize microbial molecules of bacterial origin.[52]

However, in mammals, NLRs sense several different RNA or DNA viruses, and either positively or negatively regulate the innate antiviral response.[53] The human NLR family is composed of 23 members, whereas there are at least 34 members in the mouse NLR family.[52,53] Several NLR family proteins regulate innate immunity by forming large molecular complexes called inflammasomes, which lead to the secretion of IL-1β and IL-18. Both cytokines activate NF-κB via binding their cognate receptors, leading to a caspase-dependent inflammatory cell-death program, known as pyroptosis.[54] NLRs are composed of three major domains: C-terminal leucine-rich repeats (LRR) responsible for microbe recognition, a central nucleotide-binding oligomerization (NOD) domain (also known as the NACHT cassette) that mediates self-oligomerization during activation, and a variable N-terminal protein–protein interaction domain involved in signal transduction. Based on this N-terminal effector domain, the NLRs are subdivided into four subfamilies that include: the NLRA subfamily, containing an acidic transactivating domain; the NLRB subfamily, containing a baculovirus inhibitor of apoptosis protein repeat (BIR) domain; the NLRC subfamily, containing a caspase recruitment domain (CARD); and the NLRP subfamily, containing a pyrin domain (PYD).[55] According to phylogenetic relationships, NLRs can also be categorized into three subfamilies named NODs, NLRPs (or NALPs), and IPAF.[56]

Complex NLR repertoires evolved very early in animal evolution, and NLR genes with a putative immune function are present already in basal metazoans.[57] Interestingly, three distinct NLR subfamilies were identified in the genome of various nonmammalian vertebrates, including fish, amphibians, and birds.[58] The first subfamily (NLR-A) resembles mammalian NODs, the second (NLR-B) resembles mammalian NALPs, whereas the third (NLR-C) appears to be unique to teleost fish. In zebrafish, several hundred genes belong to this unique subfamily, which is thought to have evolved from a NOD3-like molecule.[58] However, the role for these avian, amphibian, and fish NOD-like receptors in antiviral immunity is still largely unknown.

Other recently discovered IFN-inducible proteins involved in the mammalian antiviral immune system, such as the cytoplasmic dsDNA sensors DAI, AIM2, and IFI6-16,[2] have not yet been investigated in other vertebrates. AIM2 and IFI6-16 form a new family termed AIM2-like receptors (ALRs), and are both involved in inflammasome formation and apoptosis.[59–61] Future investigation is needed to provide clues as to the origin and evolution of these proteins.

3   RNA INTERFERENCE

RNA interference (RNAi) is a defense mechanism operating against RNA viruses, discovered recently, and identified as the primary and most robust antiviral response in plants and invertebrates. The mechanism consists of the cleavage of viral dsRNAs into small (20 bp) RNA fragments by an RNAase III nuclease (dicer). The small interfering RNAs (siRNAs) are then recruited into a biochemical pathway, the RNA-induced silencing complex (RISC), which unwinds the dsRNA into two ssRNA strands to be silenced and degraded.[62–65] Although it was believed at first that this RNA-based antiviral RNAi pathway had been supplanted in vertebrates with a protein-based antiviral IFN response, recent findings demonstrated the existence of a functional RNAi pathway in mammals, suggesting that both RNA and protein-based antiviral mechanisms operate simultaneously in mammalian cells.[66,67] siRNAs have been shown to inhibit viral replication in fish cells,[68,69] however, the relevance of this mechanism in the overall vertebrate antiviral response still needs to be determined.

4 TYPE I IFNs

4.1 Mammalian IFNs

The *ifn* genes have been well-characterized in mammals. Mammalian type I IFNs are encoded by genes with no introns, and can be divided into several phylogenetic groups,[70,71] consisting of IFN-α, -β, -ω/τ, -δ/limitin, -ε, and -κ (Table 7.1). They have a similar α-helical structure and all of them belong to the IL-10 cytokine family. Multiple IFN-α subtypes sharing high sequence homology are apparent within a single species, whilse IFN-β, -ω/τ, -ε, and -κ are encoded by a single copy gene. All the type I IFNs in mammals bind to the same receptor complex and exert antiviral functions via the JAK/STAT signaling pathway. The genes encoding type I IFNs are clustered in the genome; in chromosome (chro) 9 of humans and chro_4 in mouse. Interestingly, some IFN subgroups are lineage specific, and, for example, IFN-δ and limitin have been described in some species but not in humans.[72,73] On the other hand, at least 10 copies of *ifn-δ* genes have been reported in porcine species.[73]

IFN-α is predominantly expressed by activated dendritic cells and primarily participates in immune regulation by bridging innate and adaptive immunity. Conversely, IFN-β is ubiquitously produced by viral-infected cells and is the key player in promoting an antiviral state in the host. IFN-ε is constitutively produced by cells of the reproductive organs and protects the host from viral and bacterial infection.[74,75] Consequently, IFN-ε deficient mice develop severe epidermal lesions in the reproductive tissue, accompanied by high viral titer after a herpes simplex virus 2 challenge.[74] IFN-τ is limited to ruminant species, including sheep and cattle,[76] where multiple *ifn-τ* genes are found to be clustered with other type I *ifn* genes in chro_2 in sheep and in chro_8 in cattle.[77,78] Although a putative homologue has also been reported in humans,[79] it could not be confirmed in the sequenced genome by other studies. IFN-τ is closely related to IFN-ω[70] and is transiently expressed by the conceptus during early pregnancy. It is suggested to play an important role for the fetus maintenance and development, in addition to its primary antiviral function.[80,81] IFN-κ is produced by keratinocytes and certain lymphocyte subsets, and has been shown to modulate cytokine expression.[82,83]

TABLE 7.1 Vertebrate IFNs and IFN Receptors

Vertebrates	IFN	Exon/Intron	Disulfide bond	Expression	Receptor 1	Receptor 2
Mammals	IFN-α	1/0	2	Leukocytes, dendritic cells	IFNAR1	IFNAR2
	IFN-β	1/0	1	Ubiquitous expression	IFNAR1	IFNAR2
	IFN-δ	1/0	2	Reproductive and conceptus tissues		
	IFN-ε	1/0	1	Reproductive and mucosal tissues	IFNAR1	IFNAR2
	IFN-κ	1/0	2	Keratinocytes, lymphocytes	IFNAR1	IFNAR2
	IFN-ω/τ	1/0	2	Conceptus tissues, leukocytes	IFNAR1	IFNAR2
Birds	IFN-1 (IFN-α)	1/0	2	Lymphoid tissues, leukocytes	IFNAR1	IFNAR2
	IFN-2 (IFN-β)	1/0	2	Ubiquitous expression	IFNAR1	IFNAR2
Reptiles	IFN	1/0	2	NA	NA	NA
Amphibians	IFN-1-5	5/4	2	Most tissues, lungs, bone marrow, kidney cells, splenocytes	IFNAR1	IFNAR2

					IFNAR1	IFNAR2
Coelacanth	IFN-1-5	5/4	2	NA	IFNAR1	IFNAR2
Teleost fish	IFN-a	5/4	1	Ubiquitous expression	CRFB5, CRFB5a-c	CRFB1, CRFB1a
	IFN-b	5/4	2	Lymphoid tissues, leukocytes	CRFB5x	CRFB2
	IFN-c	5/4	2	Lymphoid tissues, leukocytes	CRFB5, CRFB5a, CRFB5c	CRFB2
	IFN-d	5/4	1	Ubiquitous expression	CRFB5	CRFB1
	IFN-e	5/4	1	Kidney, spleen	NA	NA
	IFN-f	5/4	2	Kidney, spleen, fibroblasts, monocytes/macrophages	NA	NA
Cartilaginous fish	IFN	4/3	2	NA	IFNAR1	IFNAR2a, IFNAR2b

NA, information not available.
See references in the text.

4.2 Avian and Reptile Type I IFNs

Avian type I IFNs have been studied mostly in chickens, where two distinct groups of type I IFNs with limited sequence identity (57%) have been found (Table 7.1), designated ChIFN1 and ChIFN2.[84] They have also been termed as IFN-α and IFN-β, mainly based on the comparison of gene copies and expression responsiveness to immune stimulants between mammalian and chicken type I IFN members. Despite this, phylogenetic analysis reveals that ChIFN1 and ChIFN2 are not 1:1 orthologues to mammalian IFN-α and IFN-β.[85] ChIFN1 exists as multiple copies sharing high sequence identities. The genes encoding these IFN molecules are located in the short arm of the sex chromosome, which also harbors the single copy of ChIFN2.[86] Both ChIFN1 and ChIFN2 contain 4 cysteines in the mature peptide, a characteristic pattern seen in mammalian IFN-αs and fish group-II IFNs.[87]

ChIFN1 and ChIFN2 are induced in response to viral infection and stimulation with viral mimics.[88] Potent inducers include Newcastle disease virus and influenza virus.[89–91] Curiously, the expression patterns of the ChIFN1 and ChIFN2 resemble that of mammalian IFN-α and IFN-β. The ChIFN1 is predominantly produced in lymphoid organs after administration of imidanoquinolines,[89] but only the ChIFN2 and not ChIFN1 can be activated by nonviral nucleotide PAMPs. Analysis of the promoter region of the *chifn2* gene revealed the presence of NF-kB binding sites, partly responsible for the observed difference in gene expression.

Reptilian IFN activities were detected three decades ago,[92] exhibiting similar chemical and antiviral properties to their avian and mammalian counterparts. However, the gene and protein sequences were only confirmed recently, when multiple genes (GenBank accession number: XM_008103493-9) were predicted in the genome of the green anole (*Anolis carolinensis*). Like birds and mammals, the green anole *ifn* genes lack introns (Ref. [87], unpublished data).

4.3 Amphibian IFNs

Type I *ifn* genes were first reported in the *X. tropicalis* genome,[87] where five were predicted in the same scaffold, all consisting of five exons and four introns (Table 7.1). The translated proteins possess four conserved cysteine residues in the mature peptides and belong to the vertebrate four cysteine containing IFN group (group II).[93] Phylogenetic tree analysis reveals two apparent groups where the IFN1 and IFN2 are related to the teleost IFNs and the IFN3–5 are related to the amniote IFNs,[93] which are believed to have diversified from a bona-fide gene shared by ray-finned fish and tetrapods. The two groups share low sequence-identities at the protein level, ranging from 15.5% to 23.7%. A homologue to the *X. tropicalis* IFN3–5 has also been sequenced in another amphibian species, *X. laevis*, and has been shown to trigger a conserved antiviral response similar to that observed in fish and amniote IFNs, protecting cells and tadpoles against ranavirus infection.[94]

4.4   Fish IFNs

Fish *ifn* genes were first identified in zebrafish,[95] Atlantic salmon (*Salmo salar*),[96] and channel catfish.[97] Later on, taking advantage of the completion of fish genomes and the vast amount of transcriptomic sequences available, significant advances have been made in discovery of *ifn* genes in other fish species. At the molecular level, the teleost type I *ifn* genes share the same genetic organization as their amphibian and sarcopterygian (coelacanth) counterparts, and are encoded by genes with a genomic structure of 5 exons and 4 introns.[93,98,99] Multiple copies are common, and, as in other vertebrates, are clustered in the genome. However, accumulating data suggest that the IFN locus may be segregated in teleosts, due to further whole genome duplications (WGD) after the second round of WGD leading to the appearance of jawed vertebrates. In the zebrafish genome, four *ifn* genes have been found, with three residing in chro_3 and one in chro_12. Interestingly, the IFN locus in chro_3 is linked with the growth hormone gene 1, a synteny also seen in the genome of elephant shark (*Callorhinchus milii*),[100] Atlantic salmon,[101] and Chinook salmon (*Oncorhynchus tshawytscha*).[102] On the other hand, several other genes, including CD79B and SCN4A, seen in the elephant shark IFN locus are also present in the IFN locus in zebrafish chro_12. It is probable that the IFN locus has been segregated into two in teleosts by the third-round WGD, which is believed to have occurred before the radiation of teleosts.

The teleost *ifn* genes are divergent in their primary sequences, and can be classified into two groups that contain two (group I) and four (group II) conserved cysteine residues in the mature peptide, and can be further divided into six phylogenetic subfamilies (IFN-a-f). In the West Indian Ocean coelacanth (*Latimeria chalumnae*), one of the two extant species of the oldest representatives of sarcopterygian lineage, all of the five IFNs identified belong to group II IFNs, and have a closer phylogenetic relationship with their counterparts from tetrapods than from teleosts.[103] Fish IFNs do not have 1:1 orthologous relationships with their counterparts in birds and mammals. Group I IFNs, consisting of IFN-a, -d and -e, are ubiquitously present in teleosts and are not the equivalent to the mammalian two-cysteine-containing IFN-β and -ε,[104] because the cysteines are paired at different positions. Group II IFNs (IFN-b, -c, and -f) are limited to some species, as of yet the cyprinids and salmonids, and contain a relatively well-conserved motif (CAWE) near the C-terminus.[87,101,104] It should be noted that the two-cysteine-containing IFNs have only been found in teleosts and mammals, whereas the four cysteine containing IFNs are present in all the jawed-vertebrate lineages.[99] Despite the limited sequence homology between fish group I and II IFNs, their overall protein structure remains similar. Hamming et al.[105] recently determined the crystal structure of zebrafish IFN-phi1 (IFN-a, group I) and IFNphi2 (IFN-c, group II), both of which display a typical structure of class II cytokines containing six α-helices. This study also provides structural evidence confirming the homologous relationship of fish IFNs to type I rather than type III IFNs in mammals.

The copy numbers of fish IFNs vary significantly among species. Salmonids have all six phylogenetic subfamilies and the largest number of gene copies in the genome. Thus in rainbow trout, at least 26 genes/pseudogenes have been identified,[104] whereas cyprinids have only three subgroups (IFN-a, -d and -c).[106] Multiple copies have also been found in some acanthopterygian species, and, in this case, all belong to one subfamily (IFN-d).[104,107–109]

Fish IFNs are produced by different cells in response to viral stimuli, suggesting distinct roles in eliciting immune responses to fend off invading pathogens during infection. The *ifn-a* genes are widely induced in different cell types, including fibroblasts, monocytes, macrophages, and lymphocytes, resembling the expression patterns of IFN-β in humans.[87,110] On the other hand, IFN-b and -c are shown to be produced primarily by limited leucocyte populations, and can be drastically upregulated in response to PAMP stimulation and viral infection.[97,110] There are contradicting reports regarding whether IFN-d is inducible by virus or by viral PAMPs in salmonids.[106,110,111] Nevertheless, acanthopterygian IFN-d is activated after viral infection.[108] Information regarding the expression of IFN-e and -f is scarce because they have only recently been described in salmonid species. Although inducible, IFN-e and -f are not upregulated to the magnitude seen for IFN-a, -b and -c during viral infection in brown trout (*Salmo trutta*).[104] All of these data demonstrate that the fish IFN response is likely to be modulated at multiple levels and may differ from species to species.

The direct antiviral activities of type I IFNs appear to be well-conserved in vertebrates. The recombinant mature peptides produced in either bacteria or mammalian cells are potent inducers of IFN-stimulated antiviral genes, including Mx, PKR/PKZ, and viperin in fish cells, and protect fish against viral infection when administered in vivo.[87,95,106,112,113] These antiviral activities of fish IFNs are in line with the observations in birds and mammals, but with some exceptions. For example, administration of recombinant IFN-a at the time of infection or postinfection does not inhibit virus replication in Atlantic salmon cells.[112] Furthermore, recombinant IFN-d from salmonids and zebrafish weakly enhances Mx/viperin gene expression, even though it is induced by both virus and viral PAMPs,[106,110,111] suggesting it may not be directly involved in activation of the cellular antiviral response. However, this observation is in contrast to other studies, where the IFN-d molecules from some acanthopterygian species are shown to trigger antiviral gene expression and protect the host against viral infection.[99,114]

IFNs are produced by viral infected cells, and activate the target cells to establish an antiviral state via cell-surface receptors in an autocrine or paracrine manner.[70] The majority of fish IFNs have a predicted hydrophobic leader peptide at the N-terminus, suggesting that their mode of action resembles that of IFNs in mammals.[98,99] However, several groups have described transcript variants generated by RNA alternative splicing in some species, including Atlantic salmon,[115] catfish,[97] and rainbow trout,[116] indicating that this might represent a common mechanism to increase the diversity of IFN function in teleosts. A later study has confirmed that some IFN transcript variants translate into functional proteins that are not secreted by the cells, and interact with intracellular receptors to induce expression of antiviral genes.[117] This intracellular IFN system has only been reported in rainbow trout and may be important for the defense of virus-infected cells at the very early stage. It would be interesting to see whether this is a common IFN feature in other fish species.

5   IFN RECEPTORS

In humans, a sole heterodimeric receptor complex consisting of IFNAR1 and IFNAR2 mediates the cellular responses triggered by all type I IFN family members, despite their low sequence homology.[70] Upon activation by the IFN ligands, IFNAR1 and IFNAR2 undergo a conformational change to facilitate a cascade of downstream signaling events leading to phosphorylation of the tyrosine kinases Tyk2 and JAK1, as well as the signal transducers and activators of transcription STAT1 and STAT2, with the subsequent formation of the IFN-stimulated gene factor 3 (ISGF3) complex, consisting of phosphorylated STAT1 and STAT2 and IFN-regulated factor 9 (IRF9). The ISGF3 complex translocates to the nucleus and binds to a specific sequence motif in the promoter region of target genes to initiate expression. To activate phosphorylation of cellular proteins, IFNs bind to the high-affinity receptor IFNAR2 and are then transported to IFNAR1, which has a weak ligand-binding affinity.[118] However, this model has been challenged by a recent study, where binding of human IFN-β to the IFNAR1 in the absence of IFNAR2 can also augment gene expression in target cells via a signaling pathway independent from the conventional JAK/STAT pathway.[119] Interestingly, Chang et al. also demonstrated that cotransfection of trout intracellular IFN-a with IFNAR1, but not IFNAR2 in human HEK293 cells, resulted in phosphorylation of STAT1.[117]

The genes encoding IFNAR1 and IFNAR2 are clustered in a single chromosome that harbors IL-10R2 and IFNγR2 in birds and mammals. The corresponding locus is also identifiable in elephant shark[100] and coelacanth,[103] and in some teleost species such as pufferfish, zebrafish, and Atlantic salmon.[107,120,121] However, recent studies have shown that the respective locus has been duplicated in several cyprinid and salmonid species. In zebrafish, IFNAR1, IFNAR2, and IL-10R2 are placed in chro_9, whereas IFNγR2 is in chro_5.[121] In contrast, four IFNAR1 genes and five IFNAR2 genes are found in two loci in chro_21 and chro_25 in the Atlantic salmon genome.[121] It must be noted that the IFNAR2 gene has expanded in all the teleost species as a result of random local-gene duplications or WGD duplications. Considering that the elephant shark genome also has duplicated copies of IFNAR2 homologues, it is difficult to ascertain whether the IFNAR2 genes have been duplicated prior to gnathostomes, or have experienced gene loss in the coelacanth/tetrapod lineage. In humans and mice, multiple forms of IFNAR2 also exist, but arise from a single gene by alternative splicing.[122,123]

Both IFNAR1 and IFNAR2 have been characterised functionally in teleost fish, including Atlantic salmon,[121] zebrafish,[106] and rainbow trout.[117] In contrast with the fact that all type I IFNs interact with a common receptor complex in mammals, emerging evidence suggests that teleost group I and II IFNs have biased receptor usage. In zebrafish, two receptor complexes, involving IFNAR1(CRFB5)/IFNAR2a(CRFB1) and IFNAR1(CRFB5)/IFNAR2b(CRFB2), were proposed (Table 7.1). The former is believed to be preferentially activated by group I IFNs, while the latter by group II IFNs.[106] In Atlantic salmon, the receptor usage seems likely to be even more complex, as there are five IFNAR2s (CRFB1–3) and four IFNAR1s (CRFB5a–c and CRFB5x).[121]

Studies in mammals demonstrate that the fibronectin (FN)-like domains in the extracellular region of IFNAR1 and IFNAR2 are indispensable for the ligand and receptor interaction, and dictate the differential roles elicited by the ligands and the species specificity seen. Human IFNAR1 comprises four tandemly assembled FNIII-like subdomains (SD1–SD4), of which SD1–SD3 have been shown to be important for IFN binding.[119,124,125] The four SD domain arrangement is also present in known IFNAR1 proteins sequenced in sarcopterygians.[103,124] However, teleost IFNAR1 proteins possess only two extracellular SD domains, suggesting that the interaction between IFN ligands and receptors may differ from that in humans. The two tandem SD structure is also present in the recently identified IFNAR1 of elephant shark.[100] These findings support the notion that the four SDs seen in sarcopterygian IFNAR1 have been duplicated in the ancestral molecule shared by coelacanths and tetrapods.[126] In the case of IFNAR2, the two extracellular FNIII-like domains (D1 and D2) are conserved across the Vertebrata phyla, with D1 being the main region interacting with the IFN ligands in humans.[125]

6 DOWNSTREAM MODULATORS OF THE INTERFERON RESPONSE

IFN signaling activates a cascade of intracellular events that leads to the formation of a multimeric complex STAT1/STAT2/IRF9, initially designated as ISGF3,[127] that translocates into the nucleus and binds specific motifs located in IFN promoters, as well as promoters of ISGs.[128,129] The elements involved in this cascade, including *stat1*, *stat2*, and *irf9* genes, have been reported in many fish species (reviewed in Ref. [130]), suggesting a conservation of the intracellular IFN signaling pathway in all vertebrates. Many of these ISGs (between 50 and 100) are believed to be directly responsible for the antiviral effects of IFNs, but only a few of them have been fully characterized in mammals. These include Myxovirus-resistance (Mx) proteins,[131] 2,5-oligoadenylate synthase (OAS),[132] protein kinase R (PKR),[133] viperin,[134] and the ubiquitin-like Interferon Stimulated Gene 15 kDa protein (ISG15).[135] Although the number of ISGs seems to be lower in fish, and also some ISGs such as OAS are missing from fish genomes,[130] it seems that some essential ISGs appeared early in vertebrate history.[130,136] Actually, Langevin et al. identified two different groups of ISGs: a family that differentiated in parallel in tetrapods and fish, which includes genes such as Mx; and a family of genes that had already diversified in the common ancestor to tetrapods and fish, which mainly includes regulatory factors and signal-transduction components such as the STATs.[130]

6.1 Mx Protein

Mx proteins are IFN-induced, dynamin-like, large GTPases, first identified in association with influenza virus-resistance in mice.[137] Since then, Mx homologs have been identified in most vertebrates examined, and even in invertebrates such as the abalone (*Haliotis discus discus*)[138]; however, their cellular location, their level of activity, and the viruses they inhibit vary widely. Mx genes have been reported in amphibians[139] and reptiles,[140] although little information regarding their functionality is available in these species. While in most species at least two Mx isoforms are present, in birds only one cytoplasmic Mx isoform exists. Furthermore, initial descriptions of duck[141] and chicken[142] Mx proteins reported a lack of antiviral activity. However, this issue is controversial since later reports suggested that certain polymorphic variants of chicken Mx were able to confer some antiviral activity,[143–145] whereas other studies with these same variants found no significant differences in viral resistance.[146,147] Furthermore, recent analyses have confirmed that some of these chicken Mx variants with suspected antiviral activity lacked GTPAse activity,[148] which is an essential requirement for antiviral activity. However, the high degree of polymorphisms in this gene observed in birds does suggest a role in antiviral immunity that is yet to be clarified.

In fish, *mx* genes have been identified in many different species,[149–161] in which usually two or three isoforms with different subcellular locations are present. Because in most fish species Mx genes were identified much earlier than IFN genes, the induction of Mx transcription has been commonly used as a marker of IFN induction. Consequently, fish Mx proteins are known to be transcriptionally modulated in response to treatment with viral mimics such as poly I:C,[149–152,154,155,157,161] diverse viral pathogens,[151–156,158–160] or antiviral vaccines, including DNA vaccines,[162–166] virus-like particles (VLPs),[167] or inactivated viruses,[168,169] demonstrating that viral replication is not required for induction of Mx. In the case of intramuscular DNA vaccination against fish rhabdovirus, Mx transcription levels induced in trout seemed to correlate with protection levels observed at early times postvaccination until adaptive immunity takes over.[163,166] Despite this, no antiviral activity has ever been reported for the trout Mx isoforms, and the bioactivity of Mx proteins in fish has only been demonstrated in a few species. In sea bream (*Sparus aurata*), a marine species naturally resistant to many viral pathogens, all three Mx isoforms showed antiviral activity against several RNA and DNA viruses.[170] Antiviral activity has also been reported for Mx proteins in species such as Atlantic salmon,[171,172] rare minnow,[173] grass carp,[174] and Senegalese sole (*Solea senegalensis*).[175] In barramundi (*Lates calcarifer*), Mx was shown to interact with the betanodavirus RNA-dependent RNA polymerase (RdRp), thus limiting viral RNA synthesis, providing for the first time in fish some insights into the possible mechanisms of action of Mx proteins.[176]

6.2 Viperin

Viperin, initially designated as vig-1 [viral hemorrhagic septicemia virus (VHSV)-induced gene 1], was identified by mRNA differential display methodology in rainbow-trout leukocytes as a major responder gene to VHSV.[177] Subsequent studies demonstrated that its transcription could also be induced by IFN in fish[178] and mammals,[134] where it was designated as viperin. Recently, a *viperin* gene has been reported in birds[179] and some other fish species.[180,181] In mammals, the antiviral activity of viperin has been revealed in several viral models when expressed in mitochondria,[134] when associated to the endoplasmatic reticulum[182] or through its interaction with lipid rafts.[183]In a respiratory syncytial virus-infection model, viperin did not affect viral protein expression or inclusion of body formation, but was associated with the inhibition of virus filament formation and reduced cell-to-cell virus transmission.[184] In contrast, equine viperin restricted equine infectious anemia virus replication at multiple steps of the replication process, including virus entry into the cells.[185] On the other hand, in humans, viperin is needed for the changes in lipid metabolism triggered during cytomegalovirus infection.[186] Although the mechanism of action against nonmammalian viral pathogens has never been reported, the antiviral activity of crucian carp (*Carassius auratus*) and rock bream (*Oplegnathus fasciatus*)[180] viperin has been revealed recently.[181]

6.3 PKR

PKR is a serine-threonine kinase that inhibits protein synthesis by phosphorylation of the eukaryotic translation initiation factor 2-alpha (eIF2α). It has also been shown to activate NFκB by inducing NFκB-inducing kinase and IκB (inhibitor of NFκB) kinase.[187] Although it has been mainly proposed as an antiviral agent in mammals that is known to limit viral translation in infections with viruses such as vesicular stomatitis virus (VSV)[188] or vaccinia virus,[189] some viruses like hepatitis C virus have developed strategies to interfere with the action of PKR, and consequently use it as a pro-infection agent.[187] The *pkr* gene has been identified in amphibians,[190] birds,[191] and in several fish species such as zebrafish,[192] Atlantic salmon,[193] rare minnow,[194] and grass carp.[195] Although these fish PKR-like proteins have Z-DNA-binding domains instead of dsRNA-binding domains in the regulatory domain, they were designated as Z-DNA-binding protein kinases (PKZs).[192] Although it was first thought that *pkz* genes were the only orthologues of mammalian *pkr* genes in fish, true *pkr* genes were later identified in several fish species, including zebrafish,[190] Japanese flounder (*Paralichthys olivaceus*),[196] fugu,[197] and rock bream.[198] Fish *pkr* genes are closer to fish *pkz* than to mammalian *pkr*, suggesting that they are paralogues that derive from an ancestral kinase gene duplicated after the divergence from the tetrapod lineage as an adaptation to specific fish viruses.[190] The salmon PKZ[193] and both fugu PKRs[197] were capable of inhibiting protein translation and activating NFκB, demonstrating equivalent roles for fish and mammalian PKRs. In Japanese flounder, PKR was also shown to phosphorylate eIF2α and to inhibit the replication of *Scophthalmus maximus* rhabdovirus (SMRV) in flounder embryonic cells,[196] also revealing a conservation of its antiviral capacities in fish.

6.4 ISG15

ISG15 is one of the most abundant transcripts after type I IFN treatment in mammals.[199] The protein has an important sequence homology to ubiquitin, and similar to ubiquitin, ISG15 is conjugated to target proteins via a pathway named "ISGylation." Both ISGylation and ubiquitination provoke posttranslational modifications that modify the stability, the function, or the localization of the targeted proteins.[200] Within the cells, ISG15 can be found either free or conjugated to target proteins. In macrophages, B and T lymphocytes and epithelial cells, an additional free form of ISG15 that functions as a cytokine is also secreted into the medium,[201,202] where it is known to activate IFN-γ production in T lymphocytes.[203] ISG15 has been shown to limit viral replication in different mammalian viral models, such as HIV-1,[204] Sindbis virus,[205] or Ebola.[206] Whereas *isg15* genes are missing in birds[207] and have not been reported in reptiles or amphibians, one or several *isg15* genes are expressed in all fish species, in which a search for these genes has been performed. These include rainbow trout,[178] goldfish,[208] Atlantic salmon,[209] crucian carp,[210] Atlantic cod (*Gadus morhua*),[211,212] and Japanese flounder[213]; all of these genes are upregulated in response to viral stimuli. In Atlantic cod, three different isoforms are present, and even though the three of them were induced in response to Poly I:C, only one of them seemed to conjugate with intracellular proteins, suggesting different functionalities for each isoform.[212] Even though the antiviral capacity of fish ISG15 has not been widely explored, results showing that Atlantic salmon ISG15 can bind an infectious salmon anemia virus (ISAV) protein as well as different cellular proteins,[209] and the fact that ISG15 is transcriptionally regulated in response to viral stimuli in all fish species examined, suggest a conservation of IFN-induced ISG15-mediated antiviral properties in fish.

6.5 TRIM

The superfamily of tripartite motif-containing (TRIM) proteins is conserved throughout the metazoan kingdom and has expanded rapidly during vertebrate evolution through gene expansion, positive selection, and alternative splicing.[214] This group of proteins is defined by the N-terminal TRIM or RBCC motif, which include in this order: a RING domain, one or two B-box domains that determine the partners of the protein and in which pathway they are involved, and an associated coiled-coil domain.[215] Interestingly, the RING domain has an E3 ubiquitin ligase activity that has the capacity to bind proteins either with ubiquitin or ubiquitin-like molecules such as ISG15,[130] suggesting a cooperative action of different ISGs. Many different mammalian *trim* genes are known to be induced by type I IFN or viral infection.[216] Additionally, many of them were shown to have direct antiviral effects through diverse mechanisms (reviewed in[214]). Several *trim* genes have been identified in birds,[217] amphibians,[218] fish, and even nematodes.[219] In teleost fish, a group of *trim* genes with variable members depending on the species was identified after viral infection.[220] Since these genes do not seem to have true orthologues in tetrapods, they were designated as finTRIMs for "fish novel TRIMs". On the other hand, while orthologues of some mammalian *trim* genes such as *trim5*, *trim22*, or *trim19* are clearly missing from fish genomes, what appear to be true counterparts of mammalian *trim* genes have also been reported in fish.[221] While the diversity of this family in fish implies an important role in antiviral immunity, the bioactivity of these proteins remains unexplored.

7 CONCLUSIONS

All vertebrates are able to mount strong and effective antiviral responses in response to pathogenic viral exposure. The first line of antiviral defense is that mediated by innate immunity through the IFN system, including recognition of viral features, induction of IFN, and translation of ISGs that directly interfere with viral replication at the cellular level. This system, conserved throughout vertebrate evolution, seems particularly important to vertebrates in which an adaptive immune system is not fully developed and/or is dependent on environmental parameters such as temperature. The variability and diversity of IFNs and ISGs illustrate the diversity of cellular mechanisms involved in antiviral responses, as well as the long term coevolutionary history of viruses and vertebrate cells. Consequently, comparing the IFN systems in the different vertebrate groups provides an evolutionary perspective to understand the basis and complexity of this remarkable system.

ACKNOWLEDGMENTS

This work was supported by Starting Grant 2011 (Project No. 280469) from the European Research Council, and the European Commission under the 7th Framework Programme for Research and Technological Development (FP7) of the European Union (Grant Agreement 311993 TARGETFISH). The authors want to thank Professor Chris Secombes for critically reviewing this chapter.

REFERENCES

1. Takeuchi O, Akira S. Innate immunity to virus infection. *Immunol Rev* 2009;**227**:75–86.
2. Gurtler C, Bowie AG. Innate immune detection of microbial nucleic acids. *Trends Microbiol* 2013;**21**:413–20.
3. Barbalat R, Ewald SE, Mouchess ML, Barton GM. Nucleic acid recognition by the innate immune system. *Annu Rev Immunol* 2011;**29**:185–214.
4. Medzhitov R. Recognition of microorganisms and activation of the immune response. *Nature* 2007;**449**:819–26.
5. Kawai T, Akira S. The role of pattern-recognition receptors in innate immunity: update on toll-like receptors. *Nat Immunol* 2010;**11**:373–84.
6. Isaacs A, Lindenmann J. Virus interference I. The interferon. *Proc R Soc Lond B Biol Sci.* 1957;**147**:258–67.
7. Gupta SL. Regulation of cellular gene expression by interferon-gamma: involvement of multiple pathways. *Int J Cell Cloning* 1990;**8**(Suppl 1):92–102.
8. Mogensen TH, Paludan SR. Reading the viral signature by toll-like receptors and other pattern recognition receptors. *J Mol Med (Berl)* 2005;**83**:180–92.
9. Gay NJ, Keith FJ. Drosophila toll and IL-1 receptor. *Nature* 1991;**351**:355–6.
10. Irazoqui JE, Urbach JM, Ausubel FM. Evolution of host innate defence: insights from *Caenorhabditis elegans* and primitive invertebrates. *Nat Rev Immunol* 2010;**10**:47–58.
11. Iwasaki A, Medzhitov R. Regulation of adaptive immunity by the innate immune system. *Science* 2010;**327**:291–5.
12. Takeda K, Akira S. Toll-like receptors in innate immunity. *Int Immunol* 2005;**17**:1–14.
13. Werling D, Jann OC, Offord V, Glass EJ, Coffey TJ. Variation matters: TLR structure and species-specific pathogen recognition. *Trends Immunol* 2009;**30**:124–30.
14. Aoki T, Hikima J, Hwang SD, Jung TS. Innate immunity of finfish: primordial conservation and function of viral RNA sensors in teleosts. *Fish Shellfish Immunol* 2013;**35**:1689–702.
15. Pietretti D, Wiegertjes GF. Ligand specificities of toll-like receptors in fish: indications from infection studies. *Dev Comp Immunol* 2014;**43**:205–22.
16. Oshiumi H, Matsuo A, Matsumoto M, Seya T. Pan-vertebrate toll-like receptors during evolution. *Curr Genomics* 2008;**9**:488–93.
17. Kasamatsu J, Oshiumi H, Matsumoto M, Kasahara M, Seya T. Phylogenetic and expression analysis of lamprey toll-like receptors. *Dev Comp Immunol* 2010;**34**:855–65.
18. Matsuo A, Oshiumi H, Tsujita T, Mitani H, Kasai H, Yoshimizu M, et al. Teleost TLR22 recognizes RNA duplex to induce IFN and protect cells from birnaviruses. *J Immunol* 2008;**181**:3474–85.
19. Chen S, Cheng A, Wang M. Innate sensing of viruses by pattern recognition receptors in birds. *Vet Res* 2013;**44**:82.
20. Liew FY, Xu D, Brint EK, O'Neill LA. Negative regulation of toll-like receptor-mediated immune responses. *Nat Rev Immunol* 2005;**5**:446–58.
21. Seya T, Matsumoto M, Ebihara T, Oshiumi H. Functional evolution of the TICAM-1 pathway for extrinsic RNA sensing. *Immunol Rev* 2009;**227**:44–53.
22. Jault C, Pichon L, Chluba J. Toll-like receptor gene family and TIR-domain adapters in *Danio rerio*. *Mol Immunol* 2004;**40**:759–71.
23. Rebl A, Goldammer T, Seyfert HM. Toll-like receptor signaling in bony fish. *Vet Immunol Immunopathol* 2010;**134**:139–50.
24. Hwang SD, Ohtani M, Hikima J, Jung TS, Kondo H, Hirono I, et al. Molecular cloning and characterization of toll-like receptor 3 in Japanese flounder *Paralichthys olivaceus*. *Dev Comp Immunol* 2012;**37**:87–96.

25. Quiniou SM, Boudinot P, Bengten E. Comprehensive survey and genomic characterization of toll-like receptors (TLRs) in channel catfish Ictalurus punctatus: identification of novel fish TLRs. *Immunogenetics* 2013;**65**:511–30.

26. Sahoo BR, Dikhit MR, Bhoi GK, Maharana J, Lenka SK, Dubey PK, et al. Understanding the distinguishable structural and functional features in zebrafish TLR3 and TLR22, and their binding modes with fish dsRNA viruses: an exploratory structural model analysis. *Amino Acids* 2015;**47**:381–400.

27. Su J, Jang S, Yang C, Wang Y, Zhu Z. Genomic organization and expression analysis of toll-like receptor 3 in grass carp (*Ctenopharyngodon idella*). *Fish Shellfish Immunol* 2009;**27**:433–9.

28. Phelan PE, Mellon MT, Kim CH. Functional characterization of full-length TLR3, IRAK-4, and TRAF6 in zebrafish (*Danio rerio*). *Mol Immunol* 2005;**42**:1057–71.

29. Castro R, Abós B, Pignatelli J, Gonzalez Granja A, Tafalla C. Short term immune responses in rainbow trout liver upon viral hemorrhagic septicemia virus (VHSV) infection. *PLoS ONE* 2014;**9**(10) e111084.

30. Abos B, Castro R, Gonzalez Granja A, Havixbeck JJ, Barreda DR, Tafalla C. Early activation of teleost B cells in response to rhabdovirus infection. *J Virol* 2015;**89**:1768–80.

31. Sundaram AY, Consuegra S, Kiron V, Fernandes JM. Positive selection pressure within teleost toll-like receptors tlr21 and tlr22 subfamilies and their response to temperature stress and microbial components in zebrafish. *Mol Biol Rep* 2012;**39**:8965–75.

32. Temperley ND, Berlin S, Paton IR, Griffin DK, Burt DW. Evolution of the chicken toll-like receptor gene family: a story of gene gain and gene loss. *BMC Genomics* 2008;**9**:62.

33. Oshiumi H, Tsujita T, Shida K, Matsumoto M, Ikeo K, Seya T. Prediction of the prototype of the human toll-like receptor gene family from the pufferfish, *Fugu rubripes*, genome. *Immunogenetics* 2003;**54**:791–800.

34. Takano T, Kondo H, Hirono I, Endo M, Saito-Taki T, Aoki T. Molecular cloning and characterization of toll-like receptor 9 in Japanese flounder *Paralichthys olivaceus*. *Mol Immunol* 2007;**44**:1845–53.

35. Barton GM. Viral recognition by toll-like receptors. *Semin Immunol* 2007;**19**:33–40.

36. Acosta F, Collet B, Lorenzen N, Ellis AE. Expression of the glycoprotein of viral haemorrhagic septicaemia virus (VHSV) on the surface of the fish cell line RTG-P1 induces type 1 interferon expression in neighbouring cells. *Fish Shellfish Immunol* 2006;**21**:272–8.

37. Verjan N, Ooi EL, Nochi T, Kondo H, Hirono I, Aoki T, et al. A soluble nonglycosylated recombinant infectious hematopoietic necrosis virus (IHNV) G-protein induces IFNs in rainbow trout (*Oncorhynchus mykiss*). *Fish Shellfish Immunol* 2008;**25**:170–80.

38. Matsumiya T, Stafforini DM. Function and regulation of retinoic acid-inducible gene-I. *Crit Rev Immunol* 2010;**30**:489–513.

39. Hornung V, Ellegast J, Kim S, Brzozka K, Jung A, Kato H, et al. 5'-triphosphate RNA is the ligand for RIG-I. *Science* 2006;**314**:994–7.

40. Pichlmair A, Schulz O, Tan CP, Naslund TI, Liljestrom P, Weber F, et al. RIG-I-mediated antiviral responses to single-stranded RNA bearing 5'-phosphates. *Science* 2006;**314**:997–1001.

41. Weber M, Gawanbacht A, Habjan M, Rang A, Borner C, Schmidt AM, Incoming RNA. et al. virus nucleocapsids containing a 5'-triphosphorylated genome activate RIG-I and antiviral signaling. *Cell Host Microbe* 2013;**13**:336–46.

42. Gack MU. Mechanisms of RIG-I-like receptor activation and manipulation by viral pathogens. *J Virol* 2014;**88**:5213–6.

43. Schlee M. Master sensors of pathogenic RNA—RIG-I like receptors. *Immunobiology* 2013;**218**:1322–35.

44. Chiu YH, Macmillan JB, Chen ZJ. RNA polymerase III detects cytosolic DNA and induces type I interferons through the RIG-I pathway. *Cell* 2009;**138**:576–91.
45. Venkataraman T, Valdes M, Elsby R, Kakuta S, Caceres G, Saijo S, et al. Loss of DExD/H box RNA helicase LGP2 manifests disparate antiviral responses. *J Immunol* 2007;**178**:6444–55.
46. Satoh T, Kato H, Kumagai Y, Yoneyama M, Sato S, Matsushita K, et al. LGP2 is a positive regulator of RIG-I- and MDA5-mediated antiviral responses. *Proc Natl Acad Sci U S A* 2010;**107**:1512–7.
47. Mukherjee K, Korithoski B, Kolaczkowski B. Ancient origins of vertebrate-specific innate antiviral immunity. *Mol Biol Evol* 2014;**31**:140–53.
48. Zou J, Chang M, Nie P, Secombes CJ. Origin and evolution of the RIG-I like RNA helicase gene family. *BMC Evol Biol* 2009;**9**:85.
49. Biacchesi S, LeBerre M, Lamoureux A, Louise Y, Lauret E, Boudinot P, et al. Mitochondrial antiviral signaling protein plays a major role in induction of the fish innate immune response against RNA and DNA viruses. *J Virol* 2009;**83**:7815–27.
50. Chang M, Collet B, Nie P, Lester K, Campbell S, Secombes CJ, et al. Expression and functional characterization of the RIG-I-like receptors MDA5 and LGP2 in rainbow trout (*Oncorhynchus mykiss*). *J Virol* 2011;**85**:8403–12.
51. Zhou ZX, Zhang BC, Sun L. Poly(I:C) induces antiviral immune responses in japanese flounder (*Paralichthys olivaceus*) that require TLR3 and MDA5 and is negatively regulated by Myd88. *PLoS ONE* 2014;**9** e112918.
52. Inohara, Chamaillard, McDonald C, Nunez G. NOD-LRR proteins: role in host-microbial interactions and inflammatory disease. *Annu Rev Biochem* 2005;**74**:355–83.
53. Muruve DA, Petrilli V, Zaiss AK, White LR, Clark SA, Ross PJ, et al. The inflammasome recognizes cytosolic microbial and host DNA and triggers an innate immune response. *Nature* 2008;**452**:103–7.
54. Jacobs SR, Damania B. NLRs, inflammasomes, and viral infection. *J Leukoc Biol* 2012;**92**:469–77.
55. Franchi L, Warner N, Viani K, Nunez G. Function of NOD-like receptors in microbial recognition and host defense. *Immunol Rev* 2009;**227**:106–28.
56. Schroder K, Tschopp J. The inflammasomes. *Cell* 2010;**140**:821–32.
57. Lange C, Hemmrich G, Klostermeier UC, Lopez-Quintero JA, Miller DJ, Rahn T, et al. Defining the origins of the NOD-like receptor system at the base of animal evolution. *Mol Biol Evol* 2011;**28**:1687–702.
58. Laing KJ, Purcell MK, Winton JR, Hansen JD. A genomic view of the NOD-like receptor family in teleost fish: identification of a novel NLR subfamily in zebrafish. *BMC Evol Biol* 2008;**8**:42.
59. Burckstummer T, Baumann C, Bluml S, Dixit E, Durnberger G, Jahn H, et al. An orthogonal proteomic-genomic screen identifies AIM2 as a cytoplasmic DNA sensor for the inflammasome. *Nat Immunol* 2009;**10**:266–72.
60. Fernandes-Alnemri T, Yu JW, Datta P, Wu J, Alnemri ES. AIM2 activates the inflammasome and cell death in response to cytoplasmic DNA. *Nature* 2009;**458**:509–13.
61. Roberts TL, Idris A, Dunn JA, Kelly GM, Burnton CM, Hodgson S, et al. HIN-200 proteins regulate caspase activation in response to foreign cytoplasmic DNA. *Science* 2009;**323**:1057–60.
62. Fire A, Xu S, Montgomery MK, Kostas SA, Driver SE, Mello CC. Potent and specific genetic interference by double-stranded RNA in *Caenorhabditis elegans*. *Nature* 1998;**391**:806–11.
63. Kingsolver MB, Huang Z, Hardy RW. Insect antiviral innate immunity: pathways, effectors, and connections. *J Mol Biol* 2013;**425**:4921–36.

64. Sagan SM, Sarnow P. Molecular biology RNAi, antiviral after all. *Science* 2013;**342**:207–8.

65. Karlikow M, Goic B, Saleh MC. RNAi and antiviral defense in *Drosophila*: setting up a systemic immune response. *Dev Comp Immunol* 2014;**42**:85–92.

66. Li Y, Lu J, Han Y, Fan X, Ding SW. RNA interference functions as an antiviral immunity mechanism in mammals. *Science* 2013;**342**:231–4.

67. Maillard PV, Ciaudo C, Marchais A, Li Y, Jay F, Ding SW, et al. Antiviral RNA interference in mammalian cells. *Science* 2013;**342**:235–8.

68. Xie JF, Lu L, Deng M, Weng SP, Zhu JY, Wu Y, et al. Inhibition of reporter gene and iridovirus-tiger frog virus in fish cell by RNA interference. *Virology* 2005;**338**:43–52.

69. Ruiz S, Schyth BD, Encinas P, Tafalla C, Estepa A, Lorenzen N, et al. New tools to study RNA interference to fish viruses: fish cell lines permanently expressing siRNAs targeting the viral polymerase of viral hemorrhagic septicemia virus. *Antiviral Res* 2009;**82**:148–56.

70. Pestka S, Krause CD, Walter MR. Interferons, interferon-like cytokines, and their receptors. *Immunol Rev* 2004;**202**:8–32.

71. Schultz U, Kaspers B, Staeheli P. The interferon system of non-mammalian vertebrates. *Dev Comp Immunol* 2004;**28**:499–508.

72. Lefevre F, Guillomot M, D'Andrea S, Battegay S, La Bonnardiere C. Interferon-delta: the first member of a novel type I interferon family. *Biochimie* 1998;**80**:779–88.

73. Cochet M, Vaiman D, Lefevre F. Novel interferon delta genes in mammals: cloning of one gene from the sheep, two genes expressed by the horse conceptus and discovery of related sequences in several taxa by genomic database screening. *Gene* 2009;**433**:88–99.

74. Fung KY, Mangan NE, Cumming H, Horvat JC, Mayall JR, Stifter SA, et al. Interferon-epsilon protects the female reproductive tract from viral and bacterial infection. *Science* 2013;**339**:1088–92.

75. Hermant P, Francius C, Clotman F, Michiels T. IFN-epsilon is constitutively expressed by cells of the reproductive tract and is inefficiently secreted by fibroblasts and cell lines. *PLoS ONE* 2013;**8**:e71320.

76. Roberts RM, Liu L, Guo Q, Leaman D, Bixby J. The evolution of the type I interferons. *J Interferon Cytokine Res* 1998;**18**:805–16.

77. Iannuzzi L, Di Meo GP, Gallagher DS, Ryan AM, Ferrara L Womack JE. Chromosomal localization of omega and trophoblast interferon genes in goat and sheep by fluorescent in situ hybridization. *J Hered* 1993;**84**:301–4.

78. Ryan AM, Gallagher DS, Womack JE. Somatic cell mapping of omega and trophoblast interferon genes to bovine syntenic group U18 and in situ localization to chromosome 8. *Cytogenet Cell Genet* 1993;**63**:6–10.

79. Whaley AE, Meka CS, Harbison LA, Hunt JS, Imakawa K. Identification and cellular localization of unique interferon mRNA from human placenta. *J Biol Chem* 1994;**269**:10864–8.

80. Leaman DW, Roberts RM. Genes for the trophoblast interferons in sheep, goat, and musk ox and distribution of related genes among mammals. *J Interferon Res* 1992;**12**:1–11.

81. Lefevre F, Boulay V. A novel and atypical type one interferon gene expressed by trophoblast during early pregnancy. *J Biol Chem* 1993;**268**:19760–8.

82. LaFleur DW, Nardelli B, Tsareva T, Mather D, Feng P, Semenuk M, et al. Interferon-kappa, a novel type I interferon expressed in human keratinocytes. *J Biol Chem* 2001;**276**:39765–71.

83. Nardelli B, Zaritskaya L, Semenuk M, Cho YH, LaFleur DW, Shah D, et al. Regulatory effect of IFN-kappa, a novel type I IFN, on cytokine production by cells of the innate immune system. *J Immunol* 2002;**169**:4822–30.

84. Sick C, Schultz U, Staeheli P. A family of genes coding for two serologically distinct chicken interferons. *J Biol Chem* 1996;**271**:7635–9.

85. Lowenthal JW, Staeheli P, Schultz U, Sekellick MJ, Marcus PI. Nomenclature of avian interferon proteins. *J Interferon Cytokine Res* 2001;**21**:547–9.
86. Nanda I, Sick C, Munster U, Kaspers B, Schartl M, Staeheli P, et al. Sex chromosome linkage of chicken and duck type I interferon genes: further evidence of evolutionary conservation of the Z chromosome in birds. *Chromosoma* 1998;**107**:204–10.
87. Zou J, Tafalla C, Truckle J, Secombes CJ. Identification of a second group of type I interferons in fish sheds light on interferon evolution in vertebrates. *J Immunol* 2007;**179**:3859–71.
88. Sekellick MJ, Ferrandino AF, Hopkins DA, Marcus PI. Chicken interferon gene: cloning, expression, and analysis. *J Interferon Res* 1994;**14**:71–9.
89. Sick C, Schultz U, Munster U, Meier J, Kaspers B, Staeheli P. Promoter structures and differential responses to viral and nonviral inducers of chicken type I interferon genes. *J Biol Chem* 1998;**273**:9749–54.
90. Liniger M, Moulin HR, Sakoda Y, Ruggli N, Summerfield A. Highly pathogenic avian influenza virus H5N1 controls type I IFN induction in chicken macrophage HD-11 cells: a polygenic trait that involves NS1 and the polymerase complex. *Virol J* 2012;**9**:7.
91. Baquero-Perez B, Kuchipudi SV, Ho J, Sebastian S, Puranik A, Howard W, et al. Chicken and duck myotubes are highly susceptible and permissive to influenza virus infection. *J Virol* 2015;**89**:2494–506.
92. Mathews JH, Vorndam AV. Interferon-mediated persistent infection of Saint Louis encephalitis virus in a reptilian cell line. *J Gen Virol* 1982;**61**(Pt 2):177–86.
93. Qi Z, Nie P, Secombes CJ, Zou J. Intron-containing type I and type III IFN coexist in amphibians: refuting the concept that a retroposition event gave rise to type I IFNs. *J Immunol* 2010;**184**:5038–46.
94. Grayfer L, De Jesus Andino F, Robert J. Prominent amphibian (*Xenopus laevis*) tadpole type III interferon response to the frog virus 3 ranavirus. *J Virol* 2015;**89**:5072–82.
95. Altmann SM, Mellon MT, Distel DL, Kim CH. Molecular and functional analysis of an interferon gene from the zebrafish *Danio rerio*. *J Virol* 2003;**77**:1992–2002.
96. Robertsen B, Bergan V, Rokenes T, Larsen R, Albuquerque A. Atlantic salmon interferon genes: cloning, sequence analysis, expression, and biological activity. *J Interferon Cytokine Res* 2003;**23**:601–12.
97. Long S, Wilson M, Bengten E, Bryan L, Clem LW, Miller NW, et al. Identification of a cDNA encoding channel catfish interferon. *Dev Comp Immunol* 2004;**28**:97–111.
98. Robertsen B. The interferon system of teleost fish. *Fish Shellfish Immunol* 2006;**20**:172–91.
99. Zou J, Secombes CJ. Teleost fish interferons and their role in immunity. *Dev Comp Immunol* 2011;**35**:1376–87.
100. Venkatesh B, Lee AP, Ravi V, Maurya AK, Lian MM, Swann JB, et al. Elephant shark genome provides unique insights into gnathostome evolution. *Nature* 2014;**505**:174–9.
101. Sun B, Robertsen B, Wang Z, Liu B. Identification of an Atlantic salmon IFN multigene cluster encoding three IFN subtypes with very different expression properties. *Dev Comp Immunol* 2009;**33**:547–58.
102. von Schalburg KR, Yazawa R, de Boer J, Lubieniecki KP, Goh B, Straub CA, et al. Isolation, characterization and comparison of Atlantic and chinook salmon growth hormone 1 and 2. *BMC Genomics* 2008;**9**:522.
103. Boudinot P, Zou J, Ota T, Buonocore F, Scapigliati G, Canapa A, et al. A tetrapod-like repertoire of innate immune receptors and effectors for coelacanths. *J Exp Zool B Mol Dev Evol* 2014;**322**:415–37.
104. Zou J, Gorgoglione B, Taylor NG, Summathed T, Lee PT, Panigrahi A, et al. Salmonids have an extraordinary complex type I IFN system: characterization of the IFN locus

in rainbow trout *Oncorhynchus mykiss*reveals two novel IFN subgroups. *J Immunol* 2014;**193**:2273–86.

105. Hamming OJ, Lutfalla G, Levraud JP, Hartmann R. Crystal structure of zebrafish interferons I and II reveals conservation of type I interferon structure in vertebrates. *J Virol* 2011; **85**:8181–7.

106. Aggad D, Mazel M, Boudinot P, Mogensen KE, Hamming OJ, Hartmann R, et al. The two groups of zebrafish virus-induced interferons signal via distinct receptors with specific and shared chains. *J Immunol* 2009;**183**:3924–31.

107. Lutfalla G, Crollius HR, Stange-Thomann N, Jaillon O, Mogensen K, Monneron D. Comparative genomic analysis reveals independent expansion of a lineage-specific gene family in vertebrates: the class II cytokine receptors and their ligands in mammals and fish. *BMC Genomics* 2003;**4**:29.

108. Casani D, Randelli E, Costantini S, Facchiano AM, Zou J, Martin S, et al. Molecular characterisation and structural analysis of an interferon homologue in sea bass (*Dicentrarchus labrax* L). *Mol Immunol* 2009;**46**:943–52.

109. Wan Q, Wicramaarachchi WD, Whang I, Lim BS, Oh MJ, Jung SJ, et al. Molecular cloning and functional characterization of two duplicated two-cysteine containing type I interferon genes in rock bream *Oplegnathus fasciatus*. *Fish Shellfish Immunol* 2012;**33**:886–98.

110. Svingerud T, Solstad T, Sun B, Nyrud ML, Kileng O, Greiner-Tollersrud L, et al. Atlantic salmon type I IFN subtypes show differences in antiviral activity and cell-dependent expression: evidence for high IFNb/IFNc-producing cells in fish lymphoid tissues. *J Immunol* 2012;**189**:5912–23.

111. Chang M, Nie P, Collet B, Secombes CJ, Zou J. Identification of an additional two-cysteine containing type I interferon in rainbow trout *Oncorhynchus mykiss* provides evidence of a major gene duplication event within this gene family in teleosts. *Immunogenetics* 2009;**61**:315–25.

112. Xu C, Guo TC, Mutoloki S, Haugland O, Marjara IS, Evensen O. Alpha interferon and not gamma interferon inhibits salmonid alphavirus subtype 3 replication in vitro. *J Virol* 2010;**84**:8903–12.

113. Sun B, Skjaeveland I, Svingerud T, Zou J, Jorgensen J, Robertsen B. Antiviral activity of salmonid gamma interferon against infectious pancreatic necrosis virus and salmonid alphavirus and its dependency on type I interferon. *J Virol* 2011;**85**:9188–98.

114. Chen YM, Kuo CE, Chen GR, Kao YT, Zou J, Secombes CJ, et al. Functional analysis of an orange-spotted grouper (*Epinephelus coioides*) interferon gene and characterisation of its expression in response to nodavirus infection. *Dev Comp Immunol* 2014;**46**:117–28.

115. Bergan V, Steinsvik S, Xu H, Kileng O, Robertsen B. Promoters of type I interferon genes from Atlantic salmon contain two main regulatory regions. *FEBS J* 2006;**273**:3893–906.

116. Purcell MK, Laing KJ, Woodson JC, Thorgaard GH, Hansen JD. Characterization of the interferon genes in homozygous rainbow trout reveals two novel genes, alternate splicing and differential regulation of duplicated genes. *Fish Shellfish Immunol* 2009;**26**:293–304.

117. Chang MX, Zou J, Nie P, Huang B, Yu Z, Collet B, et al. Intracellular interferons in fish: a unique means to combat viral infection. *PLoS Pathog* 2013;**9**:e1003736.

118. Lamken P, Gavutis M, Peters I, Van der Heyden J, Uze G, Piehler J. Functional cartography of the ectodomain of the type I interferon receptor subunit IFNAR1. *J Mol Biol* 2005;**350**:476–88.

119. de Weerd NA, Vivian JP, Nguyen TK, Mangan NE, Gould JA, Braniff SJ, et al. Structural basis of a unique interferon-beta signaling axis mediated via the receptor IFNAR1. *Nat Immunol* 2013;**14**:901–7.

120. Stein C, Caccamo M, Laird G, Leptin M. Conservation and divergence of gene families encoding components of innate immune response systems in zebrafish. *Genome Biol* 2007;**8**:R251.

121. Sun B, Greiner-Tollersrud L, Koop BF, Robertse B. Atlantic salmon possesses two clusters of type I interferon receptor genes on different chromosomes, which allows for a larger repertoire of interferon receptors than in zebrafish and mammals. *Dev Comp Immunol* 2014;**47**:275–86.

122. Lutfalla G, Holland SJ, Cinato E, Monneron D, Reboul J, Rogers NC, et al. Mutant U5A cells are complemented by an interferon-alpha beta receptor subunit generated by alternative processing of a new member of a cytokine receptor gene cluster. *EMBO J* 1995;**14**:5100–8.

123. Hardy MP, Hertzog PJ, Owczarek CM. Multiple regions within the promoter of the murine Ifnar-2 gene confer basal and inducible expression. *Biochem J* 2002;**365**:355–67.

124. Cajean-Feroldi C, Nosal F, Nardeux PC, Gallet X, Guymarho J, Baychelier F, et al. Identification of residues of the IFNAR1 chain of the type I human interferon receptor critical for ligand binding and biological activity. *Biochemistry* 2004;**43**:12498–512.

125. Thomas C, Moraga I, Levin D, Krutzik PO, Podoplelova Y, Trejo A, et al. Structural linkage between ligand discrimination and receptor activation by type I interferons. *Cell* 2011;**146**:621–32.

126. Gaboriaud C, Uze G, Lutfalla G, Mogensen K. Hydrophobic cluster analysis reveals duplication in the external structure of human alpha-interferon receptor and homology with gamma-interferon receptor external domain. *FEBS Lett* 1990;**269**:1–3.

127. Fu XY, Kessler DS, Veals SA, Levy DE, Darnell Jr JE. ISGF3, the transcriptional activator induced by interferon alpha, consists of multiple interacting polypeptide chains. *Proc Natl Acad Sci U S A* 1990;**87**:8555–9.

128. Kessler DS, Veals SA, Fu XY, Levy DE. Interferon-alpha regulates nuclear translocation and DNA-binding affinity of ISGF3, a multimeric transcriptional activator. *Genes Dev* 1990;**4**:1753–65.

129. Nagarajan U. Induction and function of IFNbeta during viral and bacterial infection. *Crit Rev Immunol* 2011;**31**:459–74.

130. Langevin C, Aleksejeva E, Passoni G, Palha N, Levraud JP, Boudinot P. The antiviral innate immune response in fish: evolution and conservation of the IFN system. *J Mol Biol* 2013;**425**:4904–20.

131. Haller O, Frese M, Kochs G. Mx proteins: mediators of innate resistance to RNA viruses. *Rev Sci Tech* 1998;**17**:220–30.

132. Silverman RH. Viral encounters with 2′,5′-oligoadenylate synthetase and RNase L during the interferon antiviral response. *J Virol* 2007;**81**:12720–9.

133. Pindel A, Sadler A. The role of protein kinase R in the interferon response. *J Interferon Cytokine Res* 2011;**31**:59–70.

134. Seo JY, Yaneva R, Cresswell P, Viperin: a multifunctional interferon-inducible protein that regulates virus replication. *Cell Host Microbe* 2011;**10**:534–9.

135. Skaug B, Chen ZJ. Emerging role of ISG15 in antiviral immunity. *Cell* 2010;**143**:187–90.

136. Collet B. Innate immune responses of salmonid fish to viral infections. *Dev Comp Immunol* 2014;**43**:160–73.

137. Horisberger MA, Hochkeppel HK. An interferon-induced mouse protein involved in the mechanism of resistance to influenza viruses Its purification to homogeneity and characterization by polyclonal antibodies. *J Biol Chem* 1985;**260**:1730–3.

138. De Zoysa M, Kang HS, Song YB, Jee Y, Lee YD, Lee J. First report of invertebrate Mx: cloning, characterization and expression analysis of Mx cDNA in disk abalone (*Haliotis discus discus*). *Fish Shellfish Immunol* 2007;**23**:86–96.

139. De Jesus Andino F, Chen G, Li Z, Grayfer L, Robert J. Susceptibility of *Xenopus laevis* tadpoles to infection by the ranavirus Frog-Virus 3 correlates with a reduced and delayed innate immune response in comparison with adult frogs. *Virology* 2012;**432**:435–43.

140. Fu JP, Chen SN, Zou PF, Huang B, Guo Z, Zeng LB, et al. IFN-gamma in turtle: conservation in sequence and signalling and role in inhibiting iridovirus replication in Chinese soft-shelled turtle *Pelodiscus sinensis*. *Dev Comp Immunol* 2014;**43**:87–95.

141. Bazzigher L, Schwarz A, Staeheli P. No enhanced influenza virus resistance of murine and avian cells expressing cloned duck Mx protein. *Virology* 1993;**195**:100–12.

142. Bernasconi D, Schultz U, Staeheli P. The interferon-induced Mx protein of chickens lacks antiviral activity. *J Interferon Cytokine Res* 1995;**15**:47–53.

143. Ko JH, Jin HK, Asano A, Takada A, Ninomiya A, Kida H, et al. Polymorphisms and the differential antiviral activity of the chicken Mx gene. *Genome Res* 2002;**12**:595–601.

144. Ko JH, Takada A, Mitsuhashi T, Agui T, Watanabe T. Native antiviral specificity of chicken Mx protein depends on amino acid variation at position 631. *Anim Genet* 2004;**35**:119–22.

145. Ewald SJ, Kapczynski DR, Livant EJ, Suarez DL, Ralph J, McLeod S, et al. Association of Mx1 Asn631 variant alleles with reductions in morbidity, early mortality, viral shedding, and cytokine responses in chickens infected with a highly pathogenic avian influenza virus. *Immunogenetics* 2011;**63**:363–75.

146. Benfield CT, Lyall JW, Kochs G, Tiley LS. Asparagine 631 variants of the chicken Mx protein do not inhibit influenza virus replication in primary chicken embryo fibroblasts or in vitro surrogate assays. *J Virol* 2008;**82**:7533–9.

147. Sironi L, Williams JL, Moreno-Martin AM, Ramelli P, Stella A, Jianlin H, et al. Susceptibility of different chicken lines to H7N1 highly pathogenic avian influenza virus and the role of Mx gene polymorphism coding amino acid position 631. *Virology* 2008;**380**:152–6.

148. Schusser B, Reuter A, von der Malsburg A, Penski N, Weigend S, Kaspers B, et al. Mx is dispensable for interferon-mediated resistance of chicken cells against influenza A virus. *J Virol* 2011;**85**:8307–15.

149. Trobridge GD, Leong JAC. Characterization of a rainbow-trout Mx-gene. *J Interferon Cytokine Res* 1995;**15**:691–702.

150. Robertsen B, Trobridge G, Leong JA. Molecular cloning of double-stranded RNA inducible Mx genes from Atlantic salmon (*Salmo salar* L). *Dev Comp Immunol* 1997;**21**:397–412.

151. Trobridge GD, Chiou PP, Kim CH, Leong JC. Induction of the Mx protein of rainbow trout *Oncorhynchus mykiss* in vitro and in vivo with poly I:C dsRNA and infectious hematopoietic necrosis virus. *DisAquat Org* 1997;**30**:91–8.

152. Jensen V, Robertsen B. Cloning of an Mx cDNA from Atlantic halibut (*Hippoglossus hippoglossus*) and characterization of Mx mRNA expression in response to double-stranded RNA or infectious pancreatic necrosis virus. *J Interferon Cytokine Res* 2000;**20**:701–10.

153. Lee JY, Hirono I, Aoki T. Cloning and analysis of expression of Mx cDNA in Japanese flounder *Paralichthys olivaceus*. *Dev Comp Immunol* 2000;**24**:407–15.

154. Plant KP, Thune RL. Cloning and characterisation of a channel catfish (*Ictalurus punctatus*) Mx gene. *Fish Shellfish Immunol* 2004;**16**:391–405.

155. Tafalla C, Aranguren R, Secombes CJ, Figueras A, Novoa B. Cloning and analysis of expression of a gilthead sea bream (*Sparus aurata*) Mx cDNA. *Fish Shellfish Immunol* 2004;**16**:11–24.

156. Zhang YB, Li Q, Gui JF. Differential expression of two *Carassius auratus* Mx genes in cultured CAB cells induced by grass carp hemorrhage virus and interferon. *Immunogenetics* 2004;**56**:68–75.

157. Abollo E, Ordas C, Dios S, Figueras A, Novoa B. Molecular characterisation of a turbot Mx cDNA. *Fish Shellfish Immunol* 2005;**19**:185–90.

158. Chen YM, Su YL, Lin JH, Yang HL, Chen TY. Cloning of an orange-spotted grouper (*Epinephelus coioides*) Mx cDNA and characterisation of its expression in response to nodavirus. *Fish Shellfish Immunol* 2006;**20**:58–71.

159. Fernandez-Trujillo MA, Porta J, Borrego JJ, Alonso MC, Alvarez MC, Bejar J. Cloning and expression analysis of Mx cDNA from Senegalese sole (*Solea senegalensis*). *Fish Shellfish Immunol* 2006;**21**:577–82.

160. Fernandez-Trujillo MA, Novel P, Manchado M, Sepulcre MP, Mulero V, Borrego JJ, et al. Three Mx genes with differential response to VNNV infection have been identified in gilthead seabream (*Sparus aurata*). *Mol Immunol* 2011;**48**:1216–23.

161. Huang B, Huang WS, Nie P. Characterization of four Mx isoforms in the European eel Anguilla anguilla. *Fish Shellfish Immunol* 2013;**35**:1048–54.

162. Kim CH, Johnson MC, Drennan JD, Simon BE, Thomann E, Leong JA. DNA vaccines encoding viral glycoproteins induce nonspecific immunity and Mx protein synthesis in fish. *J Virol* 2000;**74**:7048–54.

163. McLauchlan PE, Collet B, Ingerslev E, Secombes CJ, Lorenzen N, Ellis AE. DNA vaccination against viral haemorrhagic septicaemia (VHS) in rainbow trout: size, dose, route of injection and duration of protection-early protection correlates with Mx expression. *Fish Shellfish Immunol* 2003;**15**:39–50.

164. Purcell MK, Kurath G, Garver KA, Herwig RP, Winton JR. Quantitative expression profiling of imune response genes in rainbow trout following infectious haematopoietic necrosis virus (IHNV) infection or DNA vaccination. *Fish Shellfish Immunol* 2004;**17**:447–62.

165. Tafalla C, Chico V, Pérez L, Coll J, Estepa A. *In vitro* and *in vivo* differential expression of rainbow trout (*Oncorhynchus mykiss*) Mx isoforms in response to viral hemorrhagic septicemia virus (VHSV) G gene Poly I:C and VHSV. *Fish Shellfish Immunol* 2007;**23**:210–21.

166. Lorenzen E, Einer-Jensen K, Rasmussen JS, Kjaer TE, Collet B, Secombes CJ, et al. The protective mechanisms induced by a fish rhabdovirus DNA vaccine depend on temperature. *Vaccine* 2009;**27**:3870–80.

167. Martinez-Alonso S, Vakharia VN, Saint-Jean SR, Perez-Prieto S, Tafalla C. Immune responses elicited in rainbow trout through the administration of infectious pancreatic necrosis virus-like particles. *Dev Comp Immunol* 2012;**36**:378–84.

168. Ou-yang Z, Wang P, Huang X, Cai J, Huang Y, Wei S, et al. Immunogenicity and protective effects of inactivated Singapore grouper iridovirus (SGIV) vaccines in orange-spotted grouper *Epinephelus coioides*. *Dev Comp Immunol* 2012;**38**:254–61.

169. Munang'andu HM, Fredriksen BN, Mutoloki S, Dalmo RA, Evensen O. Antigen dose and humoral immune response correspond with protection for inactivated infectious pancreatic necrosis virus vaccines in Atlantic salmon (*Salmo salar* L). *Vet Res.* 2013;**44**:7.

170. Fernandez-Trujillo MA, Garcia-Rosado E, Alonso MC, Castro D, Alvarez MC, Bejar J. Mx1 Mx2 and Mx3 proteins from the gilthead seabream (*Sparus aurata*) show in vitro antiviral activity against RNA and DNA viruses. *Mol Immunol* 2013;**56**:630–6.

171. Larsen R, Rokenes TP, Robertsen B. Inhibition of infectious pancreatic necrosis virus replication by atlantic salmon Mx1 protein. *J Virol* 2004;**78**:7938–44.

172. Kibenge MJ, Munir K, Kibenge FS. Constitutive expression of Atlantic salmon Mx1 protein in CHSE-214 cells confers resistance to infectious salmon anaemia virus. *Virol J* 2005;**2**:75.

173. Su J, Yang C, Zhu Z, Wang Y, Jang S, Liao L. Enhanced grass carp reovirus resistance of Mx-transgenic rare minnow (*Gobiocypris rarus*). *Fish Shellfish Immunol* 2009;**26**:828–35.

174. Peng L, Yang C, Su J. Protective roles of grass carp *Ctenopharyngodon idella* Mx isoforms against grass carp reovirus. *PLoS ONE* 2012;**7**:e52142.

175. Alvarez-Torres D, Garcia-Rosado E, Fernandez-Trujillo MA, Bejar J, Alvarez MC, Borrego JJ, et al. Antiviral specificity of the Solea senegalensis Mx protein constitutively expressed in CHSE-214 cells. *Mar Biotechnol (NY)* 2013;**15**:125–32.

176. Wu YC, Lu YF, Chi SC. Anti-viral mechanism of barramundi Mx against betanodavirus involves the inhibition of viral RNA synthesis through the interference of RdRp. *Fish Shellfish Immunol* 2010;**28**:467–75.

177. Boudinot P, Massin P, Blanco M, Riffault S, Benmansour A. vig-1, a new fish gene induced by the rhabdovirus glycoprptein, has a virus-induced homologue in humans and shares conserved motifs with the MoaA family. *J Virol* 1999;**73**:1846–52.

178. O'Farrell C, Vaghefi N, Cantonnet M, Buteau B, Boudinot P, Benmansour A. Survey of transcript expression in rainbow trout leukocytes reveals a major contribution of interferon-responsive genes in the early response to a rhabdovirus infection. *J Virol* 2002;**76**:8040–9.

179. Goossens KE, Karpala AJ, Rohringer A, Ward A, Bean AG. Characterisation of chicken viperin. *Mol Immunol* 2015;**63**:373–80.

180. Zhang BC, Zhang J, Xiao ZZ, Sun L. Rock bream (*Oplegnathus fasciatus*) viperin is a virus-responsive protein that modulates innate immunity and promotes resistance against megalocytivirus infection. *Dev Comp Immunol* 2014;**45**:35–42.

181. Wang B, Zhang YB, Liu TK, Shi J, Sun F, Gui JF. Fish viperin exerts a conserved antiviral function through RLR-triggered IFN Signaling pathway. *Dev Comp Immunol* 2014;**47**:140–9.

182. Teng TS, Foo SS, Simamarta D, Lum FM, Teo TH, Lulla A, et al. Viperin restricts chikungunya virus replication and pathology. *J Clin Invest* 2012;**122**:4447–60.

183. Nasr N, Maddocks S, Turville SG, Harman AN, Woolger N, Helbig KJ, et al. HIV-1 infection of human macrophages directly induces viperin which inhibits viral production. *Blood* 2012;**120**:778–88.

184. Jumat MR, Huong TN, Ravi LI, Stanford R, Tan BH, Sugrue RJ. Viperin protein expression inhibits the late stage of respiratory syncytial virus morphogenesis. *Antiviral Res* 2015;**114**:11–20.

185. Tang YD, Na L, Zhu CH, Shen N, Yang F, Fu XQ, et al. Equine viperin restricts equine infectious anemia virus replication by inhibiting the production and/or release of viral gag, env, and receptor via distortion of the endoplasmic reticulum. *J Virol* 2014;**88**:12296–310.

186. Seo JY, Cresswell P. Viperin regulates cellular lipid metabolism during human cytomegalovirus infection. *PLoS Pathog* 2013;**9**:e1003497.

187. Dabo S, Meurs EF. dsRNA-dependent protein kinase PKR and its role in stress, signaling and HCV infection. *Viruses* 2012;**4**:2598–635.

188. Balachandran S, Roberts PC, Brown LE, Truong H, Pattnaik AK, Archer DR, et al. Essential role for the dsRNA-dependent protein kinase PKR in innate immunity to viral infection. *Immunity* 2000;**13**:129–41.

189. Lee SB, Esteban M. The interferon-induced double-stranded RNA-activated human p68 protein kinase inhibits the replication of vaccinia virus. *Virology* 1993;**193**:1037–41.

190. Rothenburg S, Deigendesch N, Dey M, Dever TE, Tazi L. Double-stranded RNA-activated protein kinase PKR of fishes and amphibians: varying the number of double-stranded RNA binding domains and lineage-specific duplications. *BMC Biol* 2008;**6**:12.

191. Ko JH, Asano A, Kon Y, Watanabe T, Agui T. Characterization of the chicken PKR: polymorphism of the gene and antiviral activity against vesicular stomatitis virus. *Jpn J Vet Res* 2004;**51**:123–33.

192. Rothenburg S, Deigendesch N, Dittmar K, Koch-Nolte F, Haag F, Lowenhaupt K, et al. A PKR-like eukaryotic initiation factor 2alpha kinase from zebrafish contains Z-DNA binding domains instead of dsRNA binding domains. *Proc Natl Acad Sci U S A* 2005;**102**:1602–7.

193. Bergan V, Jagus R, Lauksund S, Kileng O, Robertsen B. The Atlantic salmon Z-DNA binding protein kinase phosphorylates translation initiation factor 2 alpha and constitutes a unique orthologue to the mammalian dsRNA-activated protein kinase R. *FEBS J* 2008;**275**:184–97.

194. Su J, Zhu Z, Wang Y. Molecular cloning, characterization and expression analysis of the PKZ gene in rare minnow *Gobiocypris rarus*. *Fish Shellfish Immunol* 2008;**25**:106–13.

195. Hu YS, Li W, Li DM, Liu Y, Fan LH, Rao ZC, et al. Cloning, expression and functional analysis of PKR from grass carp (*Ctenopharyngodon idellus*). *Fish Shellfish Immunol* 2013;**35**:1874–81.

196. Zhu R, Zhang YB, Zhang QY, Gui JF. Functional domains and the antiviral effect of the double-stranded RNA-dependent protein kinase PKR from *Paralichthys olivaceus*. *J Virol* 2008;**82**:6889–901.

197. del Castillo CS, Hikima J, Ohtani M, Jung TS, Aoki T. Characterization and functional analysis of two PKR genes in fugu (*Takifugu rubripes*). *Fish Shellfish Immunol* 2012;**32**:79–88.

198. Zenke K, Nam YK, Kim KH. Molecular cloning and expression analysis of double-stranded RNA-dependent protein kinase (PKR) in rock bream (*Oplegnathus fasciatus*). *Vet Immunol Immunopathol* 2010;**133**:290–5.

199. Lenschow DJ. Antiviral Properties of ISG15. *Viruses* 2010;**2**:2154–68.

200. Herrmann J, Lerman LO, Lerman A. Ubiquitin and ubiquitin-like proteins in protein regulation. *Circ Res* 2007;**100**:1276–91.

201. Knight Jr E, Cordova B. IFN-induced 15-kDa protein is released from human lymphocytes and monocytes. *J Immunol* 1991;**146**:2280–4.

202. D'Cunha J, Ramanujam S, Wagner RJ, Witt PL, Knight Jr E, Borden EC. In vitro and in vivo secretion of human ISG15, an IFN-induced immunomodulatory cytokine. *J Immunol* 1996;**157**:4100–8.

203. Recht M, Borden EC, Knight Jr E. A human 15-kDa IFN-induced protein induces the secretion of IFN-gamma. *J Immunol* 1991;**147**:2617–23.

204. Okumura A, Lu G, Pitha-Rowe I, Pitha PM. Innate antiviral response targets HIV-1 release by the induction of ubiquitin-like protein ISG15. *Proc Natl Acad Sci USA* 2006;**103**:1440–5.

205. Giannakopoulos NV, Arutyunova E, Lai C, Lenschow DJ, Haas AL, Virgin HW. ISG15 Arg151 and the ISG15-conjugating enzyme UbE1L are important for innate immune control of *Sindbis virus*. *J Virol* 2009;**83**:1602–10.

206. Malakhova OA, Zhang DE. ISG15 inhibits Nedd4 ubiquitin E3 activity and enhances the innate antiviral response. *J Biol Chem* 2008;**283**:8783–7.

207. Magor KE, Miranzo Navarro D, Barber MR, Petkau K, Fleming-Canepa X, Blyth GA, et al. Defense genes missing from the flight division. *Dev Comp Immunol* 2013;**41**:377–88.

208. Liu M, Reimschuessel R, Hassel BA. Molecular cloning of the fish interferon stimulated gene 15 kDa (ISG15) orthologue: a ubiquitin-like gene induced by nephrotoxic damage. *Gene* 2002;**298**:129–39.

209. Rokenes TP, Larsen R, Robertsen B. Atlantic salmon ISG15: expression and conjugation to cellular proteins in response to interferon, double-stranded RNA and virus infections. *Mol Immunol* 2007;**44**:950–9.

210. Zhang YB, Wang YL, Gui JF. Identification and characterization of two homologues of interferon-stimulated gene ISG15 in crucian carp. *Fish Shellfish Immunol* 2007;**23**:52–61.

211. Seppola M, Stenvik J, Steiro K, Solstad T, Robertsen B, Jensen I. Sequence and expression analysis of an interferon stimulated gene (ISG15) from Atlantic cod (*Gadus morhua* L). *Dev Comp Immunol* 2007;**31**:156–71.

212. Furnes C, Kileng O, Rinaldo CH, Seppola M, Jensen I, Robertsen B. Atlantic cod (*Gadus morhua* L) possesses three homologues of ISG15 with different expression kinetics and conjugation properties. *Dev Comp Immunol* 2009;**33**:1239–46.

213. Yasuike M, Kondo H, Hirono I, Aoki T. Identification and characterization of Japanese flounder *Paralichthys olivaceus* interferon-stimulated gene 15 (Jf-ISG15). *Comp Immunol Microbiol Infect Dis* 2011;**34**:83–91.

214. Ozato K, Shin DM, Chang TH, Morse 3rd HC. TRIM family proteins and their emerging roles in innate immunity. *Nat Rev Immunol* 2008;**8**:849–60.

215. Reymond A, Meroni G, Fantozzi A, Merla G, Cairo S, Luzi L, et al. The tripartite motif family identifies cell compartments. *EMBO J* 2001;**20**:2140–51.

216. Rajsbaum R, Stoye JP, O'Garra A, Type I. interferon-dependent and -independent expression of tripartite motif proteins in immune cells. *Eur J Immunol* 2008;**38**:619–30.

217. Ruby T, Bed'Hom B, Wittzell H, Morin V, Oudin A, Zoorob R. Characterisation of a cluster of TRIM-B30 2 genes in the chicken MHC B locus. *Immunogenetics* 2005;**57**:116–28.

218. Reddy BA, Kloc M, Etkin L. The cloning and characterization of a maternally expressed novel zinc finger nuclear phosphoprotein (xnf7) in *Xenopus laevis*. *Dev Biol* 1991;**148**:107–16.

219. Genome sequence of the nematode *C. elegans*: a platform for investigating biology. *Science* 1998;282:2012–2018.

220. van der Aa LM, Levraud JP, Yahmi M, Lauret E, Briolat V, Herbomel P, et al. A large new subset of TRIM genes highly diversified by duplication and positive selection in teleost fish. *BMC Biol* 2009;**7**:7.

221. Furnes C, Robertsen B. Molecular cloning and characterization of bloodthirsty from Atlantic cod (*Gadus morhua*). *Fish Shellfish Immunol* 2010;**29**:903–9.

222. Bruns AM, Horvath CM, Antiviral RNA. recognition and assembly by RLR family innate immune sensors. *Cytokine Growth Factor Rev* 2014;**25**:507–12.

Chapter 8

Lectins as Innate Immune Recognition Factors: Structural, Functional, and Evolutionary Aspects

Gerardo R. Vasta

Department of Microbiology and Immunology, University of Maryland School of Medicine, UMB, and Institute of Marine and Environmental Technology, Columbus Center, Baltimore, MD, United States

1   INTRODUCTION

Invertebrates and protochordates rely mostly on innate immunity for defense against microbial infection.[1,2] Moreover, it has become now well-established that in vertebrates, innate immunity not only carries a substantial burden of the defense functions against infectious diseases, but it is also critical for the development of an effective adaptive immune response.[3] Although immunoglobulin superfamily members such as hemolin, FREP, and Dscam appear to mediate immune responses in selected mollusk and insect species,[4–8] true immunoglobulins, which are the typical recognition/effector components of the adaptive immunity of vertebrates, are lacking in invertebrates. Consequently, the identification and structural/functional characterization of the other recognition factors, such as lectins, toll and toll-like receptors, and other "nonself" recognition and effector mechanisms that in invertebrates may be responsible for defense against infectious disease, has generated substantial interest. Additionally, the early realization that many of these factors/mechanisms have been conserved along the vertebrate lineages leading to the mammals has expanded the interest on these studies even further.[9–11]

It is currently firmly established that soluble and cell-associated lectins play critical roles as recognition/effector factors in the immune responses of both invertebrates and vertebrates.[12] Unlike immunoglobulins, most lectins do not generate diversity in recognition by genetic recombination. Therefore, attention has focused on the potential germline-encoded diversity of the lectin repertoires, including allelic variation; the presence of multiple carbohydrate

The Evolution of the Immune System. http://dx.doi.org/10.1016/B978-0-12-801975-7.00008-6

recognition domains (CRDs) resulting from tandem gene duplications; the expression of chimeric structures housing multiple recognition and effector domains, resulting from exon shuffling; and other mechanisms, such as alternative splicing and somatic mutation that expand the lectin's structural diversity and their ligand-recognition spectrum.[12] Further, the structural basis for the specificity and potential "plasticity" of the carbohydrate-binding sites for recognition of topologically related ligands by any given lectin has recently generated great interest.[12–14]

In most lectin families, the polypeptide subunits are organized as oligomeric structures that result in increased recognition avidity for multivalent ligands displayed on soluble and cell-surface glycans. The density of the surface ligands and their scaffolding (as glycoproteins, glycolipids, or polysaccharides) modulates affinity of the CRD–ligand interaction, via negative cooperativity.[15,16] Based on their structural folds and the presence of unique sequence motifs in the CRDs, lectins have been classified within several families that considerably differ in their structural and functional aspects, as well as their evolutionary history. Among the lectin families that mediate innate immune recognition in both invertebrate and vertebrate species, the C- and F-type lectins, rhamnose-binding lectins, pentraxins, and galectins (formerly S-type lectins) have been characterized in considerable detail.[12]

Like the Toll and Toll-like receptors, those lectins that recognize microbial components have been considered as "pattern recognition receptors" (PRRs), and their binding targets, such as lipopolysaccharide, lipoteichoic acid, or peptidoglycan, have been designated as pathogen- or microbe-associated molecular patterns (PAMPs or MAMPs, respectively).[17–20] The binding of a lectin to multiple nonreducing terminal carbohydrate ligands on the microbial surface, which are not readily exposed in the host, leads to agglutination and immobilization, and potentially to the opsonization of the potential pathogen.[2] Among these lectins, the mannose-binding lectin (MBL), a member of the C-type lectin family and the collectin subfamily, has been described as the prototypical PRR.[21–23] Collectins, which also include the ficolins, conglutinin, and pulmonary surfactants, are C-type lectins with a collagenous region that, upon the CRD–ligand interaction, can recruit a serine protease (MBL-associated serine protease; MASP), and the MBL(ligand)-MASP complex can activate the complement cascade. Therefore, MBL can function not only as a recognition molecule for microbes, but also as an effector factor that triggers complement-mediated opsonization or lysis, and killing of the potential pathogen.[24–27] As the collectins and complement components are present in extant invertebrate and protochordate taxa that lack an adaptive immune system, it has been proposed that both lectins and complement played a pivotal role in both innate immune recognition and complement activation long before the emergence of adaptive immunity in vertebrates.[25,26]

The structural analysis and taxonomic distribution of selected lectins and their families have revealed key information about their evolutionary history.

For example, among the lectin families present in both invertebrate and vertebrate species, it has been concluded that galectins have been highly conserved through evolution,[12,28] whereas the F- and C-type lectins, which are largely heterogeneous from the structural standpoint, are considered as evolutionary diversified lectin families.[12,21,22,29] A comparative analysis of the structural and evolutionary aspects of galectins and F-type lectins will be discussed in this review to illustrate their functional diversification, with particular focus on their roles in innate immune recognition.

2   GALECTINS: A CONSERVED LECTIN FAMILY WITH MULTIPLE ROLES IN DEVELOPMENT AND IMMUNITY

Galectins are nonglycosylated proteins, characterized by a conserved sequence motif in their CRDs and an affinity for ß-galactosides. Some galectins, however, show a preference for *N*-acetyl-lactosamine (LacNAc; Galß1,4GlcNAc) and related disaccharides[28,30,31] (Fig. 8.1A). Most galectins are soluble proteins, although a few exceptions have transmembrane domains.[32,33] Galectins are synthesized in the cytoplasm; some family members, such as galectin 3, can be translocated into the nucleus, where they can form part of the spliceosome.[12,34] Galectins can also be secreted to the extracellular space by nonclassical mechanisms—as they lack a typical signal peptide—possibly by direct translocation across the plasma membrane.[35,36] It has been proposed that the release of galectins to the extracellular space under noninfectious stressful conditions can be perceived as a "danger-associated molecular pattern" signal that can trigger inflammatory responses.[37] In the extracellular space, galectins can not only bind to cell-surface glycans and to the extracellular matrix, but can also recognize potential pathogens and parasites.[38–44]

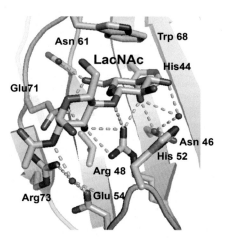

FIGURE 8.1   Structure of the galectin binding site in complex with LacNAc. Detail of the binding cleft, indicating the amino-acid residues that interact with the disaccharide.

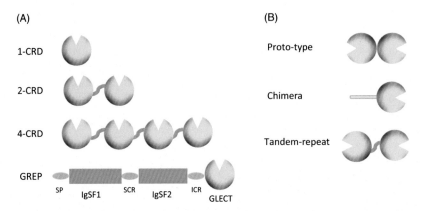

FIGURE 8.2 **Domain organization of galectins from invertebrates and vertebrates.** (A) Schematic illustration of the domain organization in the galectin types (1-CRD, 2-CRD, and 4-CRD) described in invertebrate species. GREP is the only chimeric galectin described so far. The C-terminal galectin domain (GLECT) is joined via a short interceding region (ICR) to two immunoglobulin superfamily domains (IgSF1 and IgSF2), separated by a small connecting region (SCR), and with the signal peptide (SP). (B) Schematic representation of the domain organization of the three galectin types (proto, chimera, and tandem repeat) described in vertebrate species.

2.1 Molecular, Structural, and Evolutionary Aspects

Galectins are characterized by their extensive taxonomic distribution and striking evolutionary conservation of primary structures, gene organization, and structural fold[12,28] (Fig. 8.2A, B). The identification of galectin-like proteins in the fungus *Coprinopsis cinerea* and in the sponge *Geodia cydonium*, and a protein sharing the galectin fold in the protozoan parasite *Toxoplasma gondii* revealed the early emergence and structural conservation of galectins in eukaryotic evolution.[45–47] As indicated previously, the C- and F-type lectin families are structurally diversified, and comprise numerous members that display chimeric polypeptide subunits, that, in addition to the lectin CRDs, display a variety of functionally diverse domains.[12,21–23] In contrast to C- and F-type lectins, the galectin polypeptides exhibit a relatively simple domain organization, housing one, two, or four galectin CRDs.[12,48] The only chimeric galectin described so far, is the galectin-related protein (GREP), identified in the freshwater snail *Biomphalaria glabrata*, in which a C-terminal galectin domain (GLECT) is joined via a short interceding region (ICR) to two immunoglobulin superfamily domains (IgSF1 and IgSF2), separated by a small connecting region (SCR), and with the signal peptide (SP)[49] (Fig 8.2A). Based on the CRD organization of the polypeptide monomer, mammalian galectins (and, by extension, galectins in vertebrates) have been classified into three types: "proto," "chimera," and "tandem-repeat" (TR)[50] (Fig 8.2B). Proto-type galectins, such as galectin-1, contain one CRD per subunit and are noncovalently linked homodimers. The chimera-type galectins (galectin 3) have a C-terminal CRD and an N-terminal domain rich in proline and glycine. The dimerization of proto-type galectins is critical for their function in mediating cell–cell or cell–ECM interactions,[51,52] and similar interactions via the N-terminus domain mediate oligomerization (mostly trimers and pentamers) of the chimera galectins.[53] In TR galectins such as galectin-9, two CRDs are joined by a functional linker peptide.[50] In invertebrate species, galectins that display one, two, or four tandemly arrayed CRDs have been described.[48,54–56] As in the mammalian tandem-repeat galectins, in those invertebrate galectins that carry multiple CRDs, these are similar but not identical. Based on the structure of their binding sites, they are likely to differ in their fine specificity and recognize distinct ligands.[48,57]

Analyses of the gene organization and primary structures of galectins from invertebrates and vertebrates have provided insight into their evolutionary history.[48,54–57] Among the arthropods, although the typical galectin sequence motif is present in the galectin MjGal from the shrimp *Marsupenaeus japonicus*, the primary structural organization does not fit the canonical features of either the proto- or the chimera-type galectins from vertebrates. A phylogenetic analysis indicated that MjGal clustered with galectins from invertebrates and a hemichordate, and was clearly distinct from the vertebrate galectins.[56]

Within the mollusks, the phylogenetic analysis of the full-length sequences of the 2- and 4-CRD galectins revealed that these were already present in the most recent common ancestor of both bivalves and gastropods, and that the individual CRDs in both the 2-CRD and 4-CRD galectins have been maintained in the same arrangement/sequence without domain shuffling since the divergence of these two major clades. This remarkable structural conservation of the biologically active carbohydrate-binding domains in the evolution of the mollusk taxa supports the key roles of galectins in essential biological functions related to ß-galactoside recognition.[48] How the multiple CRD galectins from invertebrates relate to the vertebrate TR galectins remains to be fully understood, but a preliminary phylogenetic analysis of the oyster galectin CvGal1 revealed that the individual CRDs cluster with the mammalian single-CRD galectins rather than with the TR galectins, suggesting that the CvGal1 gene is the product of two consecutive gene duplications of a single-CRD galectin gene.[54]

When considering the evolution of galectins along the vertebrate taxa, either prior to or early on in chordate evolution, the duplication of a mono-CRD galectin gene would have led to a bi-CRD galectin gene, in which the N- and C-terminal CRDs subsequently diverged into two different subtypes, defined by exon–intron structure (F4-CRD and F3-CRD). All vertebrate single-CRD galectins belong to either the F3- (eg, gal-1, -2, -3, -5) or F4- (eg, gal-7, -10, -13, -14) subtype, whereas the mammalian TR galectins such as gal-4, -6, -8, -9, and -12 contain both F4 and F3 subtypes.[28,57] Galectins have also been subject to evolutionary cooption. Examples of this process are the galectin-like proteins, such as the eye-lens crystallin protein GRIFIN (galectin related interfiber protein) that lack carbohydrate-binding activity in mammals, but in teleost fish display the typical galactoside-binding activity.[58,59]

The amino acid residues of the galectin 1 CRD that participate in protein–carbohydrate interactions and the hydroxyl groups recognized on the ligands have been rigorously identified by the resolution of the structure of the protein cocrystallized with LacNAc.[30,31,60] The galectin 1 subunit is a typical ß-sandwich, which contains one carbohydrate-binding site that is formed by three continuous concave strands (ß4–ß6), which in turn contains all residues involved in direct interactions with LacNac; these include histidine 44, asparagine 46, arginine 48, histidine 52, asparagine 61, tryptophan 68, glutamic acid 71, and arginine 73.[30] The higher affinity for LacNAc over Lac can be rationalized by the water-mediated interactions between His52, Asp54, and Arg73 in the galectin 1 CRD with the nitrogen of the NAc group. In galectin-3, the carbohydrate-binding site is shaped like a cleft open at both ends, exposing the GlcNAc of the LacNAc to the solvent.[61] This extended binding site in galectin 3 results in increased affinity for polylactosamines and for ABH blood-group oligosaccharides [Fucα1,2; GalNAcα1,3(Fucα1,2); and Galα1,3(Fucα1,2)]. In general, glycans that display LacNAc and polylactosamine chains [(Galβ1,4GlcNAc)n], such as laminin, fibronectin, and mucins are the preferred endogenous ligands for galectins.[62–67]

Although from the structural standpoint galectins are substantially conserved, as observed for other lectin families, the galectin repertoire is constituted by multiple galectin types, subtypes, and isoforms.[62–68] Proto- and TR-type galectins comprise several distinct subtypes: Galectins-1, -2, -5, -7, -10, -11, -13, -14, and -15 are proto-type. Galectin-3 is the only chimera-type. Galectins-4, -6, -8, -9, and -12 are TR-type. In addition, any galectin subtype may exhibit multiple isoforms in a single individual.[62] Further, because galectin types and subtypes exhibit notable differences in carbohydrate specificity, and bind a broad range of glycans that display the requisite topologies, the galectin repertoire displays considerable diversity in recognition properties that suggests functional diversification.[62–68]

2.2 Functional Aspects

The experimental evidence obtained soon after the initial identification of galectins during the early 1980s suggested that their expression was developmentally regulated, and that their functions related to embryogenesis and early development. Later studies revealed their roles in neoplastic transformation and progression, and metastasis (reviewed in Vasta and Ahmed[12]). Glycans that contain polylactosamine chains [(Galβ1,4GlcNAc)n], such as laminin, fibronectin, lysosome-associated membrane proteins, and mucins, are the preferred endogenous ligands for mammalian, bird, and amphibian galectins.[61–68] Chicken galectins have been proposed to participate in myoblast fusion, whereas murine galectin-1 and galectin-3 would have roles in notochord development, somitogenesis, and development of muscle tissue and the central nervous system.[69–72] More recently, other genetically tractable model organisms endowed with a less diversified galectin repertoire, such as *Drosophila* and zebrafish, have become attractive alternatives for functional studies.[73,74]

Since the 1990s, the roles of galectins as regulators of both innate and adaptive immune homeostasis have firmly established and characterized in detail.[75] Galectins are ubiquitously expressed and distributed in mammalian tissues, including most cells of the innate (dendritic cells, macrophages, mast cells, natural killer-cells, gamma/delta T cells, and B-1 cells) and adaptive (activated B and T cells) immune system, and in other cell types.[76,77] Endogenous glycans recognized by galectins include β-integrins, CD45, GM1, CD44, Tim3, MUC1, podoplanin, CD166, ABH-type oligosaccharides CD43, CD45, CD7, CD71, CD44, TIM3, CTLA4, MUC1, MUC16, and MerTK.[43,78–83] Although it has been proposed that a certain degree of functional redundancy exists among the members of the galectin repertoire, as the subtle aspects of their binding properties and natural ligands are characterized, and their biological roles are elucidated in increasing detail, it has become clear that this is not the case.[75]

In recent years, it has become clear that galectins can also recognize "nonself" carbohydrate moieties on the surface of microbial pathogens and parasites, and function as PRRs.[38,42] These ligands on foreign cells can be similar to those displayed on host cells such as ABH or Le blood-group oligosaccharides,[42] and LacNAc present in viral and bacterial glycans, or structurally different and absent from the host glycome, such as α1-2-mannans in *Candida*[43] and LacdiNAc in *Schistosoma*.[84] Whereas the first scenario can be rationalized as molecular mimicry by the microbial pathogens and parasites, understanding the molecular basis of galectin binding to distinct self and nonself glycans via the same CRD requires additional considerations. In this regard, galectins with tandemly arrayed CRDs such as the TR galectins from vertebrates, and the 4-CRD galectins from invertebrates, are intriguing both in their binding properties and functional aspects. Vertebrate TR galectins such as galectins-4, -8, and -9 differ from the proto- and chimera types, in that they display two tandemly arrayed CRDs (N- and C-CRDs) that are similar but not identical, suggesting that they have distinct recognition properties.[85] The structures of the TR galectins-4, -8, and -9 have been partially resolved, either by crystallization of NMR analysis of their isolated N- or C-CRDs and revealed differences in their binding specificity, or affinity for oligosaccharides or their scaffolding as glycolipids or glycoproteins.[86–88] The structure of the N-CRD of the mouse galectin-4 revealed binding sites for lactose with different affinities, whereas the galectin-8 binds preferentially to larger glycans, such as glycosphingolipids.[86–88] The capacity of TR galectins to crosslink cells with different synthetic glycoconjugates[88,89] strongly suggests significant differences in the binding properties of their N- and C-CRDs.

From the functional standpoint, galectins can function as opsonins,[56] inhibit viral adhesion to the host cell,[90] or directly kill bacteria.[42] The expression of the galectin MjGal from the kuruma shrimp *M. japonicus* is upregulated hemocytes and hepatopancreas upon bacterial challenge, and can bind to both Gram-positive and Gram-negative bacteria through the recognition of lipoteichoic acid or lipopolysaccharide, respectively. By also binding to the shrimp hemocyte surface, MjGal functions as an opsonin for microbial pathogens, promoting their phagocytosis and clearance from circulation.[56] In the zebrafish (*Danio rerio*), the extracellular proto-type galectin-1 (Drgal1-L2) and a chimera galectin-3 (Drgal3-L1) interact directly and in a carbohydrate-dependent manner with the glycosylated envelope of the infectious hematopoietic necrosis virus (IHNV), and also with the glycans on the epithelial cell surface, significantly reducing viral adhesion.[90] In mammals, the TR galectins-4 and -8 can recognize and kill *Escherichia coli* strains that display B-blood-group oligosaccharides (BGB+ *E. coli*). Mutation of key residues in either CRD revealed that the C-CRD mediates recognition of the BGB+ *E. coli,* but does not affect its viability, whereas the N-CRD was not affected, suggesting that N-CRD might be endowed with killing activity.[42] Taken together, the results of these studies indicate that galectins can function not only in immune recognition but also as effector factors.

In recent years, mounting experimental evidence has shown that some pathogens and parasites can "subvert" the roles of host or vector galectins as PRRs, to attach to or gain entry into their cells. The participation of galectin interactions in the infection mechanisms of HIV has been reported.[91,92] Galectin-1, which is abundant in organs that represent major reservoirs for HIV-1, such as the thymus and lymph nodes, promotes infection by HIV-1 by facilitating viral attachment to the CD4 receptor, and increasing infection efficiency. It is noteworthy that HIV also uses recognition by DC-SIGN, a C-type lectin, to enter dendritic cells, thereby underscoring the multiple adaptations of the viral glycome for host infection.[91,92] *Leishmania* species, which spend part of their lifecycle in phlebotomine sandflies that constitute vectors for transmission to the vertebrate hosts, attach to the insect midgut epithelium via the sandfly galectin PpGalec, to prevent their excretion along with the digested blood meal, and differentiate into free-swimming infective metacyclics.[93] The galectin is only expressed by epithelial midgut cells, is upregulated in the blood-feeding females, and binds to the Gal(ß1-3) side chains on the *Leishmania* LPG.[93] The protozoan parasite *Perkinsus marinus*, a facultative intracellular parasite that causes "Dermo" disease in the eastern oyster *Crassostrea virginica*,[94] is recognized via two 4-CRD galectins (CvGal1 and CvGal2) that are expressed by the phagocytic hemocytes.[54,95,96] The parasite is phagocytosed by the oyster hemocytes, where it inhibits respiratory burst and proliferates, eventually causing systemic infection and death of the oyster host. Thus, *P. marinus* may have evolved to adapt its glycocalyx to be selectively recognized by the oyster hemocytes CvGal1 and CvGal2, thereby subverting the oyster's innate immune/feeding recognition mechanism to gain entry into the host cells.[38,48,54,95,96] A recent study identified galectin-1 as the receptor for the protozoan parasite *Trichomonas vaginalis*,[97] the causative agent of the most prevalent nonviral sexually transmitted human infection in both women and men. As an obligate extracellular parasite, establishment and persistence of *T. vaginalis* infection requires adherence to the host epithelial cell surface. Like *Leishmania* spp, *T. vaginalis* displays a surface LPG rich in galactose and *N*-acetyl glucosamine, which is recognized in a carbohydrate-dependent manner by galectin-1 expressed by the epithelial cells in the cervical linings, as well as by placenta, prostate, endometrial, and decidual tissue, also colonized by the parasite.[97]

Recent studies in a murine model for influenza (influenza A virus, IAV) and pneumococcal pneumonia (*Streptococcus pneumoniae*) revealed that the murine lung expresses a diverse galectin repertoire, from which selected galectins, including galectin 1 (Gal1) and galectin 3 (Gal3), are released to the bronchoalveolar space upon the viral infection. In vitro studies on the human airway epithelial cell line A549 were consistent with the observations made in the mouse model, and further revealed that both Gal1 and Gal3 bind strongly to IAV and *S. pneumoniae*, and that exposure of the cells to viral neuraminidase or influenza infection increased galectin-mediated *S. pneumoniae* adhesion to the cell surface, suggesting that upon influenza infection, pneumococcal adhesion to the airway epithelial surface is enhanced by an interplay among the host galectins and viral and pneumococcal neuraminidases.[98] The combined activity of microbial neuraminidases, and the secreted Gal1 and Gal3 at the epithelial cell surface, also modulate the expression of SOCS1 and RIG1, and activation of ERK, AKT, or JAK/STAT1 signaling pathways, leading to a disregulated expression and release of proinflammatory cytokines.[99] These studies suggest that galectins released to the lung bronchoalveolar environment "fine-tune" the inflammatory response to viral and bacterial challenge.[98,99]

3 F-TYPE LECTINS: A STRUCTURALLY AND FUNCTIONALLY DIVERSIFIED LECTIN FAMILY

In contrast with the galectins, which are considered as substantially conserved in evolution, the F-type lectins, together with the C-type lectins, are characterized by their highly diversified structural organization. The F-type lectin family is the most recent to be identified, and it is characterized by a unique structural fold and a canonical sequence motif in the F-type sugar-binding domain.[12,100–102] In this family, the F-type lectin domain (FTLD) can be presented either as a single CRD, as in the European eel agglutinin (*Anguilla anguilla* agglutinin, AAA), or as tandemly arranged F-type CRD repeats, in some examples combined with unrelated domains, yielding mosaic or chimeric polypeptide subunits of variable sizes and function(s) within a single species.[12,100–102]

3.1 Molecular, Structural, and Evolutionary Aspects

The structure of the AAA/L-Fuc complex consists of a β-jellyroll sandwich composed of three- and five-stranded β-sheets (Fig. 8.3A), which interacts with the α-Fuc ligand through hydrogen bonds, established between side chains from a trio of basic amino-acid residues (Ne of His[51] and the guanidinium groups of Arg[75]

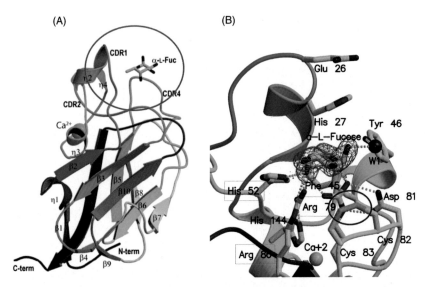

FIGURE 8.3 Structure of the F-type lectin binding site in complex with L-fuc. (A) The ribbon diagram shows the AAA in complex with L-fucose (the binding site is indicated with a *red circle*). (B) Interactions of the AAA binding site with L-fucose: the three basic amino-acid residues that interact with the axial OH on C4 are indicated with the *red boxes*. The interaction of the disulfide bond (Cys82–Cys83) with the C1—C2 bond of the L-fucose is indicated with a *circle*. *(Source: Adapted from Bianchet et al.[101])*

and Arg[103]), located in a shallow pocket, and the ring O5, and the equatorial 3- and axial 4-OH groups of the sugar (Fig. 8.3B). A van der Waals contact is established between a unique disulfide bridge, formed by contiguous cysteines (Cys[78] and Cys[79]) and the bond between ring atoms C1 and C2 of the monosaccharide, and the C6, which docks loosely in a hydrophobic pocket, stacking against the aromatic rings of two residues His[16] and Phe,[44] together with the Leu[24] and Tyr[91] residues.[105] As for most animal lectins, the specificity of AAA for a-Fuc is not absolute, but rather nominal, as carbohydrates (eg, 3-O-methyl-D-galactose and 3-O-methyl-D-fucose) that share critical configurational features of α-Fuc (ie, axial hydroxyl and hydrophobic moiety) also behave as ligands for AAA (Fig. 8.3B). Unlike C-type lectins, the role that calcium appears to play in AAA is structural stabilization, rather than participating in direct cation–saccharide interactions[101] (Fig. 8.3A). F-lectins specifically recognize selected oligosaccharides via interactions with amino-acid residues, located in what is known as an "extended binding site." For example, the recognition of H type-1 and Le[a] oligosaccharides by AAA requires additional interactions of residues in the loops (CDRs 1–5) that surround the binding pocket with subterminal sugars of the tyrisaccharides Fucα1-2 Galb1-3GlcNAcb1-3Galb1-4Glc (blood-group H type-1) and Galb1-3[Fucα1-4] GlcNAcb1-3Galb1-4Glc (Le[a]). F-lectins with a shorter CDR1 (Fig. 8.3A), such as MsFBP32 from the striped bass *Morone saxatilis* (see later in the chapter), would have a broader specificity for Le oligosaccharides.[102]

Although F-lectins such as AAA and MsFBP32 can specifically recognize a limited number of oligosaccharides, a considerable diversity in carbohydrate recognition is achieved by the presence of multiple isoforms with amino-acid substitutions at positions revealed by structural analyses.[102,104] This diversity in recognition is a critical feature for proteins that mediate immune defense. Variability of critical residues in the binding pocket and surrounding loops in the multiple isoforms, as expressed in the Japanese eel,[101,102,104] suggests that alternative interactions with terminal and subterminal sugar-units may expand the range of diverse oligosaccharides recognized by the lectin isoform repertoire.[105] Like collectins, the native structure of AAA is a homotrimer, which suggests that ligand binding is enhanced through cooperative binding to multivalent glycans. Further, the threefold cyclic symmetry of the native AAA, very similar to that observed in collectins,[106] would optimize the spacing and orientation of binding sites for recognition of glycoconjugates displayed on microbial surfaces. The distances between binding sites in the AAA trimer (26 Å) and those in MBL (45 Å) suggest that they bind to differently arrayed surface glycans on the surface of microbes. Therefore, although F- and C-type lectins may recognize the same monosaccharide (MBL also binds fucose), they may bind to different microorganisms, thereby expanding the immune recognition spectrum in those species that are endowed with both lectin types.

In contrast to AAA, the F-lectin MsFBP32 consists of two tandemly arrayed F-type CRDs. The structure of the complex of MsFBP32 with L-fucose revealed a "tail-to-tail" arrangement of three subunits.[102] Thus, the native MsBP32 trimer of approximately cylindrical shape (81-Å-long and 60-Å-wide) is divided into opposing globular structures—one containing the three N-CRDs, and the other, the three C-CRDs.[102] The resulting binding surfaces at the opposite ends of the cylindrical trimer resemble the collectin-like "bouquet" that CRD displays, and have the potential to crosslink cell surface or humoral carbohydrate ligands. The overall structure of the N-CRD is highly similar to that of the C-CRD, but significant differences between the binding sites of the MsFBP32 N- and C-CRD domains strongly suggest that the N-CRD recognizes more complex fucosylated oligosaccharides, and with a relatively higher avidity than the C-CRD.[102]

F-type lectins have been identified in a variety of taxa, from prokaryotes to amphibians (Fig. 8.4A, B). However, the F-type lectin sequence motif appears to be absent from protozoa, fungi, nematodes, ascidians, and higher vertebrates such as reptiles, birds, and mammals.[100] Despite the fact that AAA and MsFBP32 possess one and two FTLDs, respectively, substantially diverse domain topologies, in some cases lineage-related, were identified based on sequence alignments of the F-type lectin motif.[100] For example, most teleost F-type lectins contain either duplicate or quadruplicate tandem domains, whereas in *Xenopus* spp, these lectins are composed of either triplicate or quintuple tandem F-type domains. Clearly, the F-type fold with its joined N- and C-terminals favors

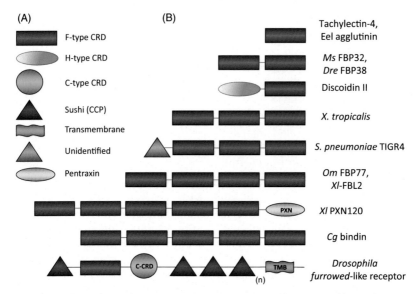

FIGURE 8.4 **Domain organization of F-type lectins from prokaryotes, invertebrates, and vertebrates.** (A) Schematic illustration of the domain types found in F-type lectins. (B) Schematic illustration of the domain organization in the F-lectin types (1-CRD, 2-CRD, 3-CRD, 4-CRD, and 5-CRD, and chimeric molecular species) described in prokaryote, invertebrate, and vertebrate species. *(Source: Adapted from Odom[107] and Odom et al.[100])*

the formation of concatenated CRD topologies in numbers that appear lineage-related. These tandem arrays may yield mosaic proteins by including pentraxin (*Xenopus laevis*) or C-type domains (*D. melanogaster* CG9095, malarial mosquito, and honey bee). The F-type sequence motif is also present in lophotrochozoan (ie, mollusks and planaria) and ecdysozoan protostomes (ie, horseshoe crabs and insects), invertebrate deuterostomes (ie, echinoderm), elasmobranchs (ie, skate), lobe- and ray-finned teleost fish, and amphibians (ie, *X. laevis* and salamander).[2,100,107]

The binary FBPLs have diversified through lineage-dependent gene duplications and speciation events, producing a combination of paralogous relationships unique to teleosts.[107] In contrast, in *Xenopus* spp., frogs are not only single-domain F-type lectins expressed, but also combinations of two, three, four, and chimeric proteincontaining five tandem F-type domains adjacent to a pentraxin domain. Clearly, *Xenopus* spp. exhibit a greater diversity of F-type lectins than the pufferfish.[107] Despite the diversity evident in this early tetrapod, no homologs are detectable in genomes of higher vertebrates, including reptile and avian representatives. This observation begs the question of whether this lectin family is uniquely restricted to invertebrates and cold-blooded vertebrates, and had been subsequently lost, as such, above the level of the amphibians. Specifically, the F-lectins may have either became truly extinct or have been coopted into other biological roles, which in the course of evolution may have imposed structural constraints, such as those proposed for the C-1 and C-2 domains of the coagulation factors V and VIII.[100–102,107]

The F-type lectin sequence motif is not restricted to eukaryotes; homologs were identified in both a Gram-positive (eg, *S. pneumoniae*)[108] and a Gram-negative (ie, *Microbulbifer degradans*)[109] eubacteria. The absence of the F-type lectin sequence motif in protozoa, fungi, nematodes, ascidians, and higher vertebrates suggests that it may have been selectively lost, even in relatively closely related lineages.[100,107] The paucity of bacteria possessing F-type CRDs suggests that it may have either been acquired through horizontal transfer from metazoans, or less likely, that most prokaryote lineages lost this CRD. Even the multiple duplicate tandem homologs present within modern teleost orders appear to be the product of independent duplications. The spotty phylogenetic distribution, diverse temporospatial expression, and varied domain architecture of the F-type family members point to a functionally plastic CRD, which has been specifically tailored in each lineage, and has apparently lost its fitness value in some taxa.[100,107] The absence of the F-type CRD in higher vertebrates is an evolutionary quandary that correlates with the appearance of cleidoic egg, and the colonization of land by vertebrates.[100,107]

3.2   Functional Aspects

The opposite orientation of the binding surfaces of the trimeric MsFBP32 supports the notion that the function of this lectin in circulation is to crosslink fucosylated glycoconjugates displayed on different cells, with an epitope separation of 25 Å on the cell surface.[102] Modeling of MsFBP32 complexed with fucosylated glycans that are widely distributed in prokaryotes and eukaryotes rationalizes the observation that binary tandem CRD F-type lectins can function as opsonins. This would take place by crosslinking "nonself" carbohydrate ligands and "self" carbohydrate ligands, such as sugar structures, displayed by microbial pathogens and glycans on the surface of phagocytic cells from the host.[102] For example, MsFBP32 may crosslink Le^a-containing glycans on the phagocytic cell surface via the N-CRD, with glycans on the microbial surface via the C-CRD, such as those containing α-linked L-Fuc, 2-acetoamido L-Fuc, 3-deoxy-L-fucose (colitose), or L-Rha (6-deoxy-L-mannose, present in *E. coli* glycans) as nonreducing terminal residues.[102] Preexposure of *E. coli* to a binary tandem F-lectin from sea bream significantly increases their phagocytosis by peritoneal macrophages relative to the unexposed bacteria,[110] confirming that F-lectins with tandemly arrayed CRDs such as MsFBP32 function as opsonins that mediate innate immune responses against microbial pathogens.

The immune-recognition functions of F-type lectins that we have identified in teleost fish are not always shared by those F-lectins expressed in other taxa. For example, the sperm "bindins" from the Japanese oyster (*Crassostrea gigas*), recently identified as F-type lectins, are polymorphic gamete-recognition proteins stored in the acrosomal rings that bind sperm to egg during fertilization.[111]

In contrast to most lectins, by mechanisms of positive selection, recombination, and alternative splicing, the single-copy bindin gene produces highly diversified transcripts, both in sequence and domain organization, within and among individuals among this species. However, only one or two polymorphic molecular species housing between one and five tandemly arrayed F-lectin domains are translated in each individual male oyster.[112] The unusually high intraspecific diversity in sequence and domain organization of the oyster bindin F-lectins could represent coevolution of sperm-gamete recognition mechanisms to "catch-up" with the high diversification of egg receptors aimed at avoiding polyspermia.[113] This diversification of the bindin F-lectins in gamete recognition resembles the eel F-lectin isoforms involved in host–pathogen interactions described previously.[104]

In other examples, the recognition properties of F-type lectins have been even more drastically modified or coopted.[100,101,107] In this regard, a structure-based search identified seven nonlectin proteins with negligible sequence similarity to the F-type lectin motif; however, they shared the same jellyroll fold with AAA.[100,101,107] These are the C domains of human blood coagulation factor V and VIII, the C-terminal domain of a bacterial sialidase, the NH2-terminal domain of a fungal galactose oxidase, a subunit of the human APC10/DOC1 ubiquitin ligase, the N-terminal domain of the XRCC1 single-strand DNA repair complex, and a yeast allantoicase.[100,101,107] Curiously, the FA58C domain of identical structure is present next to the F-type domain in the *M. bulbifer* protein previously described. In most of these proteins the AAA-like domain appears to mediate binding. However, allantoicase is the first reported analog to exhibit intrinsic enzyme activity.[100,101,107]

4 CONCLUSIONS

The structural and functional analysis of two representative families of animal lectins, such as the galectins and F-type lectins presented in this review, reveals that, in spite of their distinct evolutionary history and their structural conservation or diversification, from the functional standpoint both lectin families are mostly pleiotropic, that is, they can orchestrate an array of functions not only in innate and adaptive immunity, but also in development and homeostatic regulation of various physiological aspects. Furthermore, in recent years evidence has accumulated to support the notion that selected members of both families have been coopted to carry out other functions that, in several cases, are not dependent on their carbohydrate-binding sites, a property that is key to their definition as lectins, and appears to have been lost in the evolutionary process.

With regard to their roles in immune recognition, recent studies have firmly established that both F-type lectins and galectins can recognize self and nonself glycans. Because F-lectins and TR galectins display tandemly arrayed CRDs of similar but distinct specificity in a single polypeptide monomer, the binding and crosslinking of endogenous and exogenous glycans can be rationalized by the distinct properties of their binding sites. For other lectins, such as the single CRD F-lectins, and the proto- and chimera-type galectins that display a single binding-site per monomer, their capacity to recognize both endogenous and exogenous glycans through the same binding site can be explained by taking into consideration the multiple factors pertaining to the local lectin concentrations and oligomerization, the geometry of the presentation of the multivalent carbohydrate ligands on the host or microbial cell surface, and the properties of the microenvironment in which interactions take place.

The recent availability of genomic databases for numerous animal species has enabled greater insight into the structural complexity and functional diversity, and of lectin repertoires in invertebrates, protochordates, and ectothermic vertebrates. The identification in these taxa of members of the lectin families typical of mammals such as galectins, has resulted in the discovery of novel structural features, most likely revealing functional adaptations along the lineages leading to the higher vertebrate taxa. Further, the identification of novel lectin families such as the F-type lectins, underscores the fact that more research in nonmammalian model organisms will provide new information on all of the structural, functional, and evolutionary aspects of lectin repertoires that may not be as obvious in mouse or man. For example, structural analysis of the eel multiple isoforms as mechanisms that generate substantial diversity in oligosaccharide binding, provide the structural basis for a tantalizing novel mechanism for generating diversity for nonself recognition in innate immunity, that resembles those operative through adaptive immunity in higher vertebrates. Similarly, analysis of the genetic mechanisms that are operative in the diversification of the bindin transcripts in the Pacific oyster,[113] has contributed conceptually transformative evidence for the processes through which lectins can generate structural (and possibly, functional) diversity. The ongoing genome, transcriptome, and proteome projects on additional model organisms representative of nonmammalian taxa will reveal not only the extent of their full lectin repertoires, but, coupled to the structural analysis of selected components, has the potential to uncover novel structural features, on which a rigorous experimental assessment of their biological roles may be supported. In turn, these studies will provide greater insight into the evolutionary history of the various lectin families, from prokaryotes to the mammals.

ACKNOWLEDGMENTS

The author's research reviewed herein was supported by Grants IOS 1050518, IOB-0618409, and IOS-0822257 from the National Science Foundation, and Grant R01GM070589 from the National Institutes of Health.

REFERENCES

1. Khalturin K, et al. Recognition strategies in the innate immune system of ancestral chordates. *Mol Immunol* 2004;**41**:1077–87.
2. Vasta GR, Ahmed H, Odom EW. Structural and functional diversity of lectin repertoires in invertebrates, protochordates and ectothermic vertebrates. *Curr Opin Struct Biol* 2004;**14**:617–30.
3. Akira S, Takeda K, Kaisho T. Toll-like receptors: critical proteins linking innate and acquired immunity. *Nat Immunol* 2001;**2**:675–80.

4. Schmidt O, et al. Role of adhesion in arthropod immune recognition. *Annu Rev Entomol* 2010;**55**:485–504.

5. Zhang SM, et al. Diversification of Ig superfamily genes in an invertebrate. *Science* 2004;**305**:251–4.

6. Dishaw LJ, et al. A role for variable region-containing chitin-binding proteins (VCBPs) in host gut-bacteria interactions. *Proc Natl Acad Sci USA* 2011;**108**:16747–52.

7. Hernández Prada JA, et al. Ancient evolutionary origin of diversified variable regions demonstrated by crystal structures of an immune-type receptor in amphioxus. *Nat Immunol* 2006;**7**:875–82.

8. Watson FL, et al. Extensive diversity of Ig-superfamily proteins in the immune system of insects. *Science* 2005;**309**:1874–8.

9. Liu FT, Rabinovich GA. Galectins as modulators of tumour progression. *Nat Rev Cancer* 2005;**5**:29–41.

10. Ludwig IS, Geijtenbeek TB, van Kooyk Y. Two way communication between neutrophils and dendritic cells. *Curr Opin Pharmacol* 2006;**6**:408–13.

11. Fujita T, Matsushita M, Endo Y. The lectin-complement pathway—its role in innate immunity and evolution. *Immunol Rev* 2004;**198**:185–202.

12. Vasta GR, Ahmed H. *Animal lectins: a functional view*. Boca Raton, Florida: CRC Press; 2008.

13. Iliev DB, et al. Endotoxin recognition: in fish or not in fish? *FEBS Lett* 2005;**579**:6519–28.

14. Vasta GR, et al. Galectins in teleost fish: zebrafish (*Danio rerio*) as a model species to address their biological roles in development and innate immunity. *Glycoconj J* 2004;**21**:503–21.

15. Dam TK, Brewer CF. Effects of clustered epitopes in multivalent ligand-receptor interactions. *Biochemistry* 2008;**47**:8470–6.

16. Dam TK, Brewer CF. Effects of clustered epitopes in multivalent ligand-receptor interactions. *Biochemistry* 2008;**47**:8470–6.

17. Medzhitov R, Janeway Jr CA. Decoding the patterns of self and nonself by the innate immune system. *Science* 2002;**296**:298–300.

18. Bittel P, Robatzek S. Microbe-associated molecular patterns (MAMPs) probe plant immunity. *Curr Opin Plant Biol* 2007;**10**:335–41.

19. Seong S-Y, Matzinger P. Hydrophobicity: an ancient damage-associated molecular pattern that initiates innate immune responses. *Nat Rev Immunol* 2004;**4**:469–78.

20. Miao EA, Warren SE. Innate immune detection of bacterial virulence factors via the NLRC4 inflammasome. *J Clin Immunol* 2010;**30**:502–6.

21. Garred P, et al. Mannose-binding lectin and its genetic variants. *Genes Immun* 2006;**7**:85–94.

22. Ip WK, et al. Mannose-binding lectin and innate immunity. *Immunol Rev* 2009;**230**:9–21.

23. Zelensky AN, Gready JE. The C-type lectin-like domain superfamily. *FEBS J* 2005;**272**:6179–217.

24. Kingeter LM, Lin X. C-type lectin receptor-induced NF-kappaB activation in innate immune and inflammatory responses. *Cell Mol Immunol* 2012;**9**:105–12.

25. Weis WI, Taylor ME, Drickamer K. The C-type lectin superfamily in the immune system. *Immunol Rev* 1998;**163**:19–34.

26. Wallis R. Structural and functional aspects of complement activation by mannose-binding protein. *Immunobiology* 2002;**205**:433–45.

27. Nonaka M. The complement C3 protein family in invertebrates. *Invert Surv J* 2011;**8**:21–32.

28. Cooper DN. Galectinomics: finding themes in complexity. *Biochim Biophys Acta* 2002;**1572**:209–31.

29. Matsushita M, et al. Proteolytic activities of two types of mannose-binding lectin-associated serine protease. *J Immunol* 2000;**165**:2637–42.

30. Liao DI, et al. Structure of S-lectin, a developmentally regulated vertebrate beta-galactoside-binding protein. *Proc Natl Acad Sci USA* 1994;**91**:1428–32.

31. Bianchet MA, et al. Soluble beta-galactosyl-binding lectin (galectin) from toad ovary: crystallographic studies of two protein-sugar complexes. *Proteins* 2000;**40**:378–88.

32. Lipkowitz MS, et al. Galectin 9 is the sugar-regulated urate transporter/channel UAT. *Glycoconj J* 2004;**19**:491–8.

33. Gorski JP, et al. New alternatively spliced form of galectin-3, a member of the beta-galactoside-binding animal lectin family, contains a predicted transmembrane-spanning domain and a leucine zipper motif. *J Biol Chem* 2002;**277**:18840–8.

34. Tsay YG, et al. Export of galectin-3 from nuclei of digitonin-permeabilized mouse 3T3 fibroblasts. *Exp Cell Res* 1999;**252**:250–61.

35. Cho M, Cummings RD. Galectin-1, a beta-galactoside-binding lectin in Chinese hamster ovary cells II. Localization and biosynthesis. *J Biol Chem* 1995;**270**:5207–12.

36. Cleves AE, et al. A new pathway for protein export in *Saccharomyces cerevisiae*. *J Cell Biol* 1996;**133**:1017–26.

37. Sato S, et al. Galectins in innate immunity: dual functions of host soluble beta-galactoside-binding lectins as damage-associated molecular patterns (DAMPs) and as receptors for pathogen-associated molecular patterns (PAMPs). *Immunol Rev* 2009;**230**:172–87.

38. Vasta GR. Roles of galectins in infection. *Nat Rev Microbiol* 2009;**7**:424–38.

39. Elola MT, et al. Galectins: matricellular glycan-binding proteins linking cell adhesion, migration, and survival. *Cell Mol Life Sci* 2007;**64**:1679–700.

40. Rabinovich GA, Toscano MA. Turning 'sweet' on immunity: galectin–glycan interactions in immune tolerance and inflammation. *Nat Rev Immunol* 2009;**9**:338–52.

41. Cerliani JP, et al. Expanding the universe of cytokines and pattern recognition receptors: galectins and glycans in innate immunity. *J Clin Immunol* 2011;**31**:10–21.

42. Stowell SR, et al. Innate immune lectins kill bacteria expressing blood group antigen. *Nat Med* 2010;**16**:295–301.

43. Kohatsu L, et al. Galectin-3 induces death of Candida species expressing specific beta-1,2-linked mannans. *J Immunol* 2006;**177**:4718–26.

44. Pelletier I, et al. Specific recognition of leishmania major poly-beta-galactosyl epitopes by galectin-9: possible implication of galectin-9 in interaction between L. major and host cells. *J Biol Chem* 2003;**278**:22223–30.

45. Saouros S, Edwards-Jones B, Reiss M, Sawmynaden K, Cota E, Simpson P, Dowse TJ, Jäkle U, Ramboarina S, Shivarattan T, Matthews S, Soldati-Favre D. A novel galectin-like domain from Toxoplasma gondii micronemal protein 1 assists the folding, assembly, and transport of a cell adhesion complex. *J Biol Chem* 2005;**280**:38583–91.

46. Walser PJ1, Haebel PW, Künzler M, Sargent D, Kües U, Aebi M, Ban N. Structure and functional analysis of the fungal galectin CGL2. *Structure* 2004;**12**:689–702.

47. Stalz H, Roth U, Schleuder D, Macht M, Haebel S, Strupat K, Peter-Katalinic J, Hanisch FG. The Geodia cydonium galectin exhibits prototype and chimera-type characteristics and a unique sequence polymorphism within its carbohydrate recognition domain. *Glycobiology* 2006;**16**:402–4.

48. Vasta GR, Feng C, Bianchet MA, Bachvaroff TR, Tasumi S. Structural, functional, and evolutionary aspects of galectins in aquatic mollusks: from a sweet tooth to the Trojan horse. *Fish Shellfish Immunol* 2015;**46**(1):94–106.

49. Dheilly NM, Duval D, Mouahid G, Emans R, Allienne JF, Galinier R, et al. A family of variable immunoglobulin and lectin domain containing molecules in the snail *Biomphalaria glabrata*. *Dev Comp Immunol* 2015;**48**:234–43.

50. Hirabayashi J, Kasai K. The family of metazoan metal-independent beta-galactoside-binding lectins: structure, function and molecular evolution. *Glycobiology* 1993;**3**:297–304.

51. Gabius HJ. Animal lectins. *Eur J Biochem* 1997;**243**:543–76.

52. Colnot C, et al. Galectins in mouse embryogenesis. *Biochem Soc Trans* 1996;**24**:141–6.
53. Rabinovich GA, Rubinstein N, Toscano MA. Role of galectins in inflammatory and immuno-modulatory processes. *Biochim Biophys Acta* 2002;**1572**:274–84.
54. Tasumi S, Vasta GR. A galectin of unique domain organization from hemocytes of the Eastern oyster (*Crassostrea virginica*) is a receptor for the protistan parasite *Perkinsus marinus*. *J Immunol* 2007;**179**:3086–98.
55. Yoshino TP, et al. Molecular and functional characterization of a tandem-repeat galectin from the freshwater snail *Biomphalaria glabrata*, intermediate host of the human blood fluke *Schistosoma mansoni*. *Gene* 2008;**411**:46–58.
56. Shi XZ, Wang L, Xu S, Zhang XW, Zhao XF, Vasta GR, Wang JX. A galectin from the kuruma shrimp (*Marsupenaeus japonicus*) functions as an opsonin and promotes bacterial clearance from hemolymph. *PLoS One* 2014;**9**(3):e91794.
57. Houzelstein D, et al. Phylogenetic analysis of the vertebrate galectin family. *Mol Biol Evol* 2004;**21**:1177–87.
58. Ogden AT, Nunes I, Ko K, Wu S, Hines CS, Wang AF, et al. GRIFIN, a novel lens-specific protein related to the galectin family. *J Biol Chem* 1998;**273**:28889–96.
59. Ahmed H, Vasta GR. Unlike mammalian GRIFIN, the zebrafish homologue (DrGRIFIN) represents a functional carbohydrate-binding galectin. *Biochem Biophys Res Commun* 2008;**371**: 350–5.
60. Lobsanov YD, et al. X-ray crystal structure of the human dimeric S-Lac lectin, L-14-II, in complex with lactose at 2 9-A resolution. *J Biol Chem* 1993;**268**:27034–8.
61. Seetharaman J, et al. X-ray crystal structure of the human galectin-3 carbohydrate recognition domain at 2 1-A resolution. *J Biol Chem* 1998;**273**:13047–52.
62. Ahmed H, et al. Galectin-1 from bovine spleen: biochemical characterization, carbohydrate specificity and tissue-specific isoform profiles. *J Biochem* 1996;**120**:1007–19.
63. Sparrow CP, Leffler H, Barondes SH. Multiple soluble beta-galactoside-binding lectins from human lung. *J Biol Chem* 1987;**262**:7383–90.
64. Sato S, Hughes RC. Binding specificity of a baby hamster kidney lectin for H type I and II chains, polylactosamine glycans, and appropriately glycosylated forms of laminin and fibro-nectin. *J Biol Chem* 1992;**267**:6983–90.
65. Ahmed H, et al. Novel carbohydrate specificity of the 16-kDa galectin from *Caenorhabditis elegans*: binding to blood group precursor oligosaccharides (type 1, type 2, Talpha, and Tbeta) and gangliosides. *Glycobiology* 2002;**12**:451–61.
66. Shoji H, et al. Characterization of the *Xenopus* galectin family three structurally different types as in mammals and regulated expression during embryogenesis. *J Biol Chem* 2003;**278**:12285–93.
67. Zhou Q, Cummings RD. The S-type lectin from calf heart tissue binds selectively to the car-bohydrate chains of laminin. *Arch Biochem Biophys* 1990;**281**:27–35.
68. Fang R, Mantle M, Ceri H. Characterization of quail intestinal mucin as a ligand for endog-enous quail lectin. *Biochem J* 1993;**293**(Pt 3):867–72.
69. Cooper DN, Massa SM, Barondes SH. J Endogenous muscle lectin inhibits myoblast adhesion to laminin. *J Cell Biol* 1991;**115**:1437–48.
70. Watt DJ, Jones GE, Goldring K. The involvement of galectin-1 in skeletal muscle determina-tion, differentiation and regeneration. *Glycoconj J* 2004;**19**:615–9.
71. Georgiadis V, Stewart HJ, Pollard HJ, Tavsanoglu Y, Prasad R, Horwood J, Deltour L, Goldring K, Poirier F, Lawrence-Watt DJ. Lack of galectin-1 results in defects in myoblast fusion and muscle regeneration. *Dev Dyn* 2007;**236**:1014–24.
72. Fowlis D, Colnot C, Ripoche MA, Poirier F. Galectin-3 is expressed in the notochord, devel-oping bones, and skin of the postimplantation mouse embryo. *Dev Dyn* 1995;**203**:241–51.
73. Pace KE, Lebestky T, Hummel T, Arnoux P, Kwan K, Baum LG. Characterization of a novel *Drosophila melanogaster* galectin. *J Biol Chem* 2002;**277**:13091–8.

74. Ahmed H, Du SJ, O'Leary N, Vasta GR. Biochemical and molecular characterization of galectins from zebrafish (Danio rerio): notochord-specific expression of a prototype galectin during early embryogenesis. *Glycobiology* 2004;**14**:219–32.
75. Di Lella S, et al. When galectins recognize glycans: from biochemistry to physiology and back again. *Biochemistry* 2011;**50**:7842–57.
76. Stowell SR, Qian Y, Karmakar S, Koyama NS, Dias-Baruffi M, Leffler H, McEver RP, Cummings RD. Differential roles of galectin-1 and galectin-3 in regulating leukocyte viability and cytokine secretion. *J Immunol* 2008;**180**:3091–102.
77. Rabinovich GA, Liu FT, Hirashima M, Anderson A. An emerging role for galectins in tuning the immune response: lessons from experimental models of inflammatory disease, autoimmunity and cancer. *Scand J Immunol* 2007;**66**:143–58.
78. Guzman-Aranguez A, Mantelli F, Argueso P. Mucin-type O-glycans in tears of normal subjects and patients with non-Sjogren's dry eye. *Invest Ophthalmol Vis Sci* 2009;**50**:4581–7.
79. Hirabayashi J, et al. Oligosaccharide specificity of galectins: a search by frontal affinity chromatography. *Biochim Biophys Acta* 2002;**1572**:232–54.
80. Wu AM, et al. Fine specificity of domain-I of recombinant tandem-repeat-type galectin-4 from rat gastrointestinal tract (G4-N). *Biochem J* 2002;**367**:653–64.
81. Krzeminski M, et al. Human galectin-3 (Mac-2 antigen): defining molecular switches of affinity to natural glycoproteins, structural and dynamic aspects of glycan binding by flexible ligand docking and putative regulatory sequences in the proximal promoter region. *Biochim Biophys Acta* 2011;**1810**:150–61.
82. Functional_Glycomics. http://www.functionalglycomics.org/static/consortium/consortium.shtml
83. Caberoy NB, Alvarado G, Bigcas JL, Li W. Galectin-3 is a new MerTK-specific eat-me signal. *J Cell Physiol* 2012;**227**:401–7.
84. Stowell, SR, Arthur CM, Mehta P, Slanina KA, Blixt O, Leffler H, Smith DF, Cummings RD. Galectin-1,-2, and -3 exhibit differential recognition of sialylated glycans and blood group antigens. *J Biol Chem* 2008;**283**(15):10109–23.
85. Carlsson S, et al. Affinity of galectin-8 and its carbohydrate recognition domains for ligands in solution and at the cell surface. *Glycobiology* 2007;**17**:663–76.
86. Nagae M, et al. Structural analysis of the recognition mechanism of poly-N-acetyllactosamine by the human galectin-9 N-terminal carbohydrate recognition domain. *Glycobiology* 2009;**19**:112–7.
87. Krejcirikova V, et al. Structure of the mouse galectin-4 N-terminal carbohydrate-recognition domain reveals the mechanism of oligosaccharide recognition. *Acta Crystallogr D Biol Crystallogr* 2011;**67**:204–11.
88. Tomizawa T., et al. Solution structure of the C-terminal gal-bind lectin domain from human galectin-4. *Structural Genomics and Proteomics Initiative (RSGI), Riken*. Riken; 2005.
89. Ideo H, et al. Galectin-8-N-domain recognition mechanism for sialylated and sulfated glycans. *J Biol Chem* 2011;**286**:11346–55.
90. Nita-Lazar M, Mancini J, Feng C, Gonzalez-Montalban N, Ravindran C, Jackson S, de las Heras-Sanchez AI, Giomarelli B, Ahmed H, Wu G, Dell A, Ammayappan A, Vakharia V, Vasta GR. The zebrafish galectins Drgal1-L2 and Drgal3-L1 bind in vitro to the infectious hematopoietic necrosis virus (IHNV) glycoprotein and reduce viral adhesion to fish epithelial cells. *Dev Comp Immunol* 2016;**55**:241–52.
91. Mercier S, et al. Galectin-1 promotes HIV-1 infectivity in macrophages through stabilization of viral adsorption. *Virology* 2008;**371**:121–9.
92. Ouellet M, Mercier S, Pelletier I, Bounou S, Roy J, Hirabayashi J, Sato S, Tremblay MJ. Galectin-1 acts as a soluble host factor that promotes HIV-1 infectivity through stabilization of virus attachment to host cells. *J Immunol* 2005;**174**:4120–6.
93. Kamhawi S. Phlebotomine sand flies and Leishmania parasites: friends or foes? *Trends Parasitol* 2006;**22**:439–45.

94. Harvell CD, Kim K, Burkholder JM, Colwell RR, Epstein PR, Grimes DJ, Hofmann EE, Lipp EK, Osterhaus ADME, Overstreet RM, Porter JW, Smith GW, Vasta GR. Emerging marine diseases—climate links and anthropogenic factors. *Science* 1999;**285**:1505–10.

95. Feng C, Ghosh A, Amin MN, Giomarelli B, Shridhar S, Banerjee A, Fernández-Robledo JA, Bianchet MA, Wang LX, Wilson IB, Vasta GR. The galectin CvGal1 from the eastern oyster (*Crassostrea virginica*) binds to blood group A oligosaccharides on the hemocyte surface. *J Biol Chem* 2013;**288**(34):24394–409.

96. Feng C, Ghosh A, Amin MN, Bachvaroff TR, Tasumi S, Pasek M, Banerjee A, Shridhar S, Wang LX, Bianchet MA, Vasta GR. The galectin CvGal2 from the eastern oyster (*Crassostrea virginica*) displays unique specificity for ABH blood group oligosaccharides and differentially recognizes sympatric Perkinsus species. *Biochemistry* 2015;**54**(30):4711–30.

97. Okumura CYM, Baum LG, Johnson PJ. Galectin-1 on cervical epithelial cells is a receptor for the sexually transmitted human parasite *Trichomonas vaginalis*. *Cell Microbiol* 2008;**10**:2078–90.

98. Nita-Lazar M, Banerjee A, Feng C, Amin MN, Frieman MB, Chen WH, Cross AS, Wang LX, Vasta GR. Desialylation of airway epithelial cells during influenza virus infection enhances pneumococcal adhesion via galectin binding. *Mol Immunol* 2015;**65**(1):1–16.

99. Nita-Lazar M, Banerjee A, Feng C, Vasta GR. Galectins regulate the inflammatory response in airway epithelial cells exposed to microbial neuraminidase by modulating the expression of SOCS1 and RIG1. Mol Immunol 2015;**68**:194–202.

100. Odom EW, Vasta GR. Characterization of a binary tandem domain F-type lectin from striped bass (*Morone saxatilis*). *J Biol Chem* 2006;**281**:1698–713.

101. Bianchet MA1, Odom EW, Vasta GR, Amzel LM. A novel fucose recognition fold involved in innate immunity. *Nat Struct Biol* 2002;**9**:628–34.

102. Bianchet MA, et al. Structure and specificity of a binary tandem domain F-lectin from striped bass (*Morone saxatilis*). *J Mol Biol* 2010;**401**:239–52.

103. Zhu C, et al. The Tim-3 ligand galectin-9 negatively regulates T helper type 1 immunity. *Nat Immunol* 2005;**6**:1245–52.

104. Honda S, et al. Multiplicity, structures, and endocrine and exocrine natures of eel fucose-binding lectins. *J Biol Chem* 2000;**275**:33151–7.

105. Vasta GR, Ahmed H, Odom EW. Structural and functional diversity of lectin repertoires in invertebrates, protochordates and ectothermic vertebrates. *Curr Opin Struct Biol* 2004;**14**:617–30.

106. Weis WI, Drickamer K. Trimeric structure of a C-type mannose-binding protein. *Structure* 1994;**2**:1227–40.

107. Odom EW. F-type lectins: biochemical, genetic and structural characterization of a novel lectin family in lower vertebrates. University of Maryland, MEES Program, PhD thesis; 2004.

108. Tettelin H, Nelson KE, et al. Complete genome sequence of a virulent isolate of *Streptococcus pneumoniae*. *Science* 2001;**293**(5529):498–506.

109. Howard MB, Ekborg NA, et al. Genomic analysis and initial characterization of the chitinolytic system of *Microbulbifer degradans* strain 2-40. *J Bacteriol* 2003;**185**(11):3352–60.

110. Cammarata M, Benenati G, Odom EW, Salerno G, Vizzini A, Vasta GR, Parrinello N. Isolation and characterization of a fish F-type lectin from gilt head bream (*Sparus aurata*) serum. *Biochim Biophys Acta* 2007;**1770**:150–5.

111. Moy GW, et al. Extraordinary intraspecific diversity in oyster sperm bindin. *Proc Natl Acad Sci USA* 2008;**105**:1993–8.

112. Moy GW, Vacquier VD. Bindin genes of the Pacific oyster *Crassostrea gigas*. *Gene* 2008;**423**:215–20.

113. Springer SA, et al. Oyster sperm bindin is a combinatorial fucose lectin with remarkable intraspecies diversity. *Int J Dev Biol* 2008;**52**:759–68.

Chapter 9

Origin and Evolution of the Neuro-Immune Cross-Talk in Immunity

Enzo Ottaviani

Department of Life Sciences, University of Modena and Reggio Emilia, Modena, Italy

1 INTRODUCTION

The intercellular communication is mediated mainly by chemical signal molecules. During the course of evolution, those organisms who better developed this form of communication have increased their fitness, and thus have passed this trait on to their descendants. A plausible explanation for the emergence of a ligand-based intercellular communication can be attributed on its inherent level of sophistication, as noted by not only synaptic molecules that can enter into intercellular communication, but hormonal ones as well.[1]

Central nervous system (CNS) and immune system "talk to each other" in order to maintain the body homeostasis. In this context, lymphocyte migration, circulation, and traffic are under the influence of the CNS.[2] Studies[3,4] performed on mammals demonstrated a bidirectional communication between immune and neuroendocrine systems, and the levels of integration can be summarized as follows: (1) hormones and neurotransmitters bind to specific receptors on immune cells and modulate their activity; (2) products of the immune system, that is, cytokines, can act on cells of the neuroendocrine system, modifying their functions; (3) immune stimuli and hypothalamic releasing-factors induce the immune cells to synthesize neuropeptides, which, in turn, may influence the activity of the neuroendocrine system; and (4) cytokines able to modulate the activity of immune cells are produced by cells of the nervous system.

In higher organisms, communication between immune and neuroendocrine system is highly complex. Mammals certainly represent the most sophisticated level of complexity, but their roots must be traced back to defense mechanisms, which are also present in the simpler forms of life, such as invertebrates. In this context, the innate immune response and the neuroendocrine cross-talk of vertebrates resembles a mosaic of different invertebrate immune mechanisms toward pathogens.[5]

The Evolution of the Immune System. http://dx.doi.org/10.1016/B978-0-12-801975-7.00009-8

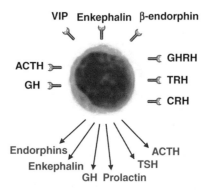

FIGURE 9.1 **Lymphocyte as a neuroendocrine cell.**

1.1 Lymphocyte as a Neuroendocrine Cell

Evidence in favor of a neuroendocrine role of the lymphocyte is well-documented, and illustrated in Fig. 9.1. Human lymphocytes are immunoreactive to neuroendocrine hormones and opioid peptides.[6,7] The opioid peptides may be classified into three families: the proopiomelanocortin (POMC), the proenkephalin (PENK), and the prodynorphin (PENK B).[8] The peptides of the POMC family derive from a single macromolecular precursor, and from the cleavage of this molecule derive hormones, such as the adrenocorticotropic hormone (ACTH) and melanocyte-stimulating hormone (MSH), as well as β-endorphin. The proteolitic cleavage of PENK produces enkephalin peptides, such as Met-enkephalin and Leu-enkephalin.[9,10]

ACTH and its receptors are reported in anuran amphibian, reptile, bird, and mouse lymphocytes.[11–15] ACTH and endorphins are encoded by the POMC gene.[16,17] The POMC gene is expressed by a variety of different cell types, which posttranslationally process the precursor protein into entirely distinct sets of peptide products.[18] In the pituitary gland, POMC mRNA transcripts are generated from the three exons of the mammalian POMC gene, but shorter transcripts are also found for extrapituitary sites of POMC gene expression.[19,20] The peptides derived from the proteolytic fragmentation of POMC undergo further modifications of utmost importance for their biological activity. Additional posttranslation modifications may include glycosylation, phosphorylation, amidation, sulfation, and acetylation, thus affecting the secretion and function of these products.[18,20–26] It is interesting to emphasize that ACTH and endorphins found in lymphocytes are identical to those produced by the pituitary.[27] Receptors for ACTH and β-endorphin have been shown in human peripheral blood lymphocytes.[3,28]

With regard to opioid peptides, PENK mRNA and PENK-derived peptides were detected in many cells of the mammalian immune system, including monocytes and lymphocytes, as well as Met-enkephalin and/or synenkephalin-containing peptides.[29,30] Furthermore, opioid peptides may specifically bind to at least four types of opioid receptors, such as μ, δ,[31,32] κ,[33] and ε,[34,35] present on the immune cells.

Furthermore, a variety of peptidic hormones, such as corticotropin-releasing hormone (CRH), thyrotropin (TSH), growth hormone (GH), vasoactive intestinal peptide (VIP), somatostatin, vasopressin, oxytocin, and so on, were also found.[4] Lastly, another group of molecules, the cytokines, play an important role in the interactions between the immune and neuroendocrine systems.[36]

1.2   Immunocyte as an Immune–Neuroendocrine Cell

Two major research groups, one in Italy (Modena) and the other in the USA (New York) found in invertebrates a correlation between immune and neuroendocrine systems similar to that observed in vertebrates. These findings emerged mainly from studies in molluscan immunocytes.[37] Using different techniques, the presence of factors similar to POMC-derived products has been found, such as ACTH-, β-endorphin-, and α-melanocyte-stimulating hormone (α-MSH)-like molecules, in the immunocytes of different molluscan species. The immunocytochemical results revealed that immunocytes were the only cell-type positive for immunocytochemical reactions for POMC-derived products (Fig. 9.2).[38] Other methods, such as flow cytometry, revealed the presence of ACTH- and β-endorphin-like molecules on the surface of immunocytes (Fig. 9.3),[39] and by radioimmunoassay (RIA) tests we have quantified these molecules both in immunocytes and in the serum.[40] In particular, the concentrations for ACTH-like molecules were 47 pg/10^3 cells in cell homogenates and 47 ± 11 pg/ml in the serum, while for β-endorphin were 39 pg/10^3 cells and 69 ± 7 pg/ml, respectively. Moreover, also quantified were the concentrations of corticotropin-releasing hormone (CRH)-like molecules, that is, 21 pg/10^3 cells and 23 ± 2.5 pg/ml, respectively.

The previous data were also confirmed by molecular biology studies. Using a probe for the human POMC gene by in situ hybridization, we showed that molluscan immunocytes were positive for POMC mRNA.[41]

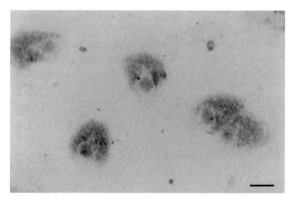

FIGURE 9.2   **Immunocytochemical staining with anti-ACTH polyclonal antibody on the immunocytes of *Viviparus ater*.** Nuclei were counterstained with hematoxylin. Scale bar = 10 μm.

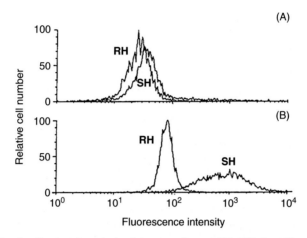

FIGURE 9.3 Cytofluorimetric analysis of the two cell types (SH, RH) from *Planorbarius corneus,* showing the presence of ACTH-like molecules only on the plasma of hemocytes endowed with phagocytic activity (SH), but not on the other (RH). A separate analysis of RH (upper) and SH (lower) was done by an electronic gate on each population. RH were not stained by the anti-ACTH polyclonal antibody (pAb), whereas SH showed a marked positivity. (A) Control; (B) anti-ACTH pAb. *(Source: Modified from Ref. [39].)*

Overall, these finding support the hypothesis[42] that the melanocortin system in vertebrates is a complex that had arisen prior to the emergence of jawless vertebrates, over 500 million of years. In this context, it should be reminded that the protozoan *Tetrahymena pyriformis* is probably the most primitive organism in which ACTH- and β-endorphin-like molecules have been detected.[43] Furthermore, ACTH-receptor-like messenger RNA was found in molluscan immunocytes.[28]

Study performed by Stefano and coworkers have demonstrated the presence of opioid-like molecules and the related opioid receptors in the hemocytes of invertebrates such as the marine mussel *Mytilus edulis*, the insect *Leucophaea Maderae,* and the leech *Theromyzon tessulatum.*[44–46]

The existence of bioactive peptides (BAPs) that function both as neurotransmitters and hormones is now accepted, and a variety of these peptides has been identified in molluscan hemocytes.[47] In this context, another important BAP such as CRH was found in hemocytes of *Planorbarius corneus, Viviparus contectus, Lymnaea stagnalis* and *M. galloprovincialis.*[48] In this last species it has also found the expression of molecules homologous to human mRNAs of the two receptor subtypes (CRH-R1 and CRH-R2).[49]

Cytokine- and growth factor-like molecules were detected in various tissues of different invertebrates, such as mollusks, insects, annelids, echinoderms, and tunicates, but immunocytes are the main source. With regard to mollusks, the presence of IL-1α-, IL-1β-, IL-2-, IL-6- and TNF-α-like molecules was detected in immunocytes and hemolymph.[1,50–54] Moreover, IL-1-, IL-6- and TNF-like molecules have been found in neurons and in a small population of glial cells in the pedal ganglia of *M. edulis*.[55–57] In the insect *Calliphora vomitoria,* the presence of TNF-α-like molecules in both plasmatocytes and granular cells has been found, and these molecules are induced in activated plasmatocytes.[58] Induction of TNF-α-like molecules has also been observed in *M. edulis* immunocytes by lipopolysaccharides (LPS).[51] IL-1α- and TNF-α-like molecules have been found in earthworm celomocytes of *Eisenia foetida,*[59] whereas IL-1α-like molecules were also detected in some small cells of the brain and in the eleocytes, a subpopulation of celomocytes of the marine worm *Nereis diversicolor.*[57] In the shrimp *Litopenaeus vannanei,* the TNF superfamily gene was isolated and characterized, and the TNF-α factor gene was LPS-induced.[60] Moreover, the TNF-receptor-like system could cooperate with the LPS-induced TNF-α factor pathway, the Toll and IMD pathways, and the JAK/STAT pathway in shrimp immune functions. Cytokine-like substances have been reported in the celomic fluid and celomocytes of the echinoderms *Pisaster ochraceus* (IL-1α)[61] and *Asterias forbesi* (IL-1, IL-6).[62,63] Studies performed in tunicates such as *Botryllus schlosserii, Styela plicata, Molugula occidentalis,* and *Ciona intestinalis* have detected IL-1-like molecules.[64] An IL-1-like fraction, designed tunicate IL-1β, has been isolated from the hemolymph of *Styela clava,* and this fraction is able to stimulate the proliferation of tunicate cells in vitro.[65]

Regarding the presence of growth factors, the majority of the available data refers to insects and mollusks. Large DNA sequence similarity has been found between the genes that encode for proteins involved in *Drosophila* embryogenesis and vertebrate growth factor, such as epidermal growth factor (EGF) and transforming growth factor (TGF)-β.[66–70] Growth-promoting factors have been found in the hemolymph of *Bombyx mori.*[71–72] *Samia cynthia*[73] and a hemolymph trophic factor has been found in *Manduca sexta.*[74] Insulin-like peptides were identified in invertebrates, such as mollusks, insects, and worms.[75–77] Blumenthal (2010)[77] surmised that the genes that encoding vertebrate insulins and insulin-like growth factors (IGFs), and invertebrate insulin-like molecules evolved from a common ancestral gene, and from the concept of an insulin superfamily of growth-promoting peptides. Moreover, the presence of platelet-derived growth factor (PDGF)-AB and TGF-β1-like molecules in immunocytes of different mollusks (*P. corneus, V. ater, V. contectus, L. stagnalis,* and *M. galloprovincialis*) has been detected.[78]

2 ROLE OF NEUROENDOCRINE HORMONES, OPIOID PEPTIDES AND CYTOKINES IN THE INVERTEBRATE IMMUNE AND NEUROENDOCRINE (STRESS RESPONSE) RESPONSES

2.1 Immune Responses

Cell-shape changes (ie, the expression of cell motility), chemotaxis (ie, the expression of cell migration), and phagocytosis are the main ancestral mechanisms used by all organisms to eliminate nonself material.[79] These defense reactions are triggered by regulatory molecules, including POMC-products, CRH, cytokines, and growth factors.

2.2 Cell-Shape Changes

ACTH,[80] PDGF, TGF-β,[81] CRH,[49] and IL-8[82] provoke changes in cellular shape affecting the locomotor activity of molluscan immunocytes. Using computer-assisted microscopic image analysis, it has been found that ACTH induces cell-shape changes via the adenylate cyclase/AMP/protein kinase A pathway, and the protein kinase C. The PDGF and TGF-β extracellular signals are transduced via the phosphoinositide signaling pathway. IL-8 provokes the cell-shape changes via protein kinase A and C pathways. Moreover, PKA, PKC, and PKB are involved in CRH-induced cell-shape changes in immunocytes, but the synergistic effect of two second messengers, that is, cAMP and inositol 1,4,5-triphosphate, is crucial.

2.3 Chemotaxis

The chamber for the study of chemotaxis is a tool that is used to measure the ability of cells to capture chemotactic stimuli. The assay was performed in 48-well microchemotaxis chambers (Nucleopore, Pleasanton, CA, USA), in which the upper and lower compartments were separated by a 5-μm pore, polycarbonate polyvinylpyrrolidone-free filter, allowing the cells to migrate actively through the pores. The cellular suspension was placed in the upper compartment and the substance to test in the lower one.

CRH and ACTH fragments (1–24), (1–4), (4–9), (1–13), (1–17), and (11–24) significantly stimulate molluscan immunocyte migration, while the whole sequence (1–39) and the fragment (4–11) have an inhibitory effect. Differences among species were found with respect to the response to individual fragments.[83] Furthermore, the whole sequence of β-endorphin, its N- and C-terminal fragments, the sequence (2–17), which lacks both N- and C-terminals, and the N-acetylated derivative are able to influence migration of molluscan immunocytes. The stimulatory effect of β-endorphin and its fragments is only partially inhibited by the antagonist naloxone.[83] Moreover, a chemotactic activity has been demonstrated against molluscan immunocytes, even by growth factors such as PDGF and TGF-β1,[84] and interleukins such as IL-1α, TNF-α, and IL-8.[82,85]

These observations probably have a general relevance, in view of the evidence that opioid neuropeptides exert stimulatory effects on locomotor activity and conformational changes of the mollusk *M. edulis* and the insect *L. maderae*. Immunocompetent immunocytes showed flattening elongation and formation of pseudopodia in the presence of opioids.[86,87]

2.4 Pagocytosis

When the chemoattractant is represented by particulate material such as bacteria, chemotaxis may be followed by engulfment and phagocytosis. All these phenomena are of pivotal importance for nutrition and defense, and are present throughout the animal kingdom. The incubation of immunocytes of *P. corneus* with bacteria (*Staphylococcus aureus*) revealed that only cells with the morphology of macrophages were able to engulf bacteria.[88] The addition of CRH, ACTH (1–4), (1–24), (4–10),[89] IL-1α, IL-2, TNF-α,[90] IL-8,[82] and PDGF-AB and TGF-β1[84] increase the phagocytic activity. ACTH fragments have different effects, depending on the concentration and the species. In particular, chemotactic and phagocytic effects are not directly correlated because peptides that influence cell migration do not always affect phagocytosis. In this context, ACTH (4–9) and (1–17), β-endorphin, and its related fragments influence the chemotactic activity, but not phagocytosis.[89] Furthermore, the mode of action of an individual peptide or growth factor could be species-specific and dose-dependent.[84,90]

Moreover, with regard to POMC-products, another important role was designed[91] in the biological system, consisting of the nematode *Schistosoma mansoni* (responsible for Schistosomiasis) by polymorphonuclear leukocytes in humans (definitive host of the parasite), and the immunocytes of the mollusk *Biomphalaria glabrata* (intermediate host). From these investigations emerged the fact that the coincubation of these cells with adult worms of *S. mansoni* gave rise to the appearance in the culture medium of α-MSH, an effect due to the conversion of the parasite ACTH by the enzyme-neutral endopeptidase 24.11, present in the molluscan immunocytes or human polymorphonuclear cells. Thanks to the inhibitory role exerted by α-MSH, these molecules are able to interfere with the immunological functions of the intermediate or final host, and favor the completion of the biological cycle of the parasite.

2.5 Stress Response

The presence of neuropeptides, and, in particular, of ACTH in immunocytes, was at first sight difficult to explain. This molecule has usually been associated with stress, that is, the complex series of responses that the body sets when its balance and internal composition are threatened. In mammals, the stress is expressed fundamentally in the production, by the paraventricular nuclei, of the hypothalamus of CRH, which induces the production of ACTH by the anterior pituitary cells. In turn, ACTH stimulates the synthesis and release of glucocorticoid hormones by the cells of the adrenal cortex. These hormones regulate the activity of the enzyme that catalyzes the final step in the biosynthesis of adrenaline from the adrenal medulla, a phenomenon that is basically under the control of the sympathetic nervous system.[92,93] What meaning could the presence of ACTH-like molecules in animals have, molecules that do not possess any of the sophisticated organs, such as the hypothalamus, pituitary, and adrenal glands that are the target points of these hormones? The first point to make in this regard is that, as previously reported, these and other molecules are found—from invertebrates to humans—in cells with phagocytic activity. Lymphocytes, though endowed with POMC-derived molecules, can be retrieved only in vertebrates, and their evolution cannot be traced back to invertebrates. These immunocytes are traceable from fish, in which the immune responses become much more complex, due to the appearance of an anticipatory immunity, characterized by the presence of a repertoire of clonotypic lymphocytes. However, ACTH-like molecules are detectable only in lymphocytes of tetrapods, whereas in teleosts ACTH-responsive corticosteroidogenic cells have been retrieved in other immune-related tissues, such as the head kidney.[13,94] The biological meaning of these observations is unknown, but potentially very exciting, as it may reflect, at the cellular level, the integration of the neuroendocrine response with adaptive immunity, in addition to the interconnection with the ancestral innate immune responses. The integration between neuroendocrine functions and adaptive immunity is present in vertebrates, but it finds its maximum expression in mammals, where lymphocytes are both immune and neuroendocrine cells. The occurrence of ACTH-like molecules in lymphocytes of anurans may not be by chance. In addition to immunoglobulin class M (IgM) already present in fish, in the amphibians a new class of antibody, IgY, is present; this is considered to be the precursor of mammalian IgG and IgE.[13,95] The presence of ACTH-like molecules in anuran lymphocytes may represent an example of how a particular gene is expressed in a new cell line, in conjunction with the emergence of a more sophisticated function.

Returning to the specific topic of the mechanisms of the stress response, it was observed that antigenic stimuli causes a release of ACTH,[96] suggesting the existence of an interconnection between stress and immune responses, even in invertebrates. In this respect, initially assessed is the presence of enzymes, such as tyrosine hydroxylase and dopamine β-hydroxylase, responsible for the synthesis of biogenic amines, the last mediators of the stress response.[97] Later, the hemolymph of mollusks was incubated with antigens, such as ACTH and CRH, and the values of biogenic amines were determined by HPCL, both in serum and in immunocytes, in a short period of time, ranging from 0 to 45 minutes. An increase was observed of biogenic amines in the serum, as well as a concomitant decrease in immunocytes, both in the presence of either ACTH or CRH.[98] This rapid phenomenon is probably due to the release of biogenic amines by immunocytes. Given that the incubation of the hemolymph with CRH increases the concentration of ACTH in immunocytes, it can be assumed that the release of biogenic amines follows the sequence CRH-ACTH-biogenic amines. However, the preincubation of the hemolymph with an anti-ACTH antibody does not abolish the phenomenon of the release of biogenic amines, suggesting that CRH could induce a direct release not mediated by ACTH, even if modest.[98] The role of ACTH in the release of biogenic amines seems to be specific because the addition to the hemolymph of other peptides, for example, the opioid β-endorphin, causes no release of amines by immunocytes.[97]

As already described in mammals,[99,100] the cytokines are involved in the stress response in invertebrates as well. The incubation of molluscan hemolymph with different cytokines, such as IL-1α and -1β, IL-2, and TNF-α and -β, provoked the release of biogenic amines from immunocytes.[90,101] It is interesting to note that the preincubation of the immunocytes, with all the cytokines tested, exerted an inhibitory effect on the CRH-induced release of biogenic amines. Immunocyto-chemical and cytofluorimetric studies have demonstrated that the cytokines and CRH probably bind to the same receptor. The competition between CRH and a large number of cytokines supports the idea that invertebrate cytokine receptors show a certain degree of promiscuity. In this context, it should be stressed that the structure of mammalian cytokine receptors has been described as multisub-units, with the same subunit shared by different cytokine receptors.[102–105] Also, the growth factors PDGF-AB and TGF-β1 have been found capable of regulating biogenic amine production: the former inhibits, whereas the latter stimulates the release of these molecules via the CRH-ACTH-biogenic amine axis.[106,107]

2.6 The Immune–Mobile Brain

The data reported in the chapter show the surprising capacity of invertebrate immunocytes to combine the typical properties of both immune and neuroen-docrine cells. This combination of functions and copresence in the most an-cestral cell, that is, the immunocyte, suggests that we use for this cell the term "immune-mobile brain," coined[108,109] for the human lymphocyte.

The immunocytes from the outset, and consistently over the course of evolu-tion, flank other nervous and endocrine cells because they form a complex network responsible for maintaining homeostasis. Moreover, these considerations allow a great unifying hypothesis between stressors and antigens, assuming that the anti-genic challenge is equivalent to a stress, and that the difference between antigen and stressor is often only quantitative and semantic, as illustrated in Fig. 9.4.

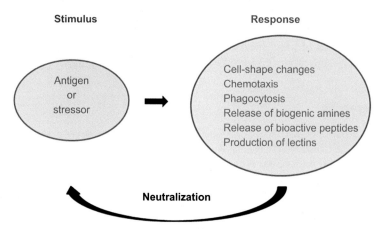

FIGURE 9.4 **Immune-neuroendocrine integration in response to stressful agents.**

3 CONCLUDING REMARKS

On the basis of the reported data, it is possible to make the following assumptions:

1. Invertebrates, despite their apparent simplicity, are capable of very refined performances, both from an immunological and neuroendocrine point of view, such as the ability to distinguish between self and nonself, and the ability to recognize extraneous stimuli and provide complex responses.

2. These animals survive in environments where there are many agents and potentially harmful substances. In this context, they show very efficient forms of defense. Indeed, a complex network of responses has been observed, comprising, among others: chemotaxis, phagocytosis, and the release of biogenic amines and other bioactive mediators. In vertebrates, the response to individual stress factors/antigens becomes more specialized and specific, but the network of responses that is activated remains essentially the same.

3. Most of the molecules that are used to perform this activity and to mediate the necessary cell–cell interactions are apparently present since ancient times, having also been described in unicellular organisms. It can be assumed that many of these molecules are considered in invertebrates to be "defensive molecules," because they are used to neutralize, directly or indirectly, agents that perturb the body homeostasis. A typical example are the ACTH-like molecules.

4. Same, or relatively similar "defensive molecules" are found in vertebrates. Even in these more advanced life forms, their function remains essentially the same. However, nature seems to have made a new use of these ancient molecules, functions, and organs while evolving toward more complex and centralized systems.

5. The neuroendocrine and immune functions in invertebrates show a partial overlap with those observed in vertebrates being assigned to the same cell type, such as the invertebrate immunocyte. This probably explains why in higher forms of life a specialized cell like the lymphocyte has retained the ability to both produce and respond to neuroendocrine signals.

REFERENCES

1. Stefano GB. Stereospecificity as a determining force stabilizing families of signal molecules within the context of evolution. In: Florey E, Stefano GB, editors. *Comparative aspects of neurendcorine functions.* Manchester (UK): Manchester University press; 1991. p. 14–28.
2. Elenkov IJ, Wilder RL, Chrousos GP, Vizi ES. The sympathetic nerve—an integrative interface between two supersystems: the brain and the immune system. *Pharmacol Rev* 2000;**52**:595–638.
3. Weigent DA, Blalock JE. Interactions between the neuroendocrine and immune systems: common hormones and receptors. *Immunol Rev* 1987;**100**:79–108.

4. Weigent DA, Blalock JE. Structural and functional relationships between the immune and neuroendocrine system. *Bull Inst Pasteur* 1989;**87**:61–92.

5. Salzet M. Vertebrate innate immunity resembles a mosaic of invertebrate immune responses. *Trends Immunol* 2001;**22**:285–8.

6. Smith EM, Blalock JE. Human lymphocyte production of corticotropin and endorphin-like substances: association with leukocyte interferon. *Proc Natl Acad Sci USA* 1981;**78**: 7530–4.

7. Smith EM. Opioid peptides in immune cells. *Adv Exp Med Biol* 2003;**521**:51–68.

8. Dores RM, Baron AJ. Evolution of POMC: origin, phylogeny, posttranslational processing, and the melanocortins. *Ann NY Acad Sci* 2011;**1220**:34–48.

9. Noda M, Teranishi Y, Takahashi H, Toyosato M, Notake M, Nakanishi S, et al. Isolation and structural organization of the human preproenkephalin gene. *Nature* 1982;**297**:431–4.

10. Jordan BA, Cvejic S, Devi LA. Opioids and their complicated receptor complexes. *Neuropsychopharmacology* 2000;**23**:S5–S18.

11. Siegel HS, Gould NR, Latimer JW. Splenic leukocytes from chickens injected with *Salmonella pullorum* antigen stimulate production of corticosteroids by isolated adrenal cells. *Proc Soc Exp Biol Med* 1985;**178**:523–30.

12. Harbour DV, Galin FS, Hughes TK, Smith EM, Blalock JE. Role of leukocyte-derived pro-opiomelanocortin peptides in endotoxic shock. *Circ Shock* 1991;**35**:181–91.

13. Ottaviani E, Franchini A, Cossarizza A, Franceschi C. ACTH-like molecules in lymphocytes A study in different vertebrate classes. *Neuropeptides* 1992;**23**:215–9.

14. Davis P, Franquemont S, Liang L, Angleson JK, Dores RM. Evolution of the melanocortin-2 receptor in tetrapods: studies on *Xenopus tropicalis* MC2R and *Anolis carolinensis* MC2R. *Gen Comp Endocrinol* 2013;**188**:175–84.

15. Dores RM, Garcia Y. Views on the co-evolution of the melanocortin-2 receptor, MRAPs, and the hypothalamus/pituitary/adrenal-interrenal axis. *Mol Cell Endocrinol* 2015;**408**:12–22.

16. Mains RE, Eipper BA, Ling N. Common precursor tocorticotropins and endorphins. *Proc Natl Acad Sci USA* 1977;**74**:3014–8.

17. Roberts JL, Herbert E. Characterization of a common precursor to corticotropin and beta-lipotrop identification of beta-lipotropin peptides their arrangement relative to corticotropin in the precursor synthesized in a cell-free F system. *Proc Natl Acad Sci USA* 1977;**74**:5300–4.

18. Eberle AN. *The melanotropins, chemistry physiology and mechanisms of action.* Karger: New York; 1988.

19. Notake M, Tobimatsu T, Watanabe Y, Takahashi H, Mishina M, Numa S. Isolation and characterization of the mouse corticotropin-beta-lipotropin precursor gene and a related pseudogene. *FEBS Lett* 1983;**156**:67–71.

20. O'Donohue TL, Handelmann GE, Chaconas T, Miller RL, Jacobowitz DM. Evidence that N-acetylation regulates the behavioral activity of alpha-MSH in the rat and human central nervous system. *Peptides* 1981;**2**:333–44.

21. O'Donohye TL, Handelmann GE, Miller RL, Jacobowitz DM. N-acetylation regulates the behavioral activity of alpha-melanotropin in a multineurotransmitter neuron. *Science* 1981;**215**:1125–7.

22. Uhler M, Herbert E, D'Eustachio P, Ruddle FD. The mouse genome contains two nonallelic pro-opiomelanocortin genes. *J Biol Chem* 1983;**258**:9444–53.

23. O'Donohue TL, Dorsa DM. The opiomelanotropinergic neuronal and endocrine systems. *Peptides* 1982;**3**:353–95.

24. Farah JM, Millington WR, O'Donohue TL. *Central action of ACTH and related peptides.* In: De Wied D, Ferrari W, editors. Padua, Berlin: Liviana Press, Springer Verlag; 1986; p. 33–52.

25. Vaudry H, Jenks BG, Verburg-Van Kemenade L, Tonon MC. Effect of tunicamycin on biosynthesis, processing and release of proopiomelanocortin-derived peptides in the intermediate lobe of the frog *Rana ridibunda*. *Peptides* 1986;**7**:163–9.

26. Burbach JPH, Wiegant WM. In: De Wied D, editor. *Neuropeptides: basic and perspectives*. Elsevier: Amsterdam; 1990. p. 45–103.

27. Blalock JE, Smith EM. Human leukocyte interferon: structural and biological relatedness to adrenocorticotropic hormone and endorphins. *Proc Natl Acad Sci USA* 1980;**77**:5972–4.

28. Ottaviani E, Franchini A, Hanukoglu I. In situ localization of ACTH receptor-like mRNA in molluscan and human immunocytes. *Cell Mol Life Sci* 1998;**54**:139–42.

29. Padrós MR, Saravia F, Vindrola O. Antibodies against the amino-terminal portion of proenkephalin inhibit DNA synthesis in human peripheral mononuclear cells. *J Neuroimmunol* 1995;**61**:79–83.

30. Hook S, Camberis M, Prout M, Konig M, Zimmer A, Van Heeke G, et al. Preproenkephalin is a Th2 cytokine but is not required for Th2 differentiation in vitro. *Immunol. Cell Biol* 1999;**77**:385–90.

31. 2Mehrishi JN, Mills IH. Opiate receptors on lymphocytes and platelets in man. *Clin Immunol Immunopathol* 1983;**27**:240–9.

32. Smith EM, Johnson NM, Blalock JE. Lymphocytes: peripheral source and target for endogenous opiates. In: Fraioli F, Mazzetti M, editors. *Opioid peptides in the periphery*. Elsevier: Amsterdam; 1984.

33. Fiorica E, Spector S. Opioid binding site in EL-4 thymoma cell line. *Life Sci* 1988;**42**:199–206.

34. Hazum E, Chang KJ, Cuatrecasas P. Role of disulphide and sulphydryl groups in clustering of enkephalin receptors in neuroblastoma cells. *Nature* 1979;**282**:626–8.

35. Schweigerer L, Schmidt W, Teschemacher H, Gramsch C. beta-Endorphin: surface binding and internalization in thymoma cells. *Proc Natl Acad Sci USA* 1985;**82**:5751–5.

36. Hughes Jr TK, Chin R. Interactions of neuropeptides and cytokines. In: Scharrer B, Smith EM, Stefano GB, editors. *Neuropeptides and immunoregulation*. Springer-Verlag: Berlin; 1994. p. 101–19.

37. Ottaviani E. Immunocyte: the invertebrate counterpart of the vertebrate macrophage. *Inv Surv J* 2011;**8**:1–4.

38. Ottaviani E, Franchini A, Franceschi C. Pro-opiomelanocortin-derived peptides, cytokines, and nitric oxide in immune responses and stress: an evolutionary approach. *Int Rev Cytol* 1997;**170**:79–141.

39. Ottaviani E, Cossarizza A, Ortolani C, Monti D, Franceschi C. ACTH-like molecules in gastropod molluscs: a possible role in ancestral immune response and stress. *Proc R Soc Lond B* 1991;**245**:215–8.

40. Ottaviani E, Petraglia F, Montagnani G, Cossarizza A, Monti D, Franceschi C. Presence of ACTH and β-endorphin immunoreactivemolecoles in the freshwater snail *Planorbarius corneus* (L.) (*Gastropoda Pulmonata*) and their possible role in phagocytosis. *Regul Pept* 1990;**27**:1–9.

41. Ottaviani E, Capriglione T, Franceschi C. Invertebrate and vertebrate immune cells express pro-opiomelanocortin (POMC) mRNA. *Brain Behav Immun* 1995;**9**:1–8.

42. Cortés R, Navarro S, Agulleiro MJ, Guillot R, García-Herranz V, Sánchez E, et al. Evolution of the melanocortin system. *Gen. Comp. Endocrinol* 2014;**209**:3–10.

43. Leroith D, Liotta AS, Roth J, Shiloach J, Lewis ME, Pert CB, et al. Corticotropin and beta-endorphin-like materials are native to unicellular organisms. *Proc Natl Acad Sci USA* 1982;**79**:2086–90.

44. Stefano GB. Role of opioid neuropeptides in immunoregulation. *Prog Neurobiol* 1989;**33**:149–59.

45. Stefano GB, Digenis A, Spector S, Leung MK, Bilfinger TV, Makman MH, et al. Opiate-like substances in an invertebrate, an opiate receptor on invertebrate and human immunocytes, and a role in immunosuppression. *Proc Natl Acad Sci USA* 1993;**90**:11099–103.

46. Salzet M, Stefano GB. Invertebrate proenkephalin: delta opioid binding sites in leech ganglia and immunocytes. *Brain Res* 1997;**768**:224–32.

47. Ottaviani E, Cossarizza A. Immunocytochemical evidence of vertebrate bioactive peptide-like molecules in the immuno cell types of the freshwater snail *Planorbarius corneus* (L.) (*Gastropoda Pulmonata*). *FEBS Lett* 1990;**267**:250–2.

48. Ottaviani E, Franchini A, Franceschi C. Presence of immunoreactivecorticotropin-releasing hormone and cortisol molecules in invertebrate haemocytes and lower and higher vertebrate thymus. *Histochem J* 1998;**30**:61–7.

49. Malagoli D, Franchini A, Ottaviani E. Synergistic role of cAMP and IP(3) in corticotropin-releasing hormone-induced cell shape changes in invertebrate immunocytes. *Peptides* 2000;**21**:175–82.

50. Hughes Jr TK, Smith EM, Chin R, Cadet P, Sinisterra J, Leung MK, et al. Interaction of immunoactivemonokines (interleukin 1 and tumor necrosis factor) in the bivalve mollusc *Mytilus edulis*. *Proc Natl Acad Sci USA* 1990;**87**:4426–9.

51. 4Hughes Jr TK, Smith EM, Barnett JA, Charles R, Stefano GB. LPS stimulated invertebrate hemocytes: a role for immunoreactive TNF and IL-1. *Dev Comp Immunol* 1991;**15**:117–22.

52. Ottaviani E, Franchini A, Franceschi C. Presence of several cytokine-like molecules in molluscan hemocytes. *Biochem Biophys Res Commun* 1993;**195**:984–8.

53. Granath Jr WO, Connors VA, Tarleton RL. Interleukin 1 activity in haemolymph from strains of the snail *Biomphalaria glabrata* varying in susceptibility to the human blood fluke, *Schistosoma mansoni*: presence, differential expression, and biological function. *Cytokine* 1994;**6**:21–7.

54. Ouwe-Missi-Oukem-Boyer O, Porchet E, Capron A, Dissous C. Characterization of immunoreactive TNF alpha molecules in the gastropod *Biomphalaria glabrata*. *Dev Comp Immunol* 1994;**18**:211–8.

55. Hughes TK, Smith EM, Stefano GB. Detection of immunoreactive interleukin 6 in invertebrate hemolymph and nervous tissue. *Prog NeuroEndocrinImmunol* 1991;**4**:234–9.

56. Stefano GB, Smith EM, Hughes TK. Opioid induction of immunoreactive interleukin-1 in *Mytilus edulis* and human immunocytes: an interleukin-1-like substance in invertebrate neural tissue. *J Neuroimmunol* 1991;**32**:29–34.

57. Paemen LR, Porchet-Hennere E, Masson M, Leung MK, Hughes Jr TK, Stefano GB. Glial localization of interleukin-1 alpha in invertebrate ganglia. *Cell Mol Neurobiol* 1992;**12**:463–72.

58. Franchini A, Miyan JA, Ottaviani E. Induction of ACTH- and TNF- α-like molecules in the hemocytes of *Calliphora vomitoria* (Insecta Diptera). *Tissue Cell* 1996;**28**:587–92.

59. Cooper EL, Franchini A, Ottaviani E. Earthworm coelomocytes possess immunoreactive cytokines and POMC-derived peptides. *Anim Biol* 1995;**4**:25–9.

60. Wang PH, Wan DH, Pang LR, Gu ZH, Qiu W, Weng SP, et al. Molecular cloning, characterization and expression analysis of the tumor necrosis factor (TNF) superfamily gene TNF receptor superfamily gene and lipopolysaccharide-induced TNF-α factor (LITAF) gene from *Litopenaeus vannamei*. *Dev Comp Immunol* 2012;**36**:39–50.

61. Burke RD, Watkins RF. Stimulation of starfish coelomocytes by interleukin-1. *Biochem Biophys Res Commun* 1991;**180**:579–84.

62. Beck G, Habicht GS. Isolation and characterization of a primitive interleukin-1-like protein from an invertebrate *Asterias forbesi*. *Proc Natl Acad Sci USA* 1986;**83**:7429–33.

63. Beck G, Habicht GS. Invertebrate cytokines. *Ann NY Acad Sci* 1994;**712**:206–12.

64. Beck G, Vasta GR, Marchalonis JJ, Habicht GS. Characterization of interleukin-1 activity in tunicates. *Comp Biochem Physiol* 1989;**92B**:93–8.
65. Raftos DA, Cooper EL, Habicht GS, Beck G. Invertebrate cytokines: tunicate cell proliferation stimulated by an interleukin 1-like molecule. *Proc Natl Acad Sci USA* 1991;**88**:9518–22.
66. Wharton KA, Johansen KM, Xu T, Artavanis-Tsakonas S. Nucleotide sequence from the neurogenic locus notch implies a gene product that shares homology with proteins containing EGF-like repeats. *Cell* 1985;**43**(3 Pt 2):567–81.
67. Kelley MR, Kidd S, Deutsch WA, Young MW. Mutations altering the structure of epidermal growth factor-like coding sequences at the *Drosophila Notch* locus. *Cell* 1987;**51**:539–48.
68. Padgett RW, St Johnston RD, Gelbart WM. A transcript from a *Drosophila* pattern gene predicts a protein homologous to the transforming growth factor-beta family. *Nature* 1987;**325**:81–4.
69. Bryant PJ. Localized cell death caused by mutations in a *Drosophila* gene coding for a transforming growth factor-beta homolog. *Dev Biol* 1988;**128**:386–95.
70. Kopczynski CC, Alton AK, Fechtel K, Kooh PJ, Muskavitch MA. Delta, a *Drosophila* neurogenic gene, is transcriptionally complex and encodes a protein related to blood coagulation factors and epidermal growth factor of vertebrates. *Genes Dev* 1988;**2**(12B):1723–35.
71. Aizawa K, Sato F. Culture de tissus de ver a soie, *Bombyx mori*, dans un milieu sans hemolymphe. *Ann Epiphyt* 1963;**14**:125.
72. Vaughn JL, Louloudes EJ. Isolation of two promoting fractions from insect hemolymph. *In Vitro* 1978;**14**:351.
73. Williams CM, Kambysellis MP. *In vitro* action of ecdisone. *Proc. Natl. Acad. Sci. USA* 1969;**63**:231.
74. Wielgus JJ, Caldwell GA, Nichols RL, White CF. Purification, properties, and titer of hemolymph trophic factor in larvae and pupae of *Manduca sexta*. *Insect Biochem* 1990;**20**:65–72.
75. Thorpe A, Duve H. Insulin-and glucagon-like peptides in insects and molluscs. *Mol Physiol* 1984;**5**:235–60.
76. Ebberink RHM, Smit AB, Van Minnen J. The insulin family: evolution of structure and function in vertebrates and invertebrates. *Biol Bull* 1989;**177**:176–82.
77. Blumenthal S. From insulin and insulin-like activity to the insulin superfamily of growth-promoting peptides: a 20th-century odyssey. *Perspect Biol Med* 2010;**53**:491–508.
78. Franchini A, Kletsas D, Ottaviani E. Immunocytochemical evidence of PDGF- and TGF-beta-like molecules in invertebrate and vertebrate immunocytes: an evolutionary approach. *Histochem J* 1996;**28**:599–605.
79. Manske M, Bade EG. Growth factor-induced cell migration: biology and methods of analysis. *Int Rev Cytol* 1994;**155**:49–96.
80. Sassi D, Kletsas D, Ottaviani E. Interactions of signaling pathways in ACTH (1-24)-induced cell shape changes in invertebrate immunocytes. *Peptides* 1998;**19**:1105–10.
81. Kletsas D, Sassi D, Franchini A, Ottaviani E. PDGF and TGF-beta induce cell shape changes in invertebrate immunocytes via specific cell surface receptors. *Eur J Cell Biol* 1998;**75**:362–6.
82. Ottaviani E, Franchini A, Malagoli D, Genedani S. Immunomodulation by recombinant human interleukin-8 and its signal transduction pathways in invertebrate hemocytes. *Cell Mol Life Sci* 2000;**57**:506–13.
83. Genedani S, Bernardi M, Ottaviani E, Franceschi C, Leung MK, Stefano GB. Differential modulation of invertebrate hemocyte motility by CRF, ACTH, and its fragments. *Peptides* 1994;**15**:203–6.
84. Ottaviani E, Franchini A, Kletsas D, Bernardi M, Genedani S. Involvement of PDGF and TGF-β1 in cell migration and phagocytosis in invertebrate and human immunocytes. *Anim Biol* 1997;**6**:95–9.

85. Ottaviani E, Franchini A, Cassanelli S, Genedani S. Cytokines and molluscan immune responses. *Biol Cell* 1995;**85**:87–91.

86. Stefano GB, Cadet P, Scharrer B. Stimulatory effects of opioid neuropeptides on locomotory activity and conformational changes in invertebrate and human immunocytes: evidence for a subtype of delta receptor. *Proc Natl Acad Sci USA* 1989;**86**:6307–11.

87. Stefano GB, Leung MK, Zhao XH, Scharrer B. Evidence for the involvement of opioid neuropeptides in the adherence and migration of immunocompetent invertebrate hemocytes. *Proc Natl Acad Sci USA* 1989;**86**:626–30.

88. Ottaviani E. The blood cells of the freshwater snail *Planorbis corneus* (*Gastropoda Pulmonata*). *Dev Comp Immunol* 1983;**7**:209–16.

89. Ottaviani E, Franchini A, Fontanili P. The effect of corticotropin-releasing factor and proopiomelanocortin-derived peptides on the phagocytosis of molluscan hemocytes. *Experientia* 1994;**50**:837–9.

90. Ottaviani E, Caselgrandi E, Franceschi C. Cytokines and evolution: in vitro effects of IL-1 alpha, IL-1 beta TNF-alpha and TNF-beta on an ancestral type of stress response. *Biochem Biophys Res Commun* 1995;**207**:288–92.

91. Duvaux-Miret O, Stefano GB, Smith EM, Dissous C, Capron A. Immunosuppression in the definitive and intermediate hosts of the human parasite *Schistosoma mansoni* by release of immunoactive neuropeptides. *Proc Natl Acad Sci USA* 1992;**89**:778–81.

92. Axelrod J, Reisine TD. Stress hormones: their interaction and regulation. *Science* 1984;**224**:452–9.

93. Bateman A, Singh A, Kral T, Solomon S. The immune-hypothalamic-pituitary-adrenal axis. *Endocr Rev* 1989;**10**:92–112.

94. Hontela A, Leblond VS, Chang JP. Purification and isolation of corticosteroidogenic cells from head kidney of rainbow trout (*Oncorhynchus mykiss*) for testing cell-specific effects of a pesticide. *Comp Biochem Physiol* 2008;**147C**:52–60.

95. Pettinello R, Dooley H. The immunoglobulins of cold-blooded Vertebrates. *Biomolecules* 2014;**4**:1045–69.

96. Ottaviani E, Caselgrandi E, Petraglia F, Franceschi C. Stress response in the freshwater snail *Planorbarius corneus* (L.) (Gastropoda, Pulmonata): interaction between CRF ACTH and biogenic amines. *Gen Comp Endocrinol* 1992;**87**:354–60.

97. Ottaviani E, Caselgrandi E, Fontanili P, Franceschi C. Evolution, immune responses and stress: studies on molluscan cells. *Acta Biol Hung* 1992;**43**:293–8.

98. Ottaviani E, Caselgrandi E, Franchini A, Franceschi C. CRF provokes the release of norepinephrine by hemocytes of *Viviparus ater* (Gastropoda Prosobranchia): Further evidence in favour of the evolutionary hypothesis of the mobile immune-brain. *Biochem Biophys Res Commun* 1993;**193**:446–52.

99. Imura H, Fukata J, Mori T. Cytokines and endocrine function: an interaction between the immune and neuroendocrine systems. *Clin Endocrinol* 1991;**35**:107–15.

100. Schöbitz B, De Kloet ER, Holsboer F. Gene expression and function of interleukin 1, interleukin 6 and tumor necrosis factor in the brain. *Prog Neurobiol* 1994;**44**:397–432.

101. Ottaviani E, Franchini A, Caselgrandi E, Cossarizza A, Franceschi C. Relationship between corticotropin-releasing factor and interleukin-2: evolutionary evidence. *FEBS Lett* 1994;**351**:19–21.

102. Taga T, Kishimoto T. Cytokine receptors and signal transduction. *FASEB J* 1992;**6**:3387–96.

103. Kondo M, Takeshita T, Ishii N, Nakamura M, Watanabe S, Arai K, et al. Sharing of the interleukin-2 (IL-2) receptor gamma chain between receptors for IL-2 and IL-4. *Science* 1993;**262**:1874–7.

104. Noguchi M, Nakamura Y, Russell SM, Ziegler SF, Tsang M, Cao X, et al. Interleukin-2 receptor gamma chain: a functional component of the interleukin-7 receptor. *Science* 1993;**262**:1877–80.

105. Russell SM, Keegan AD, Harada N, Nakamura Y, Noguchi M, Leland P, et al. Interleukin-2 receptor gamma chain: a functional component of the interleukin-4 receptor. *Science* 1993;**262**:1880–3.

106. Ottaviani E, Caselgrandi E, Kletsas D. Effect of PDGF and TGF-β on the release of biogenic amines from invertebrate immunocytes and their possible role in the stress response. *FEBS Lett* 1997;**403**:236–8.

107. Ottaviani E, Caselgrandi E, Kletsas D. The CRH-ACTH-biogenic amine axis in invertebrate immunocytes activated by PDGF and TGF-β. *FEBS Lett* 1998;**427**:255–8.

108. Blalock JE. The immune system as a sensory organ. *J Immunol* 1984;**132**:1067–70.

109. Blalock JE, Smith EM. The immune system: our mobile brain. *Immunol Today* 1985;**6**:115–7.

Chapter 10

The Immune-Related Roles and the Evolutionary History of Dscam in Arthropods

Sophie A.O. Armitage*, Daniela Brites**

*Institute for Evolution and Biodiversity, University of Münster, Münster, Germany;
**Swiss Tropical and Public Health Institute, Basel, Switzerland

1 THE DOWN SYNDROME CELL ADHESION MOLECULE

The Down syndrome cell adhesion molecule (Dscam) gene was first described in humans associated with defects in the nervous system.[1] Subsequently, several members of the Dscam family were discovered in other metazoans, in which its main described function is related to the development of the nervous system.[2–6] Both vertebrates and insects have Dscam members that have resulted from whole gene duplications, for example, DSCAM and DSCAM-like in humans,[1,5] and Dscam, Dscam2, Dscam3, and Dscam4 in *Drosophila melanogaster*.[7] These proteins are typically cell-surface receptors composed of 9(Ig)-4(FN)-1(Ig)-2(FN), where Ig stands for immunoglobulin, and FN for fibronectin type III domain (Fig. 10.1). The 16 extracellular domains are usually followed by a transmembrane domain and a cytoplasmic tail. In insects and crustaceans (pancrustaceans), one Dscam paralog is the most remarkable example known of protein diversification by duplication and alternative splicing.[2] We will refer to this gene hereafter as Dscam-hv (Dscam hypervariable).[8] Other synonymous notations have been used by different authors, that is, Dscam[2] and the most recent *D. melanogaster* notation Dscam1.[6,9] Furthermore, species-specific annotations have also been used, for example, *Anopheles gambiae* Dscam has been named AgDscam,[10] etc.

In the following sections, we will introduce the organization of the Dscam-hv gene and how protein diversity is generated from this single locus. We will also introduce what is known about the Dscam-hv protein structure and discuss the hypothetical implications of isoform diversity for immunity. Dscam-hv is part of a large gene family, which in arthropods has diversified independently through different molecular mechanisms. To better understand the origin and the importance of Dscam-hv diversity in arthropods, we will briefly review the

The Evolution of the Immune System. http://dx.doi.org/10.1016/B978-0-12-801975-7.00010-4

inferences gained on the evolutionary history of the molecule from comparative analyses.

1.1   From One Gene to Thousands of Protein Isoforms

In Dscam-hv, half of the second and third Ig domains (Ig2 and Ig3) and the complete Ig7 domain are encoded by exon duplicates arranged in three clusters in the Dscam locus (Fig. 10.1). This is made possible by a refined mechanism of mutually exclusive alternative splicing that ensures that in the mature mRNA only one exon per cluster is present (Fig. 10.1). Furthermore, in some species, the diversity of Dscam-hv Ig2, Ig3, and Ig7 domains can be coupled with diversity generated by mutually exclusive alternative splicing of two exons encoding a transmembrane domain, and by regular splicing of different cytoplasmic tails[8,12] (Fig. 10.1). In this way, one single Dscam-hv can produce thousands of protein isoforms within a single individual. The number of isoforms generated varies, depending on the species, ranging from around 10,000 in *Daphnia* species to around 100,000 in Drosophilids.

Dscam-hv plays an essential role during the development of the nervous system wiring in *D. melanogaster.* The basis of that role is the homophilic binding between identical Dscam-hv isoforms, allowing nervous cells to recognize each other, and leading to a self-avoidance behavior.[13–15] Interestingly, the large Dscam isoform diversity has been shown to be essential for the correct development of the nervous system in flies, suggesting that isoforms are not functionally redundant.[6,16] Homophilic binding between identical isoforms has been demonstrated in vitro, indicating a degree of binding specificity, in which 95% of all isoforms will bind only to other identical isoforms.[17,18]

Dscam-hv has also been shown to be involved in the immune defense of insects and crustaceans.[10,19–21] However, its role in immunity remains controversial, because, despite several lines of evidence placing Dscam-hv as a receptor contributing to immune recognition, many important questions remain open. Evidence (or lack thereof) for a role of Dscam in pancrustacean immunity will be discussed in detail in Section 2.

1.2   Structural Aspects of Dscam

The protein structure of the first eight Ig domains of Dscam has been elucidated. The first four Ig domains adopt a so-called horseshoe conformation.[22] The horseshoe conformation has a similar shape to other cell-adhesion molecules involved both in the nervous system (eg, axonin) and in the immune system (eg, hemolin).[22–24] The remaining four Ig domains (Ig5 to Ig8) provide Dscam with a serpentine shape (S-shape) (Fig. 10.1). Homophilic binding between identical isoforms occurs through the formation of Dscam dimers (Fig. 10.1). Interestingly, the dimer-binding regions are segments of Ig2, Ig3, and Ig7 domains coded by the alternative exons.[22,25] In this way the genetic diversification caused by

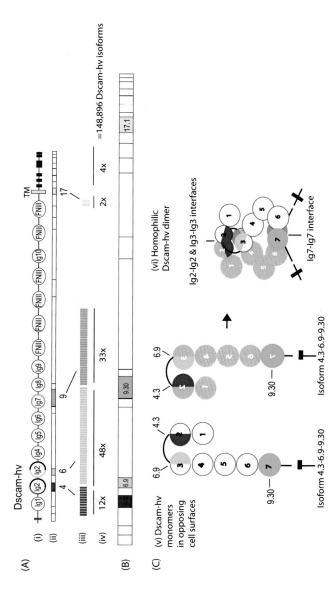

FIGURE 10.1 **Dscam-hv in *D. melanogaster*.** (A) Dscam-hv protein and mRNA; (i) protein domains. Ig stands for Immunoglobulin and FNIII stands for fibronectin domains, respectively. Colors denote part of the molecule diversified by mutually exclusive alternative splicing; (ii) mRNA, by mutually exclusive alternative splicing only one exon of array of exons 4, 6, 9, and transmembrane domain is present; (iii) arrays of duplicated exons present in the locus Dscam-hv of *D. melanogaster*; (iv) number of Dscam-hv isoforms of Dscam-hv in *D. melanogaster*, which results both from mutually alternative splicing and regular alternative splicing; (B) example of one mRNA produced by mutually exclusive alternative splicing; (C) model based on Dscam 1–8 crystal structure for the conformation of the first seven Ig domains in Dscam-hv; (v) examples of Dscam-hv monomers; the first four Ig domains form a horseshoe structure, whereas the remaining domains remain flexible; (vi) upon homophilic binding between identical isoforms, mediated by the regions of Ig2, Ig3, and Ig7 encoded by the alternative exons, the Dscam-hv dimer acquires an S shape. (*Source: Adapted from Hattori et al.[11]*)

the duplications, coupled with the strong specificity of Dscam's homophilic binding, provide a highly diverse "lock and key" system, which nerve cells exploit extensively.[11] The implications of these structural features for immunity have not been experimentally tested. Nevertheless, it has been suggested that certain variable regions within the horseshoe structure that are not involved in the formation of dimers could be responsible for recognizing pathogen-associated molecular patterns.

2 IMMUNE-RELATED ROLES OF DSCAM-HV IN ARTHROPODS

Despite lymphocytes being present only in vertebrates (see chapters: Lympho-cyte Populations in Jawless Vertebrates: Insights Into the Origin and Evolu-tion of Adaptive Immunity; The Evolution of Lymphocytes in Ectothermic Gnathostomata), there is mounting evidence that some species of pancrusta-ceans exhibit immune phenomena thought to be unique to vertebrates, that is, increased protection against pathogens upon a secondary encounter with the same pathogen[26–29] (reviewed recently).[30] In some cases, the responses found had revealed a high degree of specificity, implying the ability to distinguish be-tween Gram-positive and Gram-negative bacteria, between different species of the same genus of parasite,[27] or even between strains of the same parasite.[26,29] A comprehensive view of the immune functions underlying such responses is lacking, but there is evidence in different taxa for an involvement of phagocy-tosis.[28,29] Dscam's hypervariability, combined with the first demonstrations that it is involved in insect immunity,[10,19] has sparked a great deal of interest and discussion[31–34] about whether the variable isoforms produced by this molecule might provide antigen-receptor diversity, hypothetically allowing a host to dis-criminate between different parasites and pathogens. The same commentaries speculated that Dscam-hv could be a convergent insect example of the diversity produced by vertebrate antigen-receptors,[31–34] even though it produces diversity of many orders of magnitude lower than vertebrate antibodies, and is mechanis-tically unrelated. At present this exciting idea lacks empirical support,[20,35] and as we shall see, we are still far from understanding whether that could in fact happen.

2.1 What Is the Evidence That Dscam-hv is Involved in the Immune defence of Pancrustaceans?

There are two recent reviews on pancrustacean Dscam-hv in immunity,[20,21] and we try not to cover the same ground in detail. Similarly to Ng et al.,[21] we have taken a parasite class-based approach, although we present this information in the form of a table (Table 10.1), splitting the evidence into that which has been found on the RNA and on the protein level. We briefly discuss herein the gen-eral trends that emerge from the data in Table 10.1.

TABLE 10.1 Overview of Studies Examining Dscam-hv in Relation to Immunity, Sorted by Parasite or Immune Stimulant Used

Parasite/Stimulant		Host			Constitutive Exon mRNA Expression	Experimental Evidence			
a	Species P	b	Species	LHS		Alternatively Spliced Exon mRNA Expression	RNAi/ Mutagenesis	Cellular/ Binding Assays	R
Viruses									
	Drosophila C Virus	I	Drosophila melano- gaster	Adu		Whole body; illumina RNA sequencing of Ig2 and Ig3: no change (Inj: 6 and 30 h)			95
	P. interp. g. v.	I	D. melano- gaster	Adu		Whole body; illumina RNA sequencing of Ig2 and Ig3. No change (Inj: 6 and 30 h)			95
	White spot syndrome virus (WSSV)	C	Litopenaeus vannamei	NI		Haemocyte; Sanger sequencing cDNA: some isoforms from each Ig domain associated with different disease states (Inj: 7 days and chronic)			54
				Adu	Haemocytes; qRT-PCR; Total: ↓3 h; ↑24, 36, 48, 60 h. "tail- less": ↑1, 48, 60 h. "membrane-bound": ↓3 h. ↑24, 36, 48, 60, 72 h. (Inj): 1, 3, 12, 24, 36, 48, 60, 72 h)				41

(Continued)

TABLE 10.1 Overview of Studies Examining Dscam-hv in Relation to Immunity, Sorted by Parasite or Immune Stimulant Used (cont.)

Parasite/Stimulant		Host		Experimental Evidence				R
Species P	b	Species	LHS	Constitutive Exon mRNA Expression	Alternatively Spliced Exon mRNA Expression	RNAi/ Mutagenesis	Cellular/ Binding Assays	
a	C	P. leniusculus	Int	Hemocytes; no change; (Inj: 6, 12, 24 h)		Haematopoeic tissue cell culture; RNAi knockdown; no effect on WSSV replication		37
WSSV (Ev)	C	L. vannamei	Adu	Haemocytes; no change (Inj: 1, 2 or 3 days)				
Bacteria								
G− Al								
E. coli	I	Anopheles gambiae	Adu			RNAi knockdown; after infection ↓ adult survival; Exon 4.8 knockdown ↓ survival compared to Exon 4.1 (Inj)		10
	I	D. melanogaster	NA				Recombinantly expressed Dscam-hv bound to live E. coli	18
			Adu		Whole body (Adu: Inj: 6 and 30 h) or haemolymph, head, remainder of body (Adu: Sep: 6 h); Illumina RNA sequencing of Ig2 and Ig3; no change			95

	Pathogen		Species	Stage					Ref
	E. coli RFP	I	D. melano-gaster	Adu and Cel	No change; (Adu: Sep: 18 h; Cel: 12 and 18 h)	Whole-body minus head; PacBio RNA sequencing of Ig2, Ig3 and Ig7: no change; (Adu: Sep: 18 h; Cel: 12 and 18 h)			44
				Emb			Haemocytes of Dscam loss of function embryos bound E. coli similarly to wild type (Inj)		45
	Serratia symbiotica	I	Acyrthosi-phon pisum	Juv	Whole body; transcriptome; no changes. (stably infected aphid line)				96
	Vibrio harveyi	C	L. vannamei	NI	Haemocyte;↓1 h and ↑36 and 48 h. Cytoplasmic tail variants regulation (Inj): 0, 1, 3, 12, 18, 24, 36, 48, 72 h)	Haemocyte; Sequencing cDNA of Ig2 and Ig3; Association between sequence of isoforms and bacterial challenge (Inj: 36 h)			40
G− De	E. coli	I	A. gambiae	Adu and Cel	No change	RTqPCR of Ig2; adults and cell line: differential expression compared to control. Cells: splicing patterns at 12 and 18 h correlated with each other (Adu: NI: 12 h; Cel: 12 and 18 h)	RNAi of exon 4.8 ↓binding of Dscam-hv to the bacteria compared to exon 4.1 and GFP control	Bacteria had increased affinity to membrane-bound and secreted Dscam-hv produced by cells previously challenged with the same bacteria. Dscam-hv was highly concentrated at site of interaction with E. coli in challenged cells	10

(Continued)

TABLE 10.1 Overview of Studies Examining Dscam-hv in Relation to Immunity, Sorted by Parasite or Immune Stimulant Used (cont.)

Parasite/Stimulant		Host		Experimental Evidence				R
Species P	b	Species	LHS	Constitutive Exon mRNA Expression	Alternatively Spliced Exon mRNA Expression	RNAi/Mutagenesis	Cellular/Binding Assays	
a								
E. coli Alexa Fluor® 595	1	D. melanogaster	Adu and Cel			Dscam-hv RNAi and loss of function larvae had reduced phagocytosis	S2 cells preincubated with Dscam-hv antibody had reduced phagocytosis	18
E. coli Fluoroscein conjugate	1	A. gambiae	Cel			Dscam-hv knockdown in Sua5B cells resulted in lower phagocytosis		10
Pseudomona veronii	1	A. gambiae	Cel		RTqPCR of Ig2 variants showed they were differentially expressed compared to a naive control (12 h)	RNAi of exon 4.8 ↓binding of Dscam-hv to bacteria compared to exon 4.1 and GFP control	Bacteria had ↑ affinity to membrane-bound and secreted Dscam-hv produced by cells previously challenged with the same bacteria	10
Vibrio harveyi	C	L. vannamei	NA				1 of 2 V. harveyi-induced RE isoforms bound more strongly to V. harveyi than 2 control-induced RE isoforms. All isoforms bound (to differing degrees) to WSSV, E. coli and Staphylococcus aureus	40

G− Mi	LPS E. coli	C	Eriocheir sinensis	Adu	↑ 2 h post infection (Inj: 2, 6, 12, 24 h)		42
		C	P. leniusculus	Int	Haemocytes; ↑ 6 and 12 h (Inj: 6, 12, 24 h)		37
	LPS P. aeruginosa	I	A. gambiae	Cel		RTqPCR analysis of Ig2 variants: differentially expressed compared to control (12 h)	10
G+Al	Micrococcus luteus	I	D. melano-gaster	Adu		Illumina RNA sequencing Ig2 and Ig3: no strong treatment effects but bacteria exposure affected exon 4.9 at 6 h (Adu: Inj: 6 and 30 h); no effect on head or remainder of body, but small effect on exon 4.4 in haemolymph (Adu: Sep: 6 h)	95
	Pasteuria ramosa	C	Daphnia magna	Adu		Haemocyte cDNA sequencing Ig2, Ig3 and Ig7: variable exons expression deviated from random	8
	P. ramosa: 2 strains	C	Da. magna	Adu		Haemolymph, gut or carcass; Ilumina RNA sequencing Ig2 and Ig3: no effect (Ora: 4 h)	95

(Continued)

TABLE 10.1 Overview of Studies Examining Dscam-hv in Relation to Immunity, Sorted by Parasite or Immune Stimulant Used (cont.)

Parasite/Stimulant			Host		Experimental Evidence				R
a	Species P	b	Species	LHS	Constitutive Exon mRNA Expression	Alternatively Spliced Exon mRNA Expression	RNAi/Mutagenesis	Cellular/Binding Assays	
a	Staphylococcus aureus	I	A. gambiae	Adu			RNAi ↓ adult survival after infection. Knockdown of exon 4.1 ↓ survival after infection compared to 4.8 knockdown (Inj)		10
G+ De	S. aureus	I	A. gambiae	Adu and Cel		RTqPCR analysis of Ig2 variants in adults and cell line: differentially expressed compared to control. Cells: splicing patterns at 12 and 18 h correlated with each other (Adu: Nl: 12 h; Cel: 12 and 18 h)		Dscam-hv was highly concentrated at site of interaction with S. aureus in challenged cells	10
	S. aureus Fluoroscein conjugate	I	A. gambiae	Cel			↓ Phagocytosis in after knockdown in Sua5B cells		10
G+Mi	PGN from S. aureus	I	A. gambiae	Cel		RTqPCR of Ig2 variants: differentially expressed compared to control (12 h)			10

G− and G+ Al	E. coli and Pilibacter termitis	1	E. sinensis	Adu	↑6 h; ↓24 h (Inj: 2, 6, 12, 24 h)			37
			C	P. leniusculus	Int	Haemocytes; no change (Inj: 6, 12, 24 h)		
		1	Coptotermes formosanus	?	Whole bodies; no change (Sep: 24 h)			97
G− and G+ Mi and ?	Mixed	1	Manduca sexta	Juv	Fat body and hemocytes; whole genome transcriptome ↑ (Inj: 24 h)			98
NA	Opportunistic bacteria	1	A. gambiae	Adu			↑ In opportunistic bacteria within the mosquito haemolymph 3 days after Dscam-hv RNAi	10
		1	Anopheles stephensi	Adu			↓ in bacteria in the midgut after overexpressing splice variants from A. gambiae that are increased in expression toward bacteria and Plasmodium	46

(Continued)

TABLE 10.1 Overview of Studies Examining Dscam-hv in Relation to Immunity, Sorted by Parasite or Immune Stimulant Used (cont.)

Parasite/Stimulant			Host		Experimental Evidence				R
a	Species P	b	Species	LHS	Constitutive Exon mRNA Expression	Alternatively Spliced Exon mRNA Expression	RNAi/ Mutagenesis	Cellular/ Binding Assays	
Fungi									
Al	Beauveria bassiana	I	D. melanogaster	Adu		Whole body; illumina RNA Ig2 and Ig3: no effect (Adu: Inj: 6 and 30 h)			95
De	B. bassiana	I	A. gambiae	Adu and Cel		RTqPCR Ig2 variants showed they were differentially expressed compared to control (NI: 12 h)			10
	S. cerevisiae	I	A. gambiae	Cel				No colocalisation between Dscam-hv and S. cerevisiae	10
Mi	β-1,3-glucan S. cerevisiae	C	E. sinensis	Adu	↑2, 6 and 12 h (Inj: 2, 6, 12, 24 h)				42
Sp	Nosema ceranae	I	Apis mellifera ligustica	Adu	Abdomen: ↑6 and 72 h. Midgut to ileum: ↑3 and 5 days. (Ora: whole abdomens: 6, 12, 18, 24, 48, 72 h; midgut to ileum: 3 and 5 days)				38

Protozoa								
AI	Crithidia mellificae	1	A. mellifera ligustica	Adu	Abdomen: ↑24 h. Midgut to ileum: ↑3 days. (Ora: whole abdomens: 6, 12, 18, 24, 48, 72 hr; midgut to ileum: 3 and 5 days)			38
AI	C. mellificae and N. ceranae	1	A. mellifera ligustica	Adu	Midgut to ileum: ↑3 days. (Ora: 3 and 5 days)			38
AI	Plasmodium berghei	1	A. gambiae	Adu		RTqPCR Ig2 differential expression compared to control. (Ora: 24 h)	In Dscam-hv deficient mosquitoes number of oocysts in the midgut higher than in controls (Ora)	10
		1	A. stephensi	Adu			Infection intensity in midgut ↓ in transgenic mosquitoes over-expressing a splice variant that in A. gambiae is induced after infection with P. berghei. Splice variants induced in response to P. falciparum did not give ↑resistance to P. berghei (Ora)	46
AI	Plasmodium falciparum	1	A. gambiae	Adu		RTqPCR Ig2 differential expression compared to control. (Ora: 24 h)		10

(Continued)

TABLE 10.1 Overview of Studies Examining Dscam-hv in Relation to Immunity, Sorted by Parasite or Immune Stimulant Used (cont.)

Parasite/Stimulant			Host		Experimental Evidence				R
Species P	a	b	Species	LHS	Constitutive Exon mRNA Expression	Alternatively Spliced Exon mRNA Expression	RNAi/ Mutagenesis	Cellular/ Binding Assays	
							Dscam-hv deficient mosquitoes: number of oocysts in midgut ↑ cf. control injected mosquitoes. Knockdown of exon 4.1 ↑oocyst load, but silencing *P. berghei* infection-responsive exon 4.14 did not affect susceptibility to *P. falciparum* (Ora)		46
						Whole body cDNA sequencing; combination of Ig2 and Ig3 splice variants more diverse after infection; Multiple *P. falciparum* genotype infections meant more diverse splice variants compared to a single genotype. (Ora: 24 h)			43

	Species	LHS			Ref.
	A. stephensi	Adu		Infection intensity in midgut ↓ in transgenic mosquitoes overexpressing two splice variants that in A. gambiae are induced after infection with P. falciparum (Ora)	Antibody staining showed ↑ association of AgDscam-hv with P. falciparum ookinetes in transgenic mosquitoes expressing splice variants that in A. gambiae are induced after infection with P. falciparum (Ora)	46
Plasmodium gallinaceum	Aedes aegypti	Adu		Fat body; genome wide microarray; ↑two Dscam genes (Ora: 24 h)		39

The nature of the experimental evidence is split into four categories.

a: Phylogenetic information on parasite or immune stimulant is shown in bold. If eukaryotic or prokaryotic parasites were used, they were administered: Al, alive; De, dead; MI, microbe associated molecular pattern (MAMP); Sp, spores; and if bacteria whether: G–, Gram negative or G+, Gram positive. ?, Information regarding whether the immune stimulants used were alive or dead was not explicitly given; NA, not applicable.

Species P: The species of parasite or immune stimulant used. Abbreviations include: Ev, recombinantly expressed envelope proteins; Mixed, Curdlan (β-1,3-glucan) from Alcaligenes faecalis, E. coli and M. luteus; PGN, peptidoglycan; P. interp. g. v., Plodia interpunctella granulosis virus; P. aeruginosa, Pseudomonas aeruginosa; RFP, expressing red fluorescent protein; S. cerevisiae, Saccharomyces cerevisiae.

b: The subphyla of arthropod host used: C, crustacean; I, insect.

LHS, Life history stage; Adu, adult; Cel, cell culture; Emb, embryo; Int, intermoult; Juv, juvenile; NA, not applicable; NI, no information.

Experimental evidence: in parentheses at the end of comments, information about the way in which the parasites were administered: Inj, injection; Ora, oral infection; Sep, septic wound. Also stated, time post infection at which Dscam-hv mRNA was assayed; NI, no information. ↑ Indicates increase and ↓ indicates decrease.

R, references.

Modified from Ref. [20].

When considering functional categories of the parasite, it is only microparasites, that is, those up to a few hundred micrometers in size,[36] including viruses, bacteria, fungi, and protozoa, which have been tested in relation to Dscam-hv and immunity. The majority of the tested species are bacteria, which have been introduced into the host in either a live or a dead state, and mainly through the cuticle via injection or with a needle covered in a bacterial solution. Moving to the hosts, a handful of crustacean and insect species have been tested to date, with particular emphasis on the whiteleg shrimp, *Litopenaeus vannamei*, and the mosquito, *A. gambiae*. Furthermore, it is largely cell lines or the adult, rather than the juvenile, life-history stage that has been tested. It is not always straightforward to make generalizations on the behavior of Dscam-hv from the available data (Table 10.1); for example, if one considers whether general Dscam-hv mRNA expression changes after exposure to a parasite or immune stimulant, one observes that of the 18 examples cited (Table 10.1), 7 show no modulation (increased or decreased transcription rate) of Dscam-hv at any of the time points studied. Studies that have reported upregulation in mRNA transcripts of Dscam-hv upon pathogen exposure, have shown relatively small (<10-fold[37–40]), or sometimes stronger (10–100-fold[38,41]), changes in relative expression, in terms of effect size, when compared to control groups. Furthermore, of the species where expression is changed, this can be early (eg, 2 h[42]), or relatively late (eg, 5 days[38]), after exposure. Clearly, interpretations are limited to the time points studied; in the majority of cases, a time-span between 2 h and 5 days has been used.

It might be the case that in addition to/instead of quantitative changes in Dscam-hv transcription after infection, that there are qualitative changes in the expression of exon repertoires. To date, *A. gambiae* has shown the most promising evidence to support pathogen-specific splice-variant expression after exposure to parasites. Dead bacteria introduced into the hemocoel, as well as live-ingested *Plasmodium* species, elicited variability in the expression of different splice variants from Ig2.[10] Staying with *A. gambiae*, multiple genotype infections of live *P. falciparum* resulted in more diverse Ig2 and Ig3 variants, compared to infection with a single parasite genotype.[43] However, RNA sequencing of splice variants after exposure of *D. melanogaster* or *Daphnia magna* to live bacteria did not result in strong variation in the expression of exons from Ig2, Ig3, or Ig7.[43,44]

Dscam-hv knockdown via RNAi or mutagenesis has mainly been used in *D. melanogaster* and *A. gambiae*: in both species it has helped to elucidate the fact that Dscam-hv is involved in phagocytosis of dead bacteria.[10,19] However, it is interesting to note that *D. melanogaster* Dscam-hv loss-of-function embryos showed no impairment in binding live *E. coli* compared to wild-type embryos.[45] Once again, *A. gambiae* showed strong support for parasite-mediated responses in Dscam-hv, and indeed the highest level of specificity/involvement of particular exons to certain parasites: RNAi of *A. gambiae* exon 4.8 resulted in reduced adult survival after infection with live *E. coli*, but not after infection with *S. aureus*,[10] and vice-versa results were found for exon 4.1. This is the only published study that we are aware of to-date to have examined whether Dscam-hv is important for survival in the face of pathogen challenge. The same research group more recently inserted Dscam-hv splice variants from *A. gambiae*, which were induced after infection with *P. falciparum*, into *A. stephensi*: this resulted in a reduction of infection intensity in *A. stephensi* midgut after *P. falciparum* infection.[46] These results and similar earlier experiments on *A. gambiae*[10] are also the only data to-date indicating a direct role for Dscam-hv in parasite resistance.

Most experiments described in Table 10.1 have attempted to quantify expression of Dscam mRNA. However, it is becoming increasingly evident that the correlation between mRNA and protein abundance varies widely across genes.[47] Only a limited number of studies have addressed Dscam-hv on the protein level (Table 10.1), which we will discuss in more detail in the following section. The ways in which Dscam-hv interacts with other known molecules in the immune system[46,48,49] has been reviewed in Ref. [21] so it will not be covered here.

2.2 How Has Dscam-hv Been Predicted to Function in Arthropod Immunity?

The initial findings from *D. melanogaster* suggested that Dscam-hv is used during phagocytosis of pathogens, and it was proposed that it might be a signaling receptor or coreceptor during this process.[19] The same authors showed that when combinations of three variable Ig domains were recombinantly expressed that this was sufficient to bind live *E. coli*, which led to the hypothesis that secreted isoforms might opsonize pathogens.[19] The experiments by Dong et al.,[10] led them to the conclusion that Dscam-hv in *A. gambiae* acts as a hypervariable pattern-recognition receptor, and among many other results, they found that when confronted with a pathogen, Dscam-hv responds by producing distinctive splice variants for the different pathogens tested. In the following we discuss some of the ideas that have been stimulated from the aforementioned two studies, and discuss other more recent observations and empirical data regarding how Dscam-hv could and does function mechanistically in an immunity context.

2.3.1 Is There an Amplification of Specific Dscam-hv Isoforms in Response to an Immune Challenge?

Let us now make the assumption that Dscam-hv isoforms bind parasites with some degree of specificity. What concentrations of each isoform would be necessary to elicit an efficient immune response? The number of isoforms expressed by hemocytes and by the fat body compared to nervous system tissues is considerably reduced in *D. melanogaster*[19,50] and in *Da. magna*.[8] For instance, populations of *D. melanogaster* hemocytes can express the vast majority of alternative variants from exons 4 and 6, but unlike, for example, the larval brain, only five exons from the exon 9 cluster are highly expressed.[19,50] Our rough calculations based on the numbers of *D. melanogaster* exons from the three extracellular Ig domains that were found to be expressed by hemocytes and fat bodies in microarray studies,[19,50] suggest that a subset of just over half of the estimated 18,496 isoforms[51] would actually be found in these tissues. Individual *D. melanogaster* hemocytes subjected to RT-PCR followed by a microarray, showed that each of the limited number of hemocytes tested expressed at least two to fourteen different isoforms of Dscam-hv.[50] A restricted isoform repertoire of hemocytes could result in higher concentrations of each isoform, thus increasing their functional capacity. Yet, would a limited number of hemocytes expressing a few different isoforms have a meaningful immune action? How would this signal be amplified to reach a "critical amount"? It has been suggested that there could be proliferation of hemocytes expressing the "appropriate" Dscam-hv variants related to a particular antigen.[33] There is evidence that in *D. melanogaster* adults, hemocytes can proliferate after infection,[52] but it is unknown whether these cells would have specific properties enhanced by the elicitor. If hemocytes were to collectively change transcription, how would this be signaled? Although there is some evidence that whole-gene Dscam-hv transcription increases after immune challenge (Table 10.1), and that in mosquitoes there is amplification of specific Dscam-hv Ig2 variants,[10] amplification of specific Ig3 and Ig7 variants has not been demonstrated. Furthermore, how amplification of specific splice variants might occur remains an open question.

2.3.2 Soluble Forms of Dscam-hv Occur in the Hemolymph as the Result of an Active "Shedding" Process,[33] and These Forms Act as Opsonins

Watson et al.[19] observed a *Dscam*-hv protein of reduced molecular weight compared to the whole protein in *D. melanogaster* S2 cell conditioned-medium and in hemolymph serum, although the sizes of the proteins indicate something smaller than what might be predicted, if only the cytoplasmic tail and the transmembrane domain had been left behind after proteolytic cleavage of the extracellular domain.[35] The shrimp species, *L. vannamei* and *Penaeus monodon*, and the Chinese mitten crab, *E. sinensis*, have Dscam-hv variants that lack the transmembrane domain and cytoplasmic tail, respectively. Rather than undergoing proteolytic cleavage, they are therefore suggested to be expressed directly in a secreted form.[53–55] Interestingly, *L. vannamei* has been shown to upregulate expression of the tailless Dscam-hv form after infection with WSSV[41] (Table 10.1). In their model for how Dscam-hv may trigger phagocytosis, Ng et al[21] thus postulated that a pathogen might stimulate proteolytic cleavage, or stimulate the direct secretion of tailless Dscam.

It is unknown whether the secreted Dscam-hv acts as an opsonin, that is, binds to an antigen and in this way boosts phagocytosis,[34] although some recombinantly expressed Dscam-hv isoforms have been shown to bind to bacteria.[19,40]

2.3.3 Membrane-Bound Dscam-hv Acts as a Receptor for Phagocytosis

Dscam-hv RNAi, or incubating cells with a Dscam-hv antibody, have been shown to reduce phagocytosis of dead *E. coli* in *D. melanogaster* larvae and S2 cells[19] (Table 10.1); furthermore, mosquito Sua5B cells showed reduced phagocytosis of dead *E. coli* and *S. aureus*[10] (Table 10.1). Dscam-hv has also been implicated in phagocytosis of the same two bacteria species as in *P. leniusculus*.[37] Dscam-hv would presumably be predicted to be involved in the phagocytosis of live and nonfluorescently labeled parasites in addition to dead and labeled bacteria, although this has not yet been tested. It has been proposed that membrane-bound Dscam-hv acts as a receptor for phagocytosis, either by directly interacting with a pathogen or by interacting with a *Dscam*-hv protein that is already bound to a pathogen.[21,34]

2.3.4 How Could Dscam-hv Bind to Antigens?

The first four Ig domains of Dscam-hv have been referred to as having a horseshoe conformation (Section 1.2).[22] In the cell-adhesion molecule hemolin, the horseshoe structure has been demonstrated to create a binding site to bacterial lipopolysaccharides.[24] In Dscam-hv, parts of the Ig2 and Ig3 domains encoded by the exons 4 and 6 form two surface epitopes on either side of the horseshoe structure. One of those epitopes (epitope I) is essential for the formation of Dscam-hv dimers, that is, for homophilic binding, which mediates cell-to-cell recognition in the nervous system.[22] The other epitope (epitope II) is oriented toward the external environment of the Dscam-hv dimer.[22] When comparing individual alternatively spliced exons between *Drosophila* species (orthologous exons), the amino-acid sequence of the region involved in homophilic binding, that is, epitope I, is conserved, yet the sequences of epitope II show little conservation, suggesting faster sequence evolution, perhaps as a result of the interaction with antigens.[22] In contrast, comparisons within *D. melanogaster* duplicated exons (paralogous exons) within each cluster show that the amino-acid sequence of alternatively spliced isoforms is diverse at both epitopes I and II.[56] These two findings suggest that both epitopes I and II diverged extensively before speciation, but at some point during the evolution of Dscam-hv exons stopped diverging, with the exception of the regions encoding epitope II. If parasite-induced selection were the main reason for the sequence divergence found in epitope II regions, signatures of molecular evolution compatible with positive selection would be expected, and have indeed been found for other genes involved in insect immunity.[57,58] Such signatures have been inferred for several *Drosophila* species and for the crustaceans *Daphnia pulex* and *Da. magna* for both epitopes I and II.[56] The results did not unequivocally suggest that positive selection was the main force that maintained diversity of epitope II,[6] yet the number of available sequences was low, precluding robust tests.[6] Intraspecific comparisons denoted an excess of nonsynonymous polymorphisms in epitope II regions encoded by exon 6, which would be compatible with selection mediated by parasite recognition.[56] However, those polymorphisms were mostly present at low frequencies in the populations, and could therefore be interpreted as the result of a relaxed selection acting on epitope II coding sequences.[56]

To date, the above elegant solution for how Dscam-hv might simultaneously function in heterophilic and homophilic binding, lacks empirical evidence showing that epitope II is involved in heterophilic interactions. In the nervous system, only the molecule Netrin engaging in heterophilic interactions with Dscam-hv has been characterized,[59,60] but the exact binding sites are not known.

3 THE EVOLUTIONARY HISTORY OF DSCAM-HV IN ARTHROPODS

In this section, we will briefly review how comparative evolutionary analysis of Dscam genes across different organisms has contributed to our understanding of how Dscam-hv has evolved, and to our understanding of the parts of the molecule that seem to be under stronger functional constraints, or alternatively, evolve faster. Such insights may provide us with information regarding which parts of Dscam-hv are more likely to be important in the interaction with parasites.

3.1 The Origin of Dscam

Cell adhesion molecules were needed early in evolution for intercellular cohesion and communication in multicellular organisms.[61] Throughout the evolution of metazoans, cell adhesion molecules (CAMs) have been recruited for many different cellular functions, such as cell proliferation and differentiation, apoptosis, migration, and parasite recognition.[62,63] Many members of this family are at least in part built from Ig domains,[64] and several show relatively high molecular diversity that is also associated with alternative splicing.[65,66] Similar to Dscam, the tertiary conformation of the first four Ig domains of several CAMs is that of a horseshoe shape (Fig. 10.1), which creates, as mentioned previously, singular adhesive properties by allowing homophilic and heterophilic adhesion to similar and different proteins, respectively. The appearance of this structure might have allowed for the expansion of a subfamily of CAMs used by nervous system cells, such as, among others, axonin, roundabout, contactin, and Dscam, and by immune system cells such as hemolin and Dscam.[67] Precursors of Dscam could have been present before the evolution of the Bilateria, for example, although lacking a canonical Dscam organization, some genes in the cnidarian *Nemastostella vectensis* (Fig. 10.2) and in the sponge *Amphimedon*

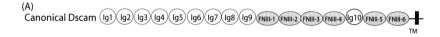

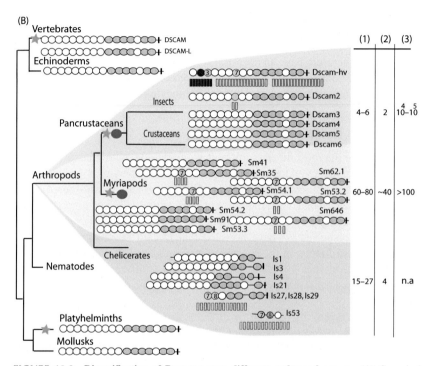

FIGURE 10.2 Diversification of Dscam across different arthropod groups. (A) Canonical composition of Dscam ectodomains; (B) general representation of Dscam molecules in different animal groups. In chelicerates and myriapods (here represented by *Ixodes scapularis* and *S. maritima*), only some representative molecules are indicated. In the cases where Ig domains are encoded by clusters of exons, the latter are represented by small rectangles using the same color code as Fig. 10.1, except for Ig8 encoding exons, which are light purple. (1) Range of number of paralogous Dscam genes present in representatives of pancrustaceans, myriapods, and chelicerates; (2) number of Dscam genes containing cluster of duplicated exons; (3) range of number of potential isoforms produced. The green stars and blue circles indicate animal groups where Dscam has been shown to be expressed or used by the nervous and immune system, respectively.

queenslandica have Ig domains with strong amino-acid conservation when compared to Dscam.[67] In addition, cytoplasmic motifs such as SH2,[2] ITIM,[68] and polyproline motifs are conserved between the NV 1 protein of *N. vectensis* and the human Dscams, indicating that they use similar signaling pathways.[67] This suggests that some of the Dscam features characteristic of complex groups such as vertebrates might have already evolved in early metazoans. The phylogenetic reconstruction of available Dscam molecules from the main animal groups suggests that the ancestral forms of Dscam were used by the nervous system and that its usage by immune cells is a derived state.[67,69] The usage by immune system cells seems to have evolved concurrently with mechanisms of molecular diversification, such as duplication and mutually exclusive alternative splicing in Dscam. However, care must be taken because this association does not necessarily imply causality. Hemocytes have several important functions unrelated to immunity throughout the embryonic development of insects.[70] Dscam could therefore have an ancestral role of mediating cellular recognition. Light will only be shed on the ancestral functions of Dscam by performing more studies addressing its role in hemocytes or hemocyte-related cells.

3.2 Dscam Radiation in Arthropods

Arthropods are the most diverse group of animal phyla, with an enormous variety of morphologies and ecological niches.[71] This diversity is grouped into four major extant groups: insects and crustaceans, which are considered sister groups (pancrustaceans),[72] myriapods and chelicerates.[73,74] The completion of genome-sequencing projects of the centipede *S. maritima*, a myriapod, and several chelicerate species[75,76] have revealed that Dscam has also diversified in these groups. Strikingly, in the species of myriapod and chelicerate studied to date, Dscam diversification has occurred through a different mechanism than that of pancrustaceans, that is, via dozens of whole-gene duplications of Dscam (Fig. 10.2).

By superimposing the genealogy of the Dscam gene family in arthropods, on the consensual reconstructions of the phylogenetic relationships between the main arthropods groups, it becomes evident that the most basal arthropod Dscams are the ones of the chelicerates.[67,77] In the tick, *I. scapularis*, there are around 27 genes with strong similarity to Dscam genes. The *I. scapularis* genes do not have a canonical domain organization but are clearly Dscam homologs, that is, they share a common ancestor with other metazoan Dscams.[67] Furthermore, the genome of *I. scapularis* has incomplete Dscam proteins containing duplicated exons coding for Ig7 and Ig8 (Fig. 10.2). Five additional chelicerate species have since been predicted to have between 4 and 35 Dscam gene copies.[76] In the myriapod *S. maritima*, 60–80 duplications of whole Dscam genes have occurred (Fig. 10.2).[67] Unlike what has been found in *I. scapularis*, a high number of these Dscam paralogs have a canonical domain organization.[67] In addition to whole-gene duplications, approximately half of the *S. maritima* paralogs have internal duplications of the exons coding Ig7, but not of exons coding for Ig2 and Ig3 Dscam domains (Figs. 10.2 and 10.3).[67] What is the relationship between Dscam-hv and the remaining paralogs of the pancrustaceans, and the Dscams of the myriapods and chelicerates? These Dscam sensu lato sequences have diverged extensively and confident phylogenetic inferences of the relationships among Dscam members of pancrustaceans and myriapods and chelicerates are difficult to infer.[67,69,77] However, some patterns can be drawn: (1) the extensive whole-gene duplications of *I. scapularis* and *S. maritima* probably originated

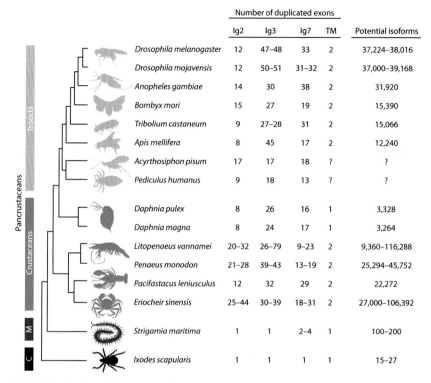

		Number of duplicated exons				
		Ig2	Ig3	Ig7	TM	Potential isoforms
	Drosophila melanogaster	12	47–48	33	2	37,224–38,016
	Drosophila mojavensis	12	50–51	31–32	2	37,000–39,168
	Anopheles gambiae	14	30	38	2	31,920
	Bombyx mori	15	27	19	2	15,390
	Tribolium castaneum	9	27–28	31	2	15,066
	Apis mellifera	8	45	17	2	12,240
	Acyrthosiphon pisum	17	17	18	?	?
	Pediculus humanus	9	18	13	?	?
	Daphnia pulex	8	26	16	1	3,328
	Daphnia magna	8	24	17	1	3,264
	Litopenaeus vannamei	20–32	26–79	9–23	2	9,360–116,288
	Penaeus monodon	21–28	39–43	13–19	2	25,294–45,752
	Pacifastacus leniusculus	12	32	29	2	22,272
	Eriocheir sinensis	25–44	30–39	18–31	2	27,000–106,392
	Strigamia maritima	1	1	2–4	1	100–200
	Ixodes scapularis	1	1	1	1	15–27

FIGURE 10.3   **Dscam-hv alternatively spliced exon radiation across the arthropods.** The number of known or putative alternatively spliced exons for Ig2, Ig3, and Ig7, as well as the transmembrane (TM) domain, are indicated for each species. Where within studies, or across studies, a range of potential alternatively spliced exon numbers has been given, this is indicated by the dashed line between numbers. "?" indicates that no information exists. Different estimates across studies may be due to, for example, lack of mRNA expression of sequenced variants (eg, *D. melanogaster* Ig3, exon 6.11), different sequence predictions in silico (eg, *T. castaneum* Ig3), and lack of full-length sequencing of the Dscam-hv loci. The maximum theoretical numbers (or range) of potential isoforms that could be produced from these alternatively spliced exons is shown to the right, assuming independent splicing. Data on exon numbers comes from Refs. [2,8,19,37,41,42,51,53–55, 69,77,79]. The tree at the left indicates the species relationships (taken from Refs. [80–84]), but the branch lengths are uninformative. *Bars* to the left indicate the four main subphyla within the arthropods, where M indicates myriapods and C indicates chelicerates.

independently, or they were inherited from a common ancestor and diverged so extensively that a common origin can no longer be ascertained; (2) the domain organization of the Dscam genes of myriapods are more similar to the ones of pancrustaceans than to the chelicerates, in agreement with the view that myriapods are a basal group to pancrustaceans, sharing a common ancestor with the latter, which is not shared by chelicerates[74,75]; (3) Dscam Ig7 domains were the first domains to engage in duplications (it is not clear whether Ig7 and Ig8 belong to functional Dscam genes in *I. scapularis*[67]); (4) the three clusters of duplicated exons coding for half of Ig2 and Ig3 domains are a derived character which appeared for the first time in pancrustaceans; (5) despite generally low conservation between the cytoplasmic tails of pancrustacean Dscam-hv paralogs, all pancrustacean Dscam-hv's and Dscam genes of *S. maritima* shown to be expressed by hemocytes, share motifs CC1 (involved in axon guidance signaling pathways and in leukocyte mobility control[78]), which are not in other Dscam paralogs.[35]

What about the origins of the Dscam mechanism of mutually exclusive alternative splicing? The Ig7 exon duplications of *S. maritima* Dscam undergo mutually exclusive alternative splicing, indicating that this character evolved before the evolution of Dscam-hv of pancrustaceans.[67] In *I. scapularis* Dscam expression has not been studied, but *I. scapularis* lacks several genes that operate as splicing factors in *D. melanogaster* Dscam.[35]

The in silico reconstruction of the Dscam genes found in *I. scapularis* and *S. maritima* suggest that many of these genes are functional.[67,77] What are the functions of this myriad of Dscam genes? In *S. maritima*, Dscam expression has been observed both in organs of the nervous systems and in hemocytes,[67] consistent with a role both in the nervous and the immune systems (but also generally in development, as referred to previously). Other interesting aspects from the in silico reconstructions are (1) that a high diversity of Dscam forms had already evolved in myriapods and chelicerates; (2) in the tick *I. scapularis* Dscam molecules with alternative transmembrane domains such as in insects were found; (3) Dscam putative soluble forms were found, as is seen in decapod crustaceans.[54,55] The genetic diversification of Dscam in arthropods might have meant that Dscam acquired new functions in these animals, but detailed functional studies in basal arthropods are needed to address this question. Based on the data available, it seems plausible that the extensive Dscam duplications as seen in chelicerates and myriapods were the raw material from which Dscam-hv evolved in the ancestors of the pancrustaceans.

3.3 The Evolutionary History of Dscam-hv in Pancrustaceans

In pancrustaceans the number of Dscam paralogs is much lower than in myriapods and chelicerates, ranging from four to six, depending on the species.[54,77] Some of these paralogs have been predicted in silico,[67,77] but expression and functional data also exists for other paralogs.[4,85] The majority of paralogs have been described for insects; in crustaceans they have only been described for *D. pulex*[67] (but no other full crustacean genome sequence is available). Of all pancrustacean Dscams, only the hypervariable gene Dscam-hv and another member called Dscam2[4] (AbSCAM in *Apis mellifera*[86]), which has two exon duplications encoded in Ig7, have duplications of alternative exons. Both Dscam-hv and Dscam2 are essential for the correct development of the nervous system in flies.[2,4,87] These are also the only two Dscam paralogs for which a common ancestry to all pancrustacean species with available genomic sequences can be found. Given the situation described for myriapods, additional Dscam genes were most likely also present in the ancestor of the pancrustaceans, but these were lost and/or diverged extensively in different pancrustacean groups, maybe because their functions are not as essential as the ones of Dscam-hv and Dscam2. The loss of Dscam paralogs in the ancestor of pancrustaceans, and the appearance of Dscam-hv seems to reflect the evolution toward a more efficient mechanism of regulating the expression of Dscam isoform diversity, that is, expression of a high repertoire of isoforms from a single gene.[35]

In Dscam-hv across pancrustaceans, the constitutive domains and the domains that result from alternatively spliced exons display considerably different levels of sequence conservation. A comparison between crustaceans and insects reveals high amino-acid conservation of the constitutive domains (around 60% identity over the complete extracellular domains), despite the fact that these groups are predicted to have last shared a common ancestor around 420 million years ago[72] The domains that result from exons that undergo alternative splicing are, on the contrary, considerably more divergent than constitutive exons when comparing crustaceans and insects, and even when comparing within certain insect groups.[67,77,88] The constitutive and alternative domains of Dscam-hv thus have had different evolutionary histories: whereas the former have evolved mainly under purifying selection probably related to the essentiality of Dscam-hv, the exons encoding the alternative domains have, at least during a certain period, diversified and expanded independently in different pancrustacean groups. It remains unclear if that diversification had been driven by positive selection (ie, was adaptive).[56,89] Alternatively, spliced exons could have diverged under a period of relative selective relaxation ("relative" because key residues remained conserved among paralogs), perhaps due to the redundancy of the duplicated sequences.[56] A recent study inferred positive selection acting to promote the divergence of Dscam-hv Ig7 orthologous domains in the social insects *A. mellifera*, *Apis florea*, *Bombus impatiens*, and *Bombus terrestris*.[88] The test was, however, based inadvertently on alignments of paralogous sequences of Ig7 coding sequences, which have diverged too extensively to be aligned reliably.

Regardless of the context in which diversity among paralogs was generated, Dscam-hv diversity became essential for survival, as referred to already. Accordingly, in extant pancrustacean species, selection acts to preserve Dscam diversity both by keeping the number and the sequences of the alternative exons unchanged, by preventing gene conversion to homogenize exon sequences.[8,56,67] However, the extent of the action of purifying selection seems to differ in the three clusters of alternative exons, as we shall discuss next.

3.4   Dscam Clusters of Duplicated Exons

The three alternative exon clusters in Dscam-hv have arisen by reiterative exon duplication and deletion.[88] For the sake of simplicity, we will use the exon nomenclature of the *D. melanogaster* Dscam-hv, that is, exons 4, exons 6, and exons 9. Generally, the exon duplications of Dscam-hv are believed to be the outcome of homologous recombination among neighboring exons with similar sequence composition.[88] A feature common to the exons of the three clusters is that exons resulting from duplication (paralogs) diverged extensively, whereas exons resulting from speciation (orthologs) are conserved. As an example, the *Drosophila* species or *Daphnia* species that have been examined have their own "set" of alternative exons, indicating that alternative exons evolved independently in different pancrustacean groups.[8,77,88] When looking within each taxonomic genus, duplicated exons (paralogs) are quite diverse, but the vast majority of paralogs have an orthologous exon in the other con-generic species (with some exceptions for clusters of exons 6 and 9).[8,77,88] This suggests that most exons duplicated and diverged by accumulating mutations in the ancestors of each genus. The high conservation of amino-acid sequences of orthologous exons indicates that they had not diverged much since the split of the extant species from their most recent common ancestor, indicating that selection acts to preserve the ancient diversity that had been created. An exception to this is amino-acid sequence variation in the orthologous regions of exons 4 and 6 that encode epitope II, as discussed previously. Despite this general pattern of sequence evolution, the three clusters of exons seem to have undergone different patterns of exon radiation.[8,69,77,88] (Fig. 10.3). The number of exons in cluster 4 tends to be more conserved among species of the same genus, whereas exons of clusters 6 and 9 seem to have higher duplication rates.[88] This could reflect that the different clusters specialized in different functions prior to species divergence, as suggested by Crayton and coworkers,[69] which is an attractive hypothesis, given the dual role of Dscam-hv in the nervous and immune systems.[31] Alternatively, it could also simply reflect protein structural constraints.[77]

3.5 Are the Patterns of Dscam-hv Molecular Evolution Compatible with a Role in Immunity?

Genes involved in the immune system typically present signatures of diversifying selection, for example, the MHC locus presents hallmarks of balancing selection, such as elevated polymorphisms and deeply diverged transpecific alleles. In Dscam-hv, strong signatures of parasite-imposed selection currently acting in populations have not been found.[56] However, perhaps such signatures will not be very apparent within a population because the variability of Dscam-hv is obtained via somatic combinatorial arrangements of variable exons and is thus not inherited. As referred to previously, selection seems to act to preserve ancient Dscam-hv diversity. It is entirely possible that such diversity has been advantageous for the nervous system, yet why would the usage of Dscam-hv in the nervous system select for different "sets" of exons in different animal groups? Why would selection imposed by the nervous system select for soluble forms of Dscam? It is now around 10 years since the discovery that Dscam-hv is involved in insect immunity, and although much progress has been made in deciphering what it might do in the face of pathogen challenge, there are abundant unanswered questions. In the following section we discuss some problems, open questions, speculations/ideas, and potential avenues for future research on Dscam-hv in immunity.

4 EXPERIMENTAL METHODOLOGY AND FUTURE PERSPECTIVES

4.1 Experimental Methodology: Choice of Experimental Host and Parasite/Antigen, and Other Experimental Parameters

Which host species should be used? This will to some degree relate to the question at hand: for example, a large crustacean would be a suitable model for testing whether specific proliferation of hemocytes occurs, and for examining whether regulation of alternative splicing occurs during an immune response since large amounts of hemolymph can be withdrawn. What is the origin of the experimental animals? It will be more controlled to use minimum laboratory F1 generation rather than directly using wild-caught animals with unknown previous exposure to parasites and pathogens. Furthermore, how do we choose the antigenic challenge? For example, does one use an off-the-shelf bacterium, or a microbial derivative that is highly controllable and has been used by others, potentially allowing for comparisons across studies? This approach relies on the assumption that Dscam-hv proteins could hypothetically react against any pathogen. Alternatively, does one use a pathogen that naturally occurs with the host, with the assumption that these pathogens might be ecologically relevant? Or does one use a pathogen that is coevolving with the host species? In this case, one might predict that other host immune-defense genes have been selected to respond to adapting parasite virulence genes. How would Dscam-hv respond in this case? Does Dscam-hv provide a certain degree of specificity toward parasites? If that is the case, then one would expect the Dscam-hv isoform repertoire to be deterministic, and therefore to be predictable in repeated experiments. If the repertoire is arbitrary then it would suggest that Dscam-hv diversity, but not the exact composition of the variable regions, is important. Conversely, if isoform variant expression is related to the infecting parasite, then it would imply that the amino-acid composition of the variable regions is important. If the latter were the case, then site-directed mutagenesis could be employed to test whether binding to the parasite is affected. Further considerations are: which infection doses should be used? This will be linked to the question at hand: to test survival after knockdown, some level of mortality would be desirable. However, when examining mRNA expression, is it more appropriate to have a nonlethal immune challenge that stimulates the immune system, or a strong challenge that causes significant mortality? Should the pathogen be administered alive or dead, and in what state would a host come across the pathogens in the wild? As touched upon previously (Section 2.1), which time point should be used postinfection to study, for example, mRNA expression, and how would Dscam-hv behave after a second challenge with the same parasite? Ideally, one would have a response profile covering a frequent and robust duration after infection, but this is often time- and financially demanding.

4.2 Future Perspectives

In Table 10.2, we have briefly summarized a few, of what we consider to be, outstanding questions relating to Dscam-hv's role in immunity.

TABLE 10.2 Some Open Questions and Avenues for Future Research on Dscam in Immunity

Question	Relevant Observations
1. Does isoform regulation occur at translation and/or secretion into the hemolymph?	The majority of studies have been done on RNA. Only one study on Dscam-hv peptide sequencing and this was not in relation to parasites.[19]
2. Which Dscam-hv epitopes interact with parasites?	
3. What is the Dscam-hv protein half-life?	
4. Why should Dscam-hv mediated cellular interactions be different in hemocytes and fat body compared to nervous-system cells?	Nervous system Dscam-hv functions in cell–cell signaling.[6] Dscam-hv could theoretically be involved in hemocyte–hemocyte, hemocyte–fat body or other cell interactions. Does knockdown affect cell–cell interactions, which secondarily affects immunity?
5. Does Dscam-hv play a role in maintaining / controlling hemolymph and gut bacterial fauna?	Dscam-hv RNAi resulted in increase in opportunistic bacteria in mosquito hemolymph.[10]
	Dscam-hv transgenic mosquitoes had reduced microbiota in gut.[46]
6. Do myriapod or chelicerate Dscam's play a role in immunity?	*S. maritima* and *I. scapularis* have multiple whole gene duplications of Dscam, but it is unknown if they have an immune role.[67] Dscam alternative splicing of Ig7 encoding exons is expressed by hemocytes of *S. maritima*.
7. Do insect Dscam-hv paralogs play a role in immunity?	Insects have multiple paralogs.[7,8,77] These have two, or no, alternatively spliced exons. Therefore, if a role in immunity exists, it would not be as a diverse pattern recognition receptor.
8. Are there specific signaling pathways activated in Dscam-hv related to immunity?	Dscam-hv has different cytoplasmic tails, which are used in different stages of nervous system morphogenesis. Furthermore, its cytoplasmic tails are rich in signaling motives, which could be related to role in immunity.[35]

5 CONCLUDING REMARKS

The immune system of arthropods is, similar to that of other invertebrates,"not homogeneous, not simple, not well understood."[90] The accumulation of genome projects from nonmodel species consistently reveals how different examples of molecular diversification have been selected for in nature.[91–94] The cells expressing diversity are in many cases not only committed to immune functions, and an understanding of how diversity is used is lacking, which complicates mechanistic inferences. Dissecting the function and evolution of the Dscam gene family in arthropods will be a challenging endeavor. However, it might be rewarded by improving considerably our understanding of the nervous and immune systems of these animals, and our understanding of how evolution has built this extremely complex solution to serve these two systems.

ACKNOWLEDGMENTS

We acknowledge Prof Louis Du Pasquier for fruitful discussions. We would like to thank Seth Barribeau and Louis du Plessis for allowing us access to their *Apis* and *Bombus* Dscam alignments and analysis.

REFERENCES

1. Yamakawa K, Huo Y-K, Haendel MA, Hubert R, Chen X-N, Lyons GE, et al. DSCAM: a novel member of the immunoglobulin superfamily maps in a Down syndrome region and is involved in the development of the nervous system. *Hum Mol Genet* 1998;**7**(2):227–37.
2. Schmucker D, Clemens JC, Shu H, Worby CA, Xiao J, Muda M, et al. *Drosophila* Dscam is an axon guidance receptor exhibiting extraordinary molecular diversity. *Cell* 2000; **101**(9):671–84.
3. Fusaoka E, Inoue T, Mineta K, Agata K, Takeuchi K. Structure and function of primitive immunoglobulin superfamily neural cell adhesion molecules: a lesson from studies on planarian. *Genes Cells* 2006;**11**(5):541–55.
4. Millard SS, Flanagan JJ, Pappu KS, Wu W, Zipursky SL. Dscam2 mediates axonal tiling in the *Drosophila* visual system. *Nature* 2007;**447**(7145):720-724.
5. Agarwala KL, Subramaniam G, Tsutsumi Y, Suzuki T, Kenji A, Yamakawa K. Cloning and functional characterization of DSCAML1, a novel DSCAM-like cell adhesion molecule that mediates homophilic intercellular adhesion. *Biochem Biophys Res Commun* 2001;**285**:760–72.
6. Zipursky SL, Grueber WB. The molecular basis of self-avoidance. *Annu Rev Neurosci* 2013;**36**:547–668.
7. Vogel C, Teichmann SA, Chothia C. The immunoglobulin superfamily in *Drosophila melanogaster* and *Caenorhabditis elegans* and the evolution of complexity. *Development* 2003;**130**(25):6317–28.
8. Brites D, McTaggart S, Morris K, Anderson J, Thomas K, Colson I, et al. The Dscam homologue of the crustacean *Daphnia* is diversified by alternative splicing like in insects. *Mol Biol Evol* 2008;**25**(7):1429–39.
9. St Pierre SE, Ponting L, Stefancsik R, McQuilton P. FlyBase 102—advanced approaches to interrogating FlyBase. *Nucleic Acids Res* 2014;**42**(Database issue):D780–8.

10. Dong Y, Taylor HE, Dimopoulos G. AgDdscam, a hypervariable immunoglobulin domain-containing receptor of the *Anopheles gambiae* innate immune system. *PLoS Biol* 2006;**4**(7):e229.
11. Hattori D, Millard SS, Wojtowicz WM, Zipursky SL. Dscam-mediated cell recognition regulates neural circuit formation. *Annu Rev Cell Dev Biol* 2008;**24**:597–620.
12. Yu HH, Yang JS, Wang J, Huang Y, Lee T. Endodoamin diversity in the *Drosophila* Dscam and its roles in neuronal morphogenesis. *J Neurosci* 2009;**29**(6):1904–14.
13. Hughes ME, Bortnick R, Tsubouchi A, Baumer P, Kondo M, Uemura T, et al. Homophilic Dscam interactions control complex dendrite morphogenesis. *Neuron* 2007;**54**(3):417–27.
14. Soba P, Zhu S, Emoto K, Younger S, Yang SJ, Yu HH, et al. *Drosophila* sensory neurons require Dscam for dendritic self-avoidance and proper dendritic field organization. *Neuron* 2007;**54**(3):403–16.
15. Matthews BJ, Kim ME, Flanagan JJ, Hattori D, Clemens JC, Zipursky SL, et al. Dendrite self-avoidance is controlled by Dscam. *Cell* 2007;**129**(3):593–604.
16. Chen BE, Kondo M, Garnier A, Watson FL, Püettmann-Holgado R, Lamar DR, et al. The molecular diversity of Dscam is functionally required for neuronal wiring specificity in *Drosophila*. *Cell* 2006;**125**:607–20.
17. Wojtowicz WM, Flanagan JJ, Millard SS, Zipursky SL. Alternative splicing of *Drosophila* Dscam generates axon guidance receptors that exhibit isoform-specific homophilic binding. *Cell* 2004;**118**(5):619–33.
18. Wojtowicz WM, Wu W, Andre I, Qian B, Baker D, Zipursky SL. A vast repertoire of Dscam binding specificities arises from modular interactions of variable ig domains. *Cell* 2007;**130**(6):1134–45.
19. Watson LF, Püttmann-Holgado FT, Thomas F, Lamar DL, Hughes M, Kondo M, et al. Extensive diversity of Ig-superfamily proteins in the immune system of insects. *Science (New York, NY)* 2005;**309**:1874–8.
20. Armitage SAO, Peuss R, Kurtz J. Dscam and pancrustacean immune memory—a review of the evidence. *Dev Comp Immunol* 2014;**19**:315–323.
21. Ng TH, Chiang YA, Yeh YC, Wang HC. Review of Dscam-mediated immunity in shrimp and other arthropods. *Dev Comp Immunol* 2014;**46**(2):129–38.
22. Meijers R, Puettmann-Holgado R, Skiniotis G, Liu J-H, Walz T, Wang J-H, et al. Structural basis of Dscam isoform specificity. *Nature* 2007;**449**:487–91.
23. Schurmann G, Haspel J, Grumet M, Erickson HP. Cell adhesion molecule L1 in folded (Horseshoe) and extended conformations. *Mol Biol Cell* 2001;**12**(6):1765–73.
24. Su XD, Gastinel LN, Vaughn DE, Faye I, Poon P, Bjorkman PJ. Crystal structure of hemolin: a horseshoe shape with implications for homophilic adhesion. *Science (New York, NY)* 1998;**281**(5379):991–5.
25. Sawaya MR, Wojtowicz WM, Andre I, Qian B, Wu W, Baker D, et al. A double S shape provides the structural basis for the extraordinary binding specificity of Dscam isoforms. *Cell* 2008;**134**(6):1007–18.
26. Kurtz J, Franz K. Evidence for memory in invertebrate immunity. *Nature* 2003;**425**:37–8.
27. Sadd BM, Schmid-Hempel P. Insect immunity shows specificity in protection upon secondary pathogen exposure. *Curr Biol* 2006;**16**(12):1206–10.
28. Pham LN, Dionne MS, Shirasu-Hiza M, Schneider DS. A specific primed immune response in *Drosophila* is dependent on phagocytes. *PLoS Pathog* 2007;**3**(3):e26.
29. Roth O, Kurtz J. Phagocytosis mediates specificity in the immune defence of an invertebrate, the woodlouse *Porcellio scaber* (Crustacea: isopoda). *Dev Comp Immunol* 2009;**33**(11):1151–5.

30. Masri L, Cremer S. Individual and social immunisation in insects. *Trends Immunol* 2014;**35**(10):471–82.
31. Pasquier LD. Insects diversify one molecule to serve two systems. *Science (New York, NY)* 2005;**309**(5742):1826–7.
32. Kurtz J, Armitage SAO. Alternative adaptive immunity in invertebrates. *Trends Immunol* 2006;**27**(11):493–6.
33. Boehm T. Two in one: dual function of an invertebrate antigen receptor. *Nat Immunol* 2007;**8**(10):1031–3.
34. Stuart LM, Ezekowitz RA. Phagocytosis and comparative innate immunity: learning on the fly. *Nat Rev Immunol* 2008;**8**(2):131–41.
35. Brites D, Du Pasquier L. Somatic and germline diversification of a putative immunoreceptor within one phylum: Dscam in arthropods. In: Hsu E, Du Pasquier L, editors. *Pathogen-host : antigenic variation v somatic adaptation*. Springer; 2015. p. 131–158.
36. Schmid-Hempel P. *Evolutionary parasitology*. Oxford: Oxford University Press; 2011.
37. Watthanasurorot A, Jiravanichpaisal P, Liu H, Soderhall I, Soderhall K. Bacteria-induced Dscam isoforms of the crustacean, *Pacifastacus leniusculus*. *PLoS Pathog* 2011;**7**(6):e1002062.
38. Schwarz RS, Evans JD. Single and mixed-species trypanosome and microsporidia infections elicit distinct, ephemeral cellular and humoral immune responses in honey bees. *Dev Comp Immunol* 2013;**40**(3–4):300–10.
39. Zou Z, Souza-Neto J, Xi Z, Kokoza V, Shin SW, Dimopoulos G, et al. Transcriptome analysis of *Aedes aegypti* transgenic mosquitoes with altered immunity. *PLoS Pathog* 2011;**7**(11):e1002394.
40. Hung HY, Ng TH, Lin JH, Chiang YA, Chuang YC, Wang HC. Properties of *Litopenaeus vannamei* Dscam (LvDscam) isoforms related to specific pathogen recognition. *Fish Shellfish Immunol* 2013;**35**(4):1272–81.
41. Chiang YA, Hung HY, Lee CW, Huang YT, Wang HC. Shrimp Dscam and its cytoplasmic tail splicing activator serine/arginine (SR)-rich protein B52 were both induced after white spot syndrome virus challenge. *Fish Shellfish Immunol* 2013;**34**(1):209–19.
42. Jin XK, Li WW, Wu MH, Guo XN, Li S, Yu AQ, et al. Immunoglobulin superfamily protein Dscam exhibited molecular diversity by alternative splicing in hemocytes of crustacean, *Eriocheir sinensis*. *Fish Shellfish Immunol* 2013;**35**(3):900–9.
43. Smith PH, Mwangi JM, Afrane YA, Yan G, Obbard DJ, Ranford-Cartwright LC, et al. Alternative splicing of the *Anopheles gambiae* Dscam gene in diverse *Plasmodium falciparum* infections. *Malaria J* 2011;**10**:156.
44. Armitage SAO, Sun W, You X, Kurtz J, Schmucker D, Chen W. Quantitative profiling of *Drosophila melanogaster* Dscam1 isoforms reveals no changes in splicing after bacterial exposure. *PLoS One* 2014;**9**(10):e108660.
45. Vlisidou I, Dowling AJ, Evans IR, Waterfield N, ffrench-Constant RH, Wood W. *Drosophila* embryos as model systems for monitoring bacterial infection in real time. *PLoS Pathog* 2009;**5**(7):e1000518.
46. Dong Y, Cirimotich CM, Pike A, Chandra R, Dimopoulos G. Anopheles NF-kappaB-regulated splicing factors direct pathogen-specific repertoires of the hypervariable pattern recognition receptor AgDscam. *Cell Host Microbe* 2012;**12**(4):521–30.
47. Maier T, Guell M, Serrano L. Correlation of mRNA and protein in complex biological samples. *FEBS Lett* 2009;**583**(24):3966–73.
48. Olson S, Blanchette M, Park J, Savva Y, Yeo GW, Yeakley JM, et al. A regulator of Dscam mutually exclusive splicing fidelity. *Nat Struct Mol Biol* 2007;**14**(12):1134–40.

49. Lee CW, Chen IT, Chou PH, Hung HY, Wang KV. Heterogeneous nuclear ribonucleoprotein hrp36 acts as an alternative splicing repressor in *Litopenaeus vannamei* Dscam. *Dev Comp Immunol* 2012;**36**(1):10–20.

50. Neves G, Zucker J, Daly M, Chess A. Stochastic yet biased expression of multiple Dscam splice variants by individual cells. *Nat Genet* 2004;**36**:240–6.

51. Sun W, You X, Gogol-Doring A, He H, Kise Y, Sohn M, et al. Ultra-deep profiling of alternatively spliced *Drosophila* Dscam isoforms by circularization-assisted multi-segment sequencing. *EMBO J* 2013;**32**(14):2029–38.

52. Ghosh S, Singh A, Mandal S, Mandal L. Active hematopoietic hubs in *Drosophila* adults generate hemocytes and contribute to immune response. *Dev Cell* 2015;**33**(4):478–88.

53. Chou PH, Chang HS, Chen IT, Lin HY, Chen YM, Yang HL, et al. The putative invertebrate adaptive immune protein *Litopenaeus vannamei* Dscam (LvDscam) is the first reported Dscam to lack a transmembrane domain and cytoplasmic tail. *Dev Comp Immunol* 2009; **33**(12):1258–67.

54. Chou PH, Chang HS, Chen IT, Lee CW, Hung HY, Han-Ching Wang KC. *Penaeus monodon* Dscam (PmDscam) has a highly diverse cytoplasmic tail and is the first membrane-bound shrimp Dscam to be reported. *Fish Shellfish Immunol* 2011;**30**(4–5):1109–23.

55. Wang J, Wang L, Gao Y, Jiang Q, Yi Q, Zhang H, et al. A tailless Dscam from *Eriocheir sinensis* diversified by alternative splicing. *Fish Shellfish Immunol* 2013;**35**(2):249–61.

56. Brites D, Encinas-Viso F, Ebert D, Du Pasquier L, Haag CR. Population genetics of duplicated alternatively spliced exons of Dscam in *Daphnia* and *Drosophila*. *PLoS One* 2011;**6**(12):e27947.

57. Obbard DJ, Welch JJ, Kim KW, Jiggins FM. Quantifying adaptive evolution in the *Drosophila* immune system. *PLoS Genet* 2009;**5**(10):e1000698.

58. Obbard DJ, Callister DM, Jiggins FM, Soares DC, Yan G, Little TJ. The evolution of TEP1, an exceptionally polymorphic immunity gene in *Anopheles gambiae*. *BMC Evol Biol* 2008;**8**:274.

59. Lai Wing Sun K, Correia JP, Kennedy TE. Netrins: versatile extracellular cues with diverse functions. *Development* 2011;**138**(11):2153–69.

60. Andrews GL, Tanglao S, Farmer WT, Morin S, Brotman S, Berberoglu MA, et al. Dscam guides embryonic axons by netrin-dependent and -independent functions. *Development* 2008;**135**(23):3839–48.

61. Hynes RO, Zhao Q. The evolution of cell adhesion. *J Cell Biol* 2000;**150**(2):F89–95.

62. Buckley CD, Rainger GE, Bradfield PF, Nash GB, Simmons DL. Cell adhesion: more than just glue (review). *Mol Membr Biol* 1998;**15**(4):167–76.

63. Humphries MJ, Newham P. The structure of cell-adhesion molecules. *Trends Cell Biol* 1998;**8**(2):78–83.

64. Chothia C, Jones EY. The molecular structure of cell adhesion molecules. *Annu Rev Biochem* 1997;**66**:823–62.

65. Kohmura N, Senzaki K, Hamada S, Kai N, Yasuda R, Watanabe M, et al. Diversity revealed by a novel family of cadherins expressed in neurons at a synaptic complex. *Neuron* 1998;**20**(6):1137–51.

66. Wu Q, Maniatis T. A striking organization of a large family of human neural cadherin-like cell adhesion genes. *Cell* 1999;**97**(6):779–90.

67. Brites D, Brena C, Ebert D, Du Pasquier L. More than one way to produce protein diversity: duplication and limited alternative splicing of an adhesion molecule gene in basal arthropods. *Evol Int J Org Evol* 2013;**67**(10):2999–3011.

68. Barrow AD, Trowsdale J. You say ITAM and I say ITIM, let's call the whole thing off: the ambiguity of immunoreceptor signalling. *Eur J Immunol* 2006;**36**(7):1646–53.

69. Crayton III ME, Powell BC, Vision TJ, Giddings MC. Tracking the evolution of alternatively spliced exons within the Dscam family. *BMC Evol Biol* 2006;**6**:16.
70. Wood W, Jacinto A. *Drosophila melanogaster* embryonic haemocytes: masters of multitasking. *Nat Rev* 2007;**8**(7):542–51.
71. Budd GE, Telford MJ. The origin and evolution of arthropods. *Nature* 2009;**457**(7231):812–7.
72. Glenner H, Thomsen PF, Hebsgaard MB, Sorensen MV, Willerslev E. The origin of insects. *Science (New York, NY)* 2006;**314**(5807):1883–4.
73. Rota-Stabelli O, Campbell L, Brinkmann H, Edgecombe GD, Longhorn SJ, Peterson KJ, et al. A congruent solution to arthropod phylogeny: phylogenomics, microRNAs and morphology support monophyletic *Mandibulata. Proc Roy Soc B* 2011;**278**(1703):298–306.
74. Rota-Stabelli O, Telford MJ. A multi criterion approach for the selection of optimal outgroups in phylogeny: recovering some support for *Mandibulata* over *Myriochelata* using mitogenomics. *Mol Phylogenet Evol* 2008;**48**(1):103–11.
75. Chipman AD, Ferrier DE, Brena C, Qu J, Hughes DS, Schroder R, et al. The first myriapod genome sequence reveals conservative arthropod gene content and genome organisation in the centipede *Strigamia maritima. PLoS Biol* 2014;**12**(11):e1002005.
76. Palmer WJ, Jiggins FM. Comparative genomics reveals the origins and diversity of arthropod immune systems. *Mol Biol Evol* 2015;**32**:2111–2129.
77. Armitage SAO, Freiburg RY, Kurtz J, Bravo IG. The evolution of Dscam genes across the arthropods. *BMC Evol Biol* 2012;**12**:53.
78. Prasad A, Qamri Z, Wu J, Ganju RK. Pivotal advance: Slit-2/Robo-1 modulates the CXCL12/CXCR4-induced chemotaxis of T cells. *J Leukocyte Biol* 2007;**82**(3):465–76.
79. Graveley B, Amardeep K, Dorian G, Lawrence ZS, Lee RcCJ. The organization and evolution of the dipteran and hymenopteran Down syndrome cell adhesion molecule (*Dscam*) genes. *RNA* 2004;**10**:1499–506.
80. Grimaldi D, Engel MS. *Evolution of the insects.* New York: Cambridge University Press; 2005.
81. Savard J, Tautz D, Richards S, Weinstock GM, Gibbs RA, Werren JH, et al. Phylogenomic analysis reveals bees and wasps (Hymenoptera) at the base of the radiation of holometabolous insects. *Genome Res* 2006;**16**(11):1334–8.
82. Wiegmann BM, Trautwein MD, Kim JW, Cassel BK, Bertone MA, Winterton SL, et al. Single-copy nuclear genes resolve the phylogeny of the holometabolous insects. *BMC Biol* 2009;**7**:34.
83. Legg DA, Sutton MD, Edgecombe GD. Arthropod fossil data increase congruence of morphological and molecular phylogenies. *Nat Commun* 2013;**4**:2485.
84. Toon A, Finley T, Staples J, Crandall K. Decapod phylogenetics and molecular evolution. In: Martin J, Crandall KA, Felder DL, editors. *Decapod Crustacean Phylogenetics.* Boca Raton, Florida: CRC Press; 2009.
85. Millard SS, Lu Z, Zipursky SL, Meinertzhagen IA. *Drosophila* dscam proteins regulate post-synaptic specificity at multiple-contact synapses. *Neuron* 2010;**67**(5):761–8.
86. Funada M, Hara H, Sasagawa H, Kitagawa Y, Kadowaki T. A honey bee Dscam family member, AbsCAM, is a brain-specific cell adhesion molecule with the neurite outgrowth activity which influences neuronal wiring during development. *Eur J Neurosci* 2007;**25**(1):168–80.
87. Lah GJ, Li JS, Millard SS. Cell-specific alternative splicing of *Drosophila* Dscam2 is crucial for proper neuronal wiring. *Neuron* 2014;**83**(6):1376–88.
88. Lee C, Kim N, Roy M, Graveley BR. Massive expansions of Dscam splicing diversity via staggered homologous recombination during arthropod evolution. *RNA* 2009;**16**(1):91–105.
89. Barribeau SM, Sadd BM, du Plessis L, Brown MJ, Buechel SD, Cappelle K, et al. A depauperate immune repertoire precedes evolution of sociality in bees. *Genome Biol* 2015;**16**(1):83.

90. Loker ES, Adema CM, Zhang SM, Kepler TB. Invertebrate immune systems—not homogeneous, not simple, not well understood. *Immunol Rev* 2004;**198**:10–24.
91. Sodergren E, Weinstock GM, Davidson EH, Cameron RA, Gibbs RA, Angerer RC, et al. The genome of the sea urchin *Strongylocentrotus purpuratus*. *Science (New York, NY)* 2006;**314**(5801):941–52.
92. Danks G, Campsteijn C, Parida M, Butcher S, Doddapaneni H, Fu B, et al. OikoBase: a genomics and developmental transcriptomics resource for the urochordate *Oikopleura dioica*. *Nucleic Acids Res* 2013;**41**(Database issue):D845–53.
93. Dehal P, Satou Y, Campbell RK, Chapman J, Degnan B, De Tomaso A, et al. The draft genome of *Ciona intestinalis*: insights into chordate and vertebrate origins. *Science (New York, NY)* 2002;**298**(5601):2157–67.
94. Zhang SM, Loker ES. The FREP gene family in the snail *Biomphalaria glabrata*: additional members, and evidence consistent with alternative splicing and FREP retrosequences fibrinogen-related proteins. *Dev Comp Immunol* 2003;**27**(3):175–87.
95. Smith P. Dscam gene expression in invertebrate immunity: alternative splicing in response to diverse pathogens PhD; [2012]
96. Burke GR, Moran NA. Responses of the pea aphid transcriptome to infection by facultative symbionts. *Insect Mol Biol* 2011;**20**(3):357–65.
97. Husseneder C, Simms DM. Effects of caste on the expression of genes associated with septic injury and xenobiotic exposure in the Formosan subterranean termite. *PLoS One* 2014;**9**(8):e105582.
98. Gunaratna RT, Jiang H. A comprehensive analysis of the *Manduca sexta* immunotranscriptome. *Dev Comp Immunol* 2012;**39**(4):388–98.

Chapter 11

Structural and Functional Diversity of Fibrinogen-Related Domains

Russell F. Doolittle

Departments of Chemistry & Biochemistry and Molecular Biology, University of California, San Diego, La Jolla, CA, United States

1 INTRODUCTION

Fibrinogen-related domains (FReDs) were named and defined for the globular portions of vertebrate fibrinogen,[1] the precursor molecule of fibrin blood clots. As will happen, the first instance of a protein domain being found may not be representative of its general function, and the vast majority of FReDs in the animal world have nothing to do with blood clotting. Rather, these domains are found in numerous extracellular proteins with widely different functions, a substantial number of which appear to be associated with innate immunity.

In this chapter, an attempt is made to weave together phylogenetic occurrence, structural features, rates of change, and function. In keeping with the general theme of this book, the emphasis will be on the diversity of some putative immune-related FRePs (FReD-containing proteins), eschewing, except for brief mention, those others with more specialized functions like the clotting of blood, or the stimulation of neurite development, or blood vessel growth, and so on, although these latter are included in a "time-line" of when various FReDs first appear in the chordate lineage.

2 STRUCTURAL FEATURES

FReDs actually consist of three subdomains,[2] usually denoted A, B, and P (Fig. 11.1). The amino-terminal subdomain ("A domain") consists of about 50 amino-acid residues and a single disulfide bond. The B and P subdomains are closely associated, the middle strand of the central β sheet in the B subdomain being provided by a segment that originates after the third subdomain. The B and P subdomains together amount to 150–200 residues.

The Evolution of the Immune System. http://dx.doi.org/10.1016/B978-0-12-801975-7.00011-6

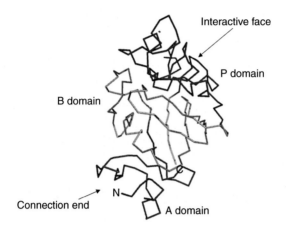

FIGURE 11.1 **Backbone structure of a typical FReD (human H-ficolin), showing three sub-domains (A, violet; B, brown; P, blue).** The amino-terminal (N) is usually preceded by one of a variety of connecting domains of various sorts. Interactions usually occur on the outer face of the third subdomain ("P domain"). Note how the central strand of the main sheet *(green)* is provided by a sequence segment that occurs after the third subdomain. *(Reprinted from Ref. [3].)*

The carboxy-terminal P domain invariably contains a disulfide bond, almost always with 12 residues between the two cysteines. The peptide bond between the second cysteine and its amino-terminal neighbor is in the *cis* configuration, a feature that is important to the architecture of this region, and especially in maintaining a cavity that is, in most instances, the binding site by which FReDs interact with other entities. Remarkably, the same natural binding cavity is used to bind a sugar derivative to a horseshoe-crab lectin as is used to bind amino-terminal peptide "knobs" on fibrinogen molecules during fibrin formation (Fig. 11.2).

A bound calcium is also an integral feature of the P domain. In line with the fact that FReDs, with rare exception, occur in extracellular environments, many are glycosylated, carbohydrate clusters occurring sporadically on any of the three subdomains.

As it happens, the A (amino-terminal) subdomain often occurs in many other settings, in which cases it is usually referred to as a NEC domain (an acronym based on the neuro- and collagenous environments in which they are found). In FReDs, these subdomains are more or less accessory in nature and do not participate directly in ligand binding. Because genuine FReDs consist of all three subdomains, NEC occurrences will not be considered further, except to discount irrelevant observations.

3 PHYLOGENETIC OCCURRENCE

We recently conducted a comprehensive bioinformatics survey of the occurrence of FReD genes in a wide assortment of animal genomes—from very early diverging phyletic groups like sponge and sea anemone, to crown protostomes

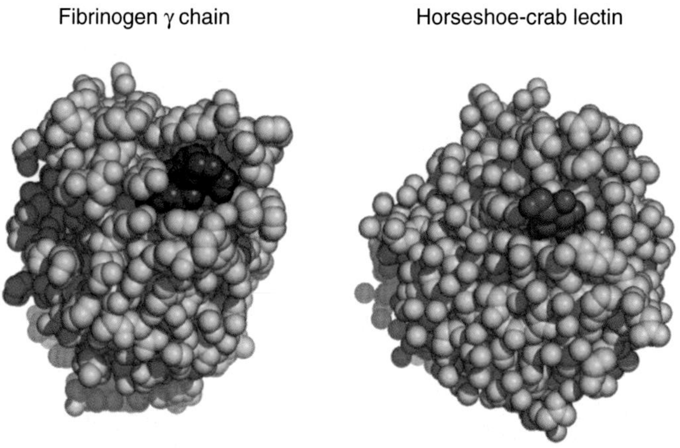

Fibrinogen γ chain   Horseshoe-crab lectin

FIGURE 11.2   **Comparison of γC domain from human fibrinogen with a tachylectin from horseshoe crab, each with a bound ligand** *(shown in red).* The ligand in the fibrinogen "hole" is a tetrapeptide, and the one in tachylectin is a sugar (*N*-acetyl glucosamine). *(Reprinted from Ref. [4].)*

and deuterostomes like insects and mammals.[3] In line with using past experimental data together with sequence searching regimens, those data have served as the raw material for proposals and inferences made in this chapter. The survey was sufficiently broad that the first appearance—in a phylogenetic sense—of various types of FReP can be gauged.

In this regard, FReDs are very much restricted to animals, making their first evolutionary appearance in sponges (Fig. 11.3). Contrary to what is often reported,[5,6] no gene for a full-length FReD can be found in the genome of the choanoflagellate *Monosiga brevicollis*,[7] generally regarded as the closest extant organism sharing common ancestry with animals. The mistaken reports are the unfortunate result of the National Center for Biotechnology Information (NCBI) referring to the 50-residue NEC domains—which *do* occur in several choanoflagellate proteins—as FReDs. In our 2012 survey, a FReD was found in a single bacterium, *Bacteriovorax marinus*, and an updated search now reveals one more such occurrence, this time in the proteobacterium *Cupriavidus metallidurans*. Both of these instances appear to be the result of horizontal transfers from an animal genome to the bacterium.

As a reminder, phylogenetic trees have two important features: branching order and branch lengths. The branching order depicts the temporal order in which gene duplications or speciation events occur; the branch lengths reflect the amount of change along each interval. A long branch-length indicates faster change for a particular interval than would a short one. As we shall see, occasionally variations in rates of change can lead to mistaken branching orders. Matters can sometimes be resolved by a consideration of unique indels (insertion/deletion events).

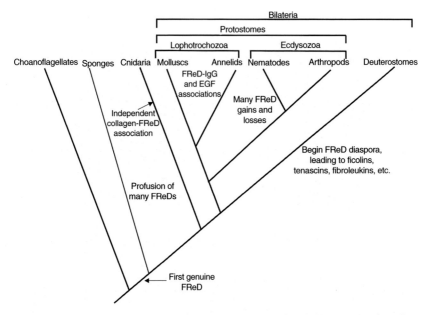

FIGURE 11.3   Simplified time-line for organisms mentioned in this chapter, showing where different FRePs had first made their evolutionary appearance. Deuterostomes are detailed in Fig. 11.5.

The vocabulary of phylogenies and gene duplication is important. Gene or protein sequences from different organisms that play the same roles as a result of simple parent to progeny passage are said to be *orthologs*, whereas homologous proteins that are the result of gene duplications are said to be *paralogs*. One of the purposes of tracking the evolution of protein domains like FReDs that are shuffled around in genomes is to sort out the orthologs from the paralogs. All 23 FReDs in Fig. 11.4 are paralogs, because they occur in the same organism (human) and must be the result of gene duplications.

4   FReDs AND NEIGHBOR DOMAINS

FReDs often, but not always, occur in the accompaniment of other domains, like immunoglobulin (Ig) or fibronectin type III (Fn3) or collagen or coiled-coil domains; when they do, the FReD is invariably at the carboxy-terminal domain of the cluster. The nature of these accompanying domains can bear heavily on the function of the FReP, especially with regard to the valence of ligand binding.

For example, the tight triple-helix nature of an adjacent collagen segment insures that three terminal FReDs are packed together as a symmetrical homotrimer, a feature with obvious advantage for binding to surfaces with numerous, uniformly distributed ligands, as might be expected to occur on the cell walls of bacteria. In some other FRePs, two-stranded coiled-coils are important

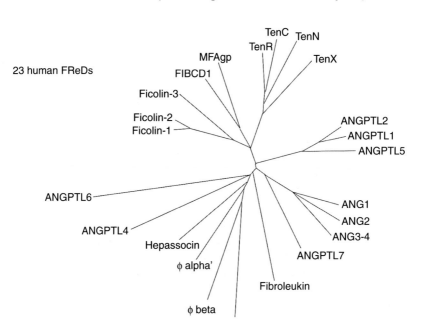

FIGURE 11.4 **Phylogenetic tree (unrooted), constructed from 23 FReD sequences found in human genome.** Designations for angiopoietins and angioarrestins are those used by the NCBI. Φ denotes fibrinogen and the Φ' denotes the minor form of the alpha chain called alpha-prime. *(Reprinted from Ref. [3].)*

for orienting identical pairs of FReDs side-by-side so that they can bind to and bring together diffusible entities on cell surfaces. In contrast, the FReDs in tenascins are only loosely associated, operating more or less independently at the ends of long, flexible tethers composed of Fn3 and/or EGF domains. These examples illustrate how identifying neighbor domains during a bioinformatic analysis can provide critical information for the inference of function.

Importantly, FReDs can also occur by themselves with no neighbor domains, in which case we will refer to them as "stand-alone FReDs." It must be clear, however, that these solitary FreDs can associate with each other to form dimers, trimers, and higher oligomers, without the aid of neighbor domains, thereby achieving the benefits of polyvalence that can aid pattern recognition.

5 HUMAN FRePs

Genes for 23 different FReDs (in 23 different FRePs) were identified in the human genome, including four for tenascins, three for ficolins, nine for angiopoietin or angiopoietin-like proteins, three that give rise to fibrinogen, and four others: fibroleukin, hepassocin, microfibril-associated protein (MFAP), and the FIBCD1 protein (Fig. 11.4).

Although FRePs in humans are arguably the most studied, the functions of the 23 kinds are not all known with the same degree of certainty. On the secure side, tenascins have been researched intensely for several decades; it is well established that they are part of the fabric of the extracellular matrix (ECM) and have a variety of regulatory and developmental functions. They attract and interact with numerous cell-surface proteins, including those of leucocytes and neurites.[8,9]

Another case where function is not in question involves the FReDs in the β and γ chains of fibrinogen, the protein for which FReDs were named. The "holes" in these FReDs unequivocally bind "knobs" from other fibrinogen molecules, causing the polymerization that is at the heart of fibrin blood clots. In contrast, the closely related FReD that occurs in an alternative form of the fibrinogen α chain does not seem to play a role in polymerization events, and remains mysterious.[10] And although the liver-specific FReP called hepassocin is clearly a mitogen,[11] the evidence for fibroleukin being an immuno-procoagulant with prothrombinase activity remains tenuous.[12] Indeed, early claims about possible immunofunctions for fibroleukins were dealt a serious blow by a study with knockout mice in which the fibroleukin gene was deleted but no differences in any immune-related phenomena could be detected.[13]

Angiopoietins are well-characterized proteins that stimulate blood vessel growth;[14] the related angioarrestins are paralogs that act antagonistically.[15] On another front, the FReP called "fibrinogen C domain connecting 1" (FIBCD1) occurs in the intestinal brush border, as well as some airway and salivary gland cells, and is well known to bind chitin, an entity that is indigestible in most animals.[16] The mature protein contains a transmembrane segment at its amino-terminus that holds it bound to the component cell membrane. The function of the closely related—in a phylogenetic sense—microfibril(lar)-associated proteins (MFAPs) remains vague, however.[17] MFAPs are "stand-alone" FRePs without accompanying domains, and it is not impossible that their binding to microfibrils accords them a kind of polyvalence that would aid in recognizing repetitive patterns on the surfaces of pathogens. The association of a serious developmental syndrome in persons with a deleted gene for MFAP4 argues for something more profound, however.[18,19]

Finally, the human genome encodes three different ficolins,[20–22] designated M-, L- and H- (also called ficolin-1, -2 and -3). In addition to having different amino-acid sequences, the three types differ with regard to the number of collagen triplets (GXX-) in their amino-terminal segments, leading to slightly different molecular weights. These are well-studied proteins with similar but different capabilities for binding ligands that have a number of attributes associated with immunity, and we will need to revisit them during our discussion of FReDs with apparent immune-related functions. Interestingly, recombinant forms in which the collagen segments are omitted still form trimers.[22]

Homologs for the 23 human FRePs are found in most mammals, but strict orthologs, as we will now try to demonstrate, appear at distinctly different stages during chordate evolution. Moreover, the survey of FReD occurrences revealed a surprising amount of gain and loss, with closely related groups having different numbers of FReDs, both in general and of particular kinds. As an example, although human and chicken genomes both have 23 FReP genes, they are not the same 23. Gains and losses were sustained along both lineages on the way to birds and mammals.

In explanation, defense mechanisms in animals tend to be highly redundant and genetically "backed up," even in the face of the evolutionary dictum "use it or lose it." In the course of the never-ending war against pathogens, the challenge of expecting the unexpected from an ever-changing enemy may require numerous copies of a defensive agent. But such genes are readily lost, perhaps accounting for why frogs have four MFAPs and lizards and humans only one, and chickens none at all. Another possibility is that on occasion a particular FReD may develop the capability for binding a broader array of ligands, thus lowering the number of genomic versions needed for responding to potential adversaries. As an example, human L-ficolin has been reported to bind a much more diverse collection of ligands than M-ficolins or H-ficolin.[23]

6   EVOLUTION OF FUNCTIONAL DIVERSITY IN CHORDATES

Because FReDs occur in a very wide range of proteins with very different functions, we need to inquire: when and under what circumstances during evolution did these diverse functionalities arise? The newly engendered FReDs need to adapt to two quite different needs depending on whether they are recognizing endogenous entities, like proteins of the extracellular matrix, or components of developmental networks, and so on, or whether the function at hand is to fend off exogenous, alien materials, like microorganisms or indigestible foreign substances. The first category would include tenascins, angiopoietins, hepassocin, and so on; the second should include ficolins and FIBCD1, although it should be noted that it has been suggested that some ficolins may also recognize endogenous materials from disrupted cells.[23]

Let us begin with tenascins, the evolution of which has been thoroughly reviewed in the past.[8,9] If the presence of an Fn3 neighbor domain is regarded as diagnostic, then it is generally accepted that tenascins occur in all chordates, making their first appearance in protochordates such as amphioxus.[24] Next, angiopoietin and angiopoietin-like proteins, which, as we noted, are involved in the development of the vascular system, make their first appearance in jawless fish like the lamprey,[3] coincident with the development of a closed vascular system (Fig. 11.5). We can feel confident about this identification because genuine angiopoietins have a unique signature in the way of an additional disulfide bond. There is no sign of these entities among those protochordates whose genome sequences are available.

The intestinal chitin-binding protein known as FIBCD1 protein is more problematic. The NCBI lists two entries from the protochordate *Ciona intestinalis* labeled as "FIBCD1-like," but neither has the obligatory membrane-spanning

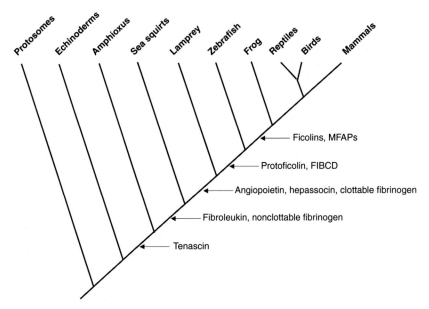

FIGURE 11.5 **Simplified time-line showing where different FRePs had first made their evolutionary appearance along the deuterostome lineage.**

sequence needed for localizing in the intestinal wall. In fact their sequences are much more "ficolin-like" than they are FIBCD1-like. Nor has an authentic FIBCD1 yet been identified in the jawless vertebrates. The problem in this case is that a high-quality genome assembly for neither the lamprey nor the hagfish (the only two genera of jawless fish extant) is yet available. It is possible that one or both may have such a gene, but it has not yet been found. In our recent review[3] based on a fragmentary finding, we thought the lamprey might have such a gene, but that conclusion may have been premature.

Genes for fibroleukin and the liver mitogen hepassocin, like the three genes encoding FReDs that occur in fibrinogen, are found in all vertebrates. This includes jawless fish. Indeed, a gene for fibroleukin is present in the protochordate *Ciona intestinalis*.[3] More remarkably, genes for a protofibrinogen have also been found in those creatures, even though the hemolymph of protochordates does not clot.[25]

Authentic MFAPs, of the type designated MFAP4 in humans, make their first appearance in amphibians. There are four in the frog, and one each in lizard, opossum, and human. None was found in the chicken or in a draft genome of the basal mammalian platypus.[3] It has been reported that asparagine-linked carbohydrate in MFAP plays a role in their binding to integrins,[9] and indeed a specific glycosylation site is found in these proteins in all of the sequences available, as well as in the intestinal chitin-binding protein, consistent with the close relationship of these two FReDs (Fig. 11.6).

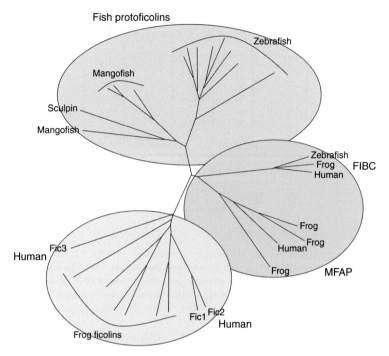

FIGURE 11.6 **Phylogenetic tree (unrooted) for 29 FReDs (ficolins, MFAPs, and FIBCDs) found in zebrafish, mangofish, sculpin, frog, and human.** Members of the group labeled "protoficolins" are called MFAP-like by the NCBI.

Ficolins of the kind found in mammals with collagen domains adjacent to FReDs also make their first appearance among the Amphibia (Fig. 11.5). Indeed, the African clawed frog has 25 verifiable ficolins. Four of these do not have collagen segments, but phylogenetic trees show that they have lost those segments, as opposed to never having had them.[3] The number of collagen-triplets in the remaining 21 ficolins ranges from 2 to 36. These fluctuations are in accord with the old maxim that "gene duplication begets more gene duplication," the consequence of the increasing opportunity for mismatching of similar DNA sequences during meiotic divisions.[26]

Although jawed fish have an abundance of proteins labeled as MFAP-like by the NCBI, these are not orthologs of the MFAPs found in tetrapods. They are apparently absent from jawless ones like lamprey. We suggested that in fish these proteins are playing the same role as ficolins,[3] and indeed, the notion was promptly confirmed when it was found that in a fish called the sculpin (*Trachidermus fasciatus*) a protein, the amino-acid sequence of which clearly shows it to be "MFAP-like" (Fig. 11.6), is expressed in response to challenge by the bacterial parasite *Vibrio anguillarum*.[27] Even more convincing, a recombinant version of the same protein agglutinated the bacteria.[27] We propose that

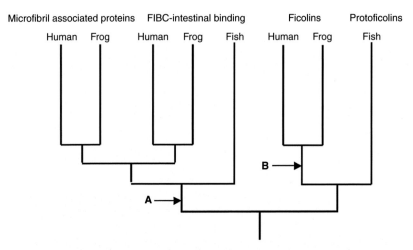

FIGURE 11.7   **Phylogeny showing evolutionary relationships for FIBCD1, MFAPs, ficolins, and protoficolins for zebrafish, mangofish, sculpin, frog, and human.** The arrow labeled A shows where a unique 5-amino-acid insertion took place that remains in all known FIBCDs and MFAPs. At about the same time, a new glycosylation site appears in these same taxa. The arrow labeled B shows where a collagen domain was genetically joined with a FReD at the dawn of tetrapods.

all these fish proteins might better be called "collagen-free" ficolins, or, perhaps more reasonably, "protoficolins" (Fig. 11.7).

The NCBI probably denoted these fish proteins as "MFAP-like" because simple amino-acid sequence comparisons show them to be more similar to tetrapod MFAP sequences than to tetrapod ficolins. The average similarity for zebrafish entries with frog MFAPs is about 50%, but the same proteins are only about 45% identical to frog ficolins. Nonetheless, as we will show here, there is good reason to think that the fish proteins are really orthologs of tetrapod ficolins and not of frog or human MFAPs.

Pointedly, the FIBC proteins from zebrafish, frog, and human and the MFAP proteins from frog and human all have a unique 5-amino-acid insert that is lacking in other FreDs (Fig. 11.6), the presence of which indicates that tetrapod MFAPs diverged from FIBCD1 after the separation of fish from other vertebrates. The discrepant relationship of the MFAP-like and MFAPs is the combined result of very rapid change among the ficolins and very slow change for the FIBC–MFAP group, making the distances between paralogs seem less than between orthologs. Evidence for such confounding comparisons has been noted in the past[28]; the phenomenon is the flip-side of well-known systematic errors attributable to "long branch attraction."[29]

7   RATES OF SEQUENCE CHANGE

Perhaps not unexpectedly, it was found that FReDs with different functions have changed at different rates, with ficolins being by far the fastest-changing group. Significantly, the greatest amount of change in ficolin FReDs occurs in

TABLE 11.1 Different Rates of Change for FReD Subdomains, as Reflected in Ratio of %IDs: (AB Domains)/(P Domain)

FRePs	#Seqs	#Comps	(AB)/P (frac IDs + SD)
Chordates			
Angiopoietins	9	36	0.87 + 0.08
Angioarrestins	5	10	0.85 + 0.12
FIBCD1	8	28	0.90 + 0.05
Tenascins	10	45	0.90 + 0.05
Fibroleukins	12	66	0.87 + 0.07
Fibrin-gamma	6	15	0.90 + 0.06
Fibrin-beta	6	15	0.75 + 0.08
Fibrin-alpha′	6	15	0.82 + 0.08
Hepassocin	6	15	0.83 + 0.05
Ficolins			
Not frog	7	21	1.16 + 0.28
Frog	25	276	1.42 + 0.24
Sea squirt	6	15	1.08 + 0.13
Protoficolins	9	36	1.28 + 0.20
Nonchordates			
Paralogs			
Sponges	14	91	1.57 + 0.25
Jellyfish	19	171	1.33 + 0.29
Snail	6	15	1.46 + 0.15
Mosquito	6	15	1.17 + 0.20
Orthologs (insects)			
Scabrous	3	3	0.81 + 0.02
Unknown protein	3	3	0.92 + 0.03

the third subdomain ("P domain" in Fig. 11.1), the very opposite of the situation in FReDs with either singular or more specialized functions like blood clotting or angiogenesis, in which cases the P domain sequences are locked into more conserved modes. The different patterns are readily codified as the ratio of percent identities of the A and B domains relative to the percent identities of P domains (Table 11.1). Ficolins, for example, have ratios greater than 1.0, whereas tenascins, angiopoietins, and other FReDs have ratios less than 1.0.

Not coincidentally, similar patterns of unbalanced sequence change occur among the fish proteins mistakenly labeled "MFAP-like," and, as we shall see, the unbalanced style of change is also observed in FReDs from nonchordates, the rapid change in the P domain being observed in many FRePs that have been implicated in innate immunity. All indications are that the significantly different rates of change in the subdomains of FReDs with putative immune functions are the result of positive selection.

8   FReDs IN PROTOCHORDATES

At this point, two protochordates have had their whole genomes sequenced. One is a urochordate called the sea squirt (*Ciona intestinalis*), and the other is the earlier diverging cephalochordate amphioxus (*Branchiostoma floridae*). Both genomes encode numerous FReDs, and experiments on closely related species have implicated some of them with immune functions. In the amphioxus, *B. belcheri*, bacteriolytic activity has been reported for a FReD described as a multivalent pattern-recognition receptor,[30] and a novel ficolin has been cloned from the urochordate, *Halocynthia roretzi*.[31] Sequence-based phylogenetic trees showed this ficolin to be the result of a genetic joining of a collagen domain and a FReD independent of the one that had led to ficolins in tetrapods.[3]

Beyond that, the genome of the sea squirt contains a remarkable set of evolutionary innovations involving FReDs, including self-incompatibility factors,[32] a nonclottable protofibrinogen,[25] and a putative transcription factor.[33] None of these appear to have a counterpart in the amphioxus genome.

9   EXTENDING THE DEUTEROSTOME TIME-LINE

Echinoderms are early diverging deuterostomes and a reasonable place to search for ancestors of chordate FRePs (Fig. 11.5). The common sea urchin (*Strongylocentrotus purpuratus*) has 35 identified FReDs, several of which tend to cluster with human ficolins and tenascins, but none of them have collagen segments or any hint of domains found in combination with vertebrate tenascins.[3] So far it has not been possible to place any of these FReDs as orthologs with chordate counterparts.

Recently, it was reported that a FReP in a different echinoderm, the sea cucumber *Apostichopus japonicus*, is involved in tissue regeneration as determined by expression levels in various tissues.[34] This may be so, but it seems a remarkable coincidence that several decades ago the same gene product had been cloned from another sea cucumber species as part of a general search for nonvertebrate FReDs, simply on the basis of its abundance.[35] These are "standalone" proteins without any accompanying domain, and, as a result, that attribute cannot be used as an aid in defining function.

10   NONDEUTEROSTOME ANIMALS

Although FReDs from nondeuterostome animals (Fig. 11.3) are frequently called "ficolin-like," or "tenascin-like," and so on, mostly these are not genuine ficolins (no collagen domains), nor are they authentic tenascins (no Fn3 domains), nor any of the other types of FReD found in deuterostomes. Nonetheless, the conventions of current nomenclature are such that many FRePs from nondeuterostome animals have been named "angiopoietin-like" and some other ones "FReD-like" based on the kind of sequence they tend most to resemble.

In the past we have cautioned that it would be unwise to infer any commonality of function from these names.[3] Even so, I am now going to suggest, cautiously, that the majority of FReDs found in early diverging organisms like sponges and jellyfish may actually be involved with a kind of immune response similar to that reported for chordate ficolins, probably antibacterial in nature. As in the case of a group of fish FReDs discussed previously, I will use the term *protoficolins* for these collagen-free entities.

11 SPONGES AND JELLYFISH

Sponges (phylum Porifera) and jellyfish (phylum Cnidaria) are the earliest diverging animals (Fig. 11.3) and where one might logically look for new physiological functions. Immune phenomena in sponges have long been a matter of discussion, especially with intrinsic activity directed against bacteria.[36] Although the molecular details of most of these interactions remain to be studied, there is one case of a particular sponge, *Suberites domuncula*, where a FReD has been implicated as part of a system for fending off fungi.[37]

Given that limited experimental background, the completion of the genome DNA sequence for the sponge, *Amphimedon queenslandica*,[38] presents an opportunity for testing a strict bioinformatics approach for assigning functions to FReDs for which no experimental data are yet in hand. Partial sequences aside, 92 full-length FReDs were identified in the sponge genome, the majority of which have short uncharacterized sequences on their amino-terminal sides (< 60 residues between the signal sequence and the FReD).[3] None have collagen-like sequences nor any of the domains associated with FRePs found in chordates. However, 41 of the 106 had an approximately 50-residue motif containing five or six cysteines, consistent with a tightly folded, disulfidebonded domain. The motif was not found in any other proteins in the NCBI protein database.

When included in phylogenetic trees with FReDs from other phyla, sponge entries invariably cluster separately, indicating an independent diaspora that has been occurring since the time of the last common ancestor of sponges and other animals. That said, and neighbor domains aside, sponge FReD sequences tend to most resemble chordate ficolins and tenascins. The question is, are any, all, or most of these FReDs involved with binding to bacteria or other pathogens?

Indeed, a case for sponge FReDs being involved in some kind of immune function can be made on the following counts: (1) the number of related FReD genes is extensive; (2) among these, the interactive P subdomain changes at a much faster rate than the A and B subdomains, just as it occurs in chordate ficolins and protoficolins (Table 11.1); and (3) the key residues known to be involved in binding to N-acetylated small molecules in ficolins,[39–41] FIBCD1,[42,43]

```
F101Sponge      ..SAHNGMKFSTKNQDN-DAASGNCAIVYKGAWWYRACHASNLNGLYLVGHHSS-YANGVNWYHFKGHYYSLKT..
F102Sponge      ..GHHNNMKFSTHDHDN-DIYDGNCALAYKGAWWYSKCHASNLNGWYLAGTHST-YADGVMWAHFKGLHYSLKV..
P10Jelly        ..AYHNNFAFSTKDQDNDDKTDESCAVTFKGAWWYGGCHHSNLNGFYFVNSQSP-YGQGINWLDWKGYDYSLKR..
P12Jelly        ..SDHRGAPFSTKDRDN-DSAGASCAIIYKGAWWYTACHSSNLNGKYYHGSHAS-YADGVNWRAWKGYHYSLKH..
P22Jelly        ..SFHQNMTFSTIDHDSDAMEDESCAQMFTGAWWYKNCHEANLNGRYRHGPHKT-FADGINWKTFRGYYYSLKS..
                                     o          o              o            o
*Tachylectin    ..GRHNGHNFSTIDKDH-DTHETHCAQTYKGGWWYDRCHESNLNGLYLNGEHNS-YADGIEWRAWKGYHYSLPQ..
                                     o          o              o            o
*Fic1Human      ..TGHNNNFFSTKDQDN-DVSSSNCAEKFQGAWWYADCHASSLNGLYLMGPHES-YANGINWSAAKGYKYSYKV..
*Fic2Human      ..TFHNNQSFSTKDQDN-DLNTGNCAVMFQGAWWYKNCHVSNLNGRYLRGTHGS-FANGINWKSGKGYNYSYKV..
*Fic3Human      ..SLHSGRPFTTYDADH-DSSNSNCAVIVHGAWWYASCYRSNLNGRYAVSEAAA-HKYGIDWASGRGVGHPYRR..
PFICMango       ..SYHSGQKFSTFDKDQ-DNWSGNCAKTYLGAFWYNTCHYANPNGVYRWGADGTIFAVGVAWHQWKGHDYSLKT..
PFICMango       ..NSHNRQKFTTFDKDQ-DSSSGNCAKTYLGAFWYNSCHHANPNGVYRWGADGTIFAVGVAWHQWKGHDYSLKT..
                                     o          o              o            o
*FibCHuman      ..LKHSGMRFTTKDRDS-DHSENNCAAFYRGAWWYRNCHTSNLNGQYLRGAHAS-YADGVEWSSWTGWQYSLKF..
MFAgpHuman      ..SYHSGQKFSTFDRDQ-DLFYQNCAALSSGAFWFRSCHFANLNGFYLGGSHLS-YANGINWAQWKGFYYSLKR..
```

FIGURE 11.8 **Alignment of key interfacial region (P subdomain) from a series of FReDs from sponges, jellyfish, horseshoe crab, mangofish, and humans.** Residues known to be involved in ligand contacts are denoted by o (X-ray structures are available for the sequences marked with *). Rapidly changing residues are in red; conserved residues are in blue. Note that similar matches occur in human ficolins and the horseshoe crab tachylectin, as well as among several sponge and jellyfish FReDs.

and an arthropod lectin,[44] vary in a similar way against a background of a conserved structural core (Fig. 11.8).

A similar case can be made for the jellyfish *Nematostella vectensis* (more formally, the sea anemone, a cnidarian), with the added observation that among its 25 full-length FReDs there is one with an adjacent collagen segment, its position high in the phylogenetic tree, which is clear evidence of an independently evolved ficolin, but true to the original acronym based on FIbrinogen and COLlagen (Fig. 11.3).

12 BILATERIANS

12.1 Phylum Mollusca

Inquiries into possible immune responses for molluscs go way back,[45] and as a result of these longstanding interests, FReDs were long ago found in the snail *Biomphalaria glabrata*.[46] That discovery has been greatly exploited in the intervening years,[47–49] and we will not dwell on this work beyond noting that a convincing case has been made for snail FRePs having a role in immunity, particularly with regard to resistance to infection by trematode parasites. Neighboring domains in these FRePs include immunoglobulin domains, and, occasionally, EGF domains.[49]

FReDs with putative immune-related properties have also been identified in other mollusks, including the scallop, *Argopectin irradians*, in which studies have demonstrated the ability of these FRePs to agglutinate or otherwise immobilize specific bacteria.[50] Moreover, in the case of the slug, *Limax flavus*, a FReP has been thoroughly characterized and shown to bind sialic acid.[51,52]

12.2 Phylum Arthropoda

Defense mechanisms in the horseshoe crab *Tachypleus tridentatus* have been subjected to intense scrutiny over the past several decades, during the course of which a series of lectins was isolated that bind to and agglutinate bacteria and other foreign materials. Quite unexpectedly, two of these, tachylectin 5A and 5B, were found to be FRePs.[53] Remarkably, an X-ray structure showed that these proteins bound N-acetylated small molecule ligands at a site coincident with the peptide-binding holes on vertebrate fibrinogen (Fig. 11.2).[44] Even though the horseshoe crab tachylectins 5A and 5B are "stand-alone" proteins, evidence was provided that showed that the solitary proteins tend to form hexamers and octamers,[54] demonstrating that their binding capabilities could be polyvalent and well-adapted for recognizing patterned repeats. As such, it was suggested that these proteins were the functional equivalent of ficolins found in vertebrates.[54]

12.3 Pancrustacea—Crustaceans

A situation similar to that described in the horseshoe crab was found more recently in a crustacean, the kuruma shrimp, *Marsupenaeus japonicus*, where a stand-alone FReD has been found to agglutinate the bacterium *Vibrio anguillarum*.[55]

12.4 Insects

Insect FRePs have also been the subject of numerous inquiries in the past.[56–59] The possibility of FRePs playing a role in fending off infection by malarial parasites as well as bacteria has spurred these studies in mosquitoes especially.[56] The point must be underscored that, like the situation in chordates, there is great variation in numbers of FReDs from one organismic group to another, ranging from upwards of 30 in some mosquitoes to only 2 in the honeybee, *Apis mellifera*. Even within a single genus there is great diversity, as a dozen different fruit-fly species, for example, having anywhere from 14 to 43 FReDs.[59]

In the case of the honeybee, both FRePs appear to be orthologs of proteins found in other insects with specific functions, one being the well-known *scabrous* protein originally found in *Drosophila melanogaster*.[60] It is significant that once a specific nonimmune function is acquired by one of these genes, the rate and pattern of sequence change becomes greatly moderated.[3]

13 FReD-BASED IMMUNITY AND THE RECOGNITION PROBLEM

Given that an assortment of FReDs from across the entire animal spectrum has been found to bind bacteria, it is tempting to think that their initial appearance in sponges heralded that phenomenon. We have already pointed out those features of sponge FReDs in accordance with that notion, particularly the rapid and unbalanced nature of amino-acid sequence change. The obvious center of interest is the binding cavity on the P subdomain. The fact that so many extant FReDs bind to acetylated small molecules argues that the original cavity likely had that capability also. The still unanswered question is, how did the binding site on the P-domain originate?

The binding sites of human ficolins and FIBCD1, which bind similar sets of acetylated entities, have been scrutinized with great care,[40–43] and several important observations have emerged. For one, it is surprising how many different small molecules, sugars (or not), and acetylated (or not), are bound to various different FReDs.[40] For another, it is now clear that the same ligand can be bound in slightly different ways in different FReDs. Unexpectedly, also, the binding site can be expanded in some instances, as occurs in human L-ficolin, where a set of subsites has been found.[23,41] With regard to fine-tuning, adjustments to how the cavities in a single FReP cluster may be arrayed have been attributed to small shifts in the P-domain, relative to the adjacent B-domain.[23]

Despite all the attention to structural detail, several questions linger about the nature of recognition and about the rapid rate of change, as well as the multiplicity of FReDs in some organisms compared to a paucity in others. Why does a frog have 25 ficolins and a chicken only one? Perhaps this reflects two different strategies of defense, in the one case, maintaining a diverse inventory of FReDs, each with different binding potential, and, in the second case, having a specialized FReD that can somehow recognize a diverse set of pathogens.

There are other problems to contemplate, beginning with the fact that *N*-acetylated small molecules are ubiquitous. How does a FReD distinguish between friend and foe? The glib explanation is that alien ligands often come in regularized patterns, like the peptido-glycans found in bacteria capsules. In these cases an intrinsically weak binding becomes amplified (exponentially) by having more interactive sites (polyvalence). But pattern recognition, often mentioned but seldom spelled out, has its limits. Bacterial mimicry of animal surfaces is another circumstance where distinguishing self from nonself remains an issue. The simple observation that a FReD can agglutinate a bacterium always deserves further contemplation.

Finally, we need to inquire where those original sponge FReDs with putative magical binding-sites came from. It seems unlikely that they were fashioned *de novo* in a primitive sponge. More likely, a gene for the more widely occurring NEC domain found itself adjacent to one resembling a B–P subdomain combination, the origins of which remain unknown. At this point, it is an open question.

14 CONCLUDING REMARKS

In conclusion, FReDs are widely distributed in the animal kingdom, almost entirely as extracellular, diffusible proteins, the interactive sites of which typically involve the carboxyl-terminal subdomain. The broad diversity of functions exhibited by these structures range from the binding of dangerous pathogens to endogenous cell signaling and fibrin gel formation. I have tried to make the case that it is the potential for binding and neutralizing bacteria that is reflected by a very rapid change in the P subdomain—clearly manifested in vertebrate ficolins and protoficolins—as well as numerous and as yet uncharacterized FReDs in sponges where the system had its start. This unusual and uneven kind of variability has to be the result of positive selection. During the course of evolution, advantage was taken of gene duplications, sometimes with the accompaniment of new neighbor domains, which led to new capabilities, derived from a deformable and easily tweaked binding site, to adopt new and singular nonimmune functions.

REFERENCES

1. Doolittle RF. A detailed consideration of a principal domain of vertebrate fibrinogen and its relatives. *Protein Sci* 1992;**1**:1563–77.
2. Yee VC, Pratt KP, Cote HCF, LeTrong I, Chung D, Davie EW, Stenkamp RE, Teller DC. Crystal structure of a 30 kDa fragment from the gamma chain of human fibrinogen. *Structure* 1997;**5**:125–38.
3. Doolittle RF, Mcnamara, Lin K. Correlating structure and function during the evolution of fibrinogen-related domains. *Protein Sci* 2012;**21**:1808–23.
4. Doolittle RF. *The evolution of vertebrate blood clotting*. Mill Valley, CA: University Science Books; 2012.
5. Williams F, Tew HA, Paul CE, Adams JC. The predicted secretomes of Monosiga brevicollis and *Capsaspora owczarzaki*, close unicellular relatives of metazoans, reveal new insights into the evolution of the metazoan extracellular matrix. *Matrix Biol* 2014;**37**:60–8.
6. Gordy MA, Pila EA, Hannington PC. The role of fibrinogen-related proteins in the gastropod immune response. *Fish Shellfish Immunol* 2015;**46**(1):39–49.
7. King N, and 34 other authors. The genome of the choanoflagellate *Monosiga brevicollis* and the origin of metazoans. *Nature* 2008;**451**:783–8.
8. Erickson H. Evolution of the tenascin family—implications for function of the C-terminal fibrinogen-like domain. *Perspect Dev Neurobiol* 1994;**2**:9–19.
9. Adams JC, Chiquet-Ehrismann R, Tucker RP. The evolution of tenascins and fibronectin. *Cell Adh Migr* 2015;**9**:22–33.
10. Lishko VK, Yakubenko VP, Hertzberg KM, Grieninger G, Ugarova TP. The alternatively spliced alpha(E)C domain of human fibrinogen-420 is a novel ligand for leukocyte integrins $\alpha_M\beta_2$ and $\alpha_X\beta_2$. *Blood* 2001;**98**:2448–55.
11. Hara H, Yoshimura H, Uchida S, Toyoda Y, Aoki M, Sakai S, Morimoto S, Shiokawa K. Molecular cloning and functional expression analysis of cDNA for human hepassocin, a liver-specific protein with hepatocyte mitogenic activity. *Biochim Biophys Acta* 2001;**1520**:45–53.
12. Yuwaraj S, Ding JW, Liu M, Marsden PA, Levy GA. Genomic characterization, localization, and functional expression of FGL2, the human gene encoding fibroleuk: a novel human procoagulant. *Genomics* 2001;**71**:330–8.
13. Hancock WW, Szaba FM, Berggren KN, Parent MA, Mullarky IK, Pearl J, Cooper AM, Ely KH, Woodland DL, Kim IJ, Blackman MA, Johnson LL, Smiley ST. Intact type 1 immunity and immune-associated coagulative responses in mice lacking IFN gamma-inducible fibringen-like protein 2. *Proc Natl Acad Sci USA* 2004;**101**:3005–10.
14. Fagiani E, Christofori G. Angiopoietins in angiogenesis. *Cancer Lett* 2013;**328**:18–26.
15. Dhanabal M, Jeffers M, LaRochelle WJ, Lichenstein HS. Angioarrestin: a unique angiopoietin-related protein with anti-angiogenic properties. *Biochem Biophys Res Comm* 2005;**333**:308–15.

16. Schlosser A, Thomsen T, Moeller JB, Nielsen O, Tornoe I, Mollenhauer J, Moestrup SK, Holmskov U. Characterization of FIBCD1 as an acetyl group-binding receptor that binds chitin. *J Immunol* 2009;**183**:3800–9.

17. Kobayashi R, Mizutani A, Hidaka H. Isolation and characterization of a 36-kDa microfibril-associated glycoprotein by the newly synthesized isoquinolinesulfonamide affinity chromatography. *Biochem Biophys Res Comm* 1994;**198**:1262–6.

18. Zhao Z, Lee C-C, Jiralerspong S, Juyal RC, Lu F, Baldoini A, Greenberg F, Caskey CT, Patel PI. The gene for a human microfibril-associated glycoprotein is commonly deleted in Smith-Magenis syndrome patients. *Hum Mol Genet* 1995;**4**:589–97.

19. Wulf-Johansson H, Johansson SL, Schlosser A, Holm AT, Rasmussen LM, Mickley H, Diederischsen ACP, Munkholm H, Poulsen TS, Tornoe I, Bielsen V, Marcussen N, Vestbo J, Saekmose SG, Holmskov U, Sorenson GL. Localization of microfibrillar-associated protein 4 (MFAP4) in human tissues: clinical evaluation of serum MFAP4 and its association with various cardiovascular conditions. *PLoS ONE* 2013;**8**(12):e82243.

20. Ichijo H, Hellman U, Wernstedt C, Gonez LJ, Claesson-Welsh L, Heldin C-H, Miyazono K. Molecular cloning and characterization of ficolin, a multimeric protein with fibrinogen- and collagen-like domains. *J Biol Chem* 1993;**268**:14505–13.

21. Garlatti V, Belloy N, Martin L, Lacroix M, Matsushita M, Endo Y, Fujita T, Fontecilla-Camps JC, Arlaud GJ, Thielens NM, Gaboriaud C. Structural insights into the innate immune recognition specificities of L- and H- ficolin. *EMBO J* 2007;**26**:623–33.

22. Tanio M, Kondo S, Sugio S, Kohno T. Trivalent recognition unit of innate immunity system: crystal structure of trimeric human M-ficolin fibrinogen-like domain. *J Biol Chem* 2007;**282**:3889–95.

23. Garlatti V, Martin L, Lacroix M, Gout E, Arlaud GJ, Thielens NM, Gaboriaud C. Structural insights into the recognition properties of human ficolins. *J Innate Immunity* 2010;**2**:17–23.

24. Tucker RP, Chiquet-Ehrismann R. Evidence for the evolution of tenascin and fibronectin early in the chordate lineage. *Int J Biochem Cell Biol* 2009;**41**:424–34.

25. Doolittle RF. The protochordate *Ciona intestinalis* has a protein like full-length vertebrate fibrinogen. *J Innate Immunity* 2012;**4**:219–22.

26. Doolittle RF. Protein Evolution. Neurath H, Hill R, editors. *The proteins*, vol. 4. New York: Academic Press; 1979.

27. Chai Y, Yu S, Liu Y, Zhu Q. A fibrinogen-related protein (TfFREP2) gene involving in the immune response of *Trachidermus fasciatus* against *Vibrio anguillarum*. *Fish Shellfish Immunol* 2013;**35**:1988–92.

28. Doolittle RF, Jiang Y, Nand J. Genomic evidence for a simpler clotting scheme in jawless vertebrates. *J Mol Evol* 2008;**66**:185–96.

29. Felsenstein J. Cases in which parsimony or compatability methods will be positively misleading. *Systematic Biol* 1978;**27**:401–10.

30. Fan C, Zhang S, Li L, Chou Y. Fibrinogen-related protein from amphioxus *Branchiostoma belcheri* is a multivalent pattern recognition receptor with a bacteriolytic activity. *Mol Immunol* 2008;**45**:3338–46.

31. Kenjo A, Takahashi M, Matsushita M, Endo Y, Nakata M, Mizuochi T, Fujita T. Cloning and characterization of novel ficolins from the solitary ascidian *Halocynthia roretzi*. *J Biol Chem* 2001;**276**:19959–65.

32. Harada Y, Takagaki Y, Sunagawa M, Saito T, Yamada Y, Taniguchi H, Shoguchi E, Sawada H. Mechanism of self-sterility in a hermaphroditic chordate. *Science* 2008;**320**:548–50.

33. Miwata K, Chiba T, Horii R, Yamada L, Kubo A, Miyamura D, Satoh N, Satou Y. Systematic analysis of embryonic expression profiles of zinc finger genes in *Ciona intestinalis*. *Dev Biol* 2006;**292**:546–54.

34. Wu Y, Yao F, Mei Y, Chu B, Cheng C, Liu Y, Li X, Zou X, Hou L. Cloning and expression of the gene encoding fibrinogen-like protein. A novel regeneration-related protein from *Apostichopus japonicus*. *Mol Biol Rep* 2014;**41**:2617–27.

35. Xu X, Doolittle RF. Presence of a vertebrate fibrinogen-like sequence in an echinoderm. *Proc Natl Acad Sci USA* 1990;**87**:2097–101.

36. Bohm M, Hentschel U, Friedrich AB, Fiesler L, Steffen R, Gamulin V, Muller IM, Muller WEG. Molecular response of the sponge *Suberites domuncula* to bacterial infection. *Marine Biol* 2001;**139**:1037–45.

37. Perovic-Ottstadt S, Adell T, Proksch P, Wiens M, Korzhev M, Gamulin V, Muller IM, Muller WEG. A (1- > 3)-β-D-glucan recognition protein from the sponge *Suberites domuncula*. *Eur J Biochem* 2001;**271**:1924–37.

38. Srivastava M, et al. The *Amphimedon queenslandica* genome and the evolution of animal complexity. *Nature* 2010;**466**:720–6.

39. Krarup A, Thiel S, Hansen A, Fujita T, Jensenius JC. L-ficolin is a pattern recognition molecule specific for acetyl groups. *J Biol Chem* 2004;**279**:47513–9.

40. Gout E, Garlatti V, Smith DF, Lacroix M, Dumestre-Perard C, Lunardi T, Martin L, Cesbron J-Y, Arlaud GJ, Gaboriaud C, Thielens NM. Carbohydrate recognition properties of human ficolins. Glycan array screening reveals the sialic acid binding specificity. *J Biol Chem* 2010;**285**:6612–22.

41. Laffly E, Lacroix M, Maertin L, Vassal-Stermann E, Thielens NM, Gaboriaud C. Human ficolin-2 recognition versatility extended: an update on the binding of ficolin-2 to sulfated/phosphated carbohydrates. *FEBS Lett* 2014;**588**:4694–700.

42. Shrive AK, Moeller JB, Burns I, Paterson JM, Shaw AJ, Schlosser A, Sorenson GL, Greenhough TJ, Holmskov U. Crystal structure of the tetrameric fibrinogen-like recognition domain containing 1 (FIBCD1) protein. *J Biol Chem* 2014;**289**:2880–7.

43. Thomsen T, Moeller JB, Schlosser A, Sorenson GL, Moestrup SK, Palaniyar N, Wallis R, Mollenhauer J, Holmskov U. The recognition unit of FIBCD1 organizes into a noncovalently linked tetrameric structure and uses a hydrophobic funnel (S1) for acetyl group recognition. *J Biol Chem* 2010;**285**:1229–38.

44. Kaires N, Beisel H-G, Fuentes-Prior P, Tsuda R, Muta T, Iwanaga S, Bode W, Huber R, Kawabata S. The 2.0-Å crystal structure of tachylectin 5A provides evidence for the common origin of the innate immunity and blood coagulation systems. *Proc Natl Acad Sci USA* 2001;**98**:13519–24.

45. Tripp MR. Molluscan immunity. *Ann NY Acad Sci* 1974;**234**:23–7.

46. Adema CM, Hertel LA, Miller RD, Loker ES. A family of fibrinogen-related proteins that precipitates parasite-derived molecules is produced by an invertebrate after infection. *Proc Natl Acad Sci USA* 1997;**94**:8691–6.

47. Zhang SM, Adema CM, Kepler TB, Loker ES. Diversification of Ig superfamily genes in an invertebrate. *Science* 2004;**305**:251–4.

48. Leonard PM, Adema CM, Zhang S-M, Loker ES. Structure of two FREP genes that combine IgSF and fibrinogen domains, with comments on diversity of the FREP gene family in the snail *Biomphalaria glabrata*. *Gene* 2001;**269**:155–65.

49. Zhang S-M, Nian H, Zeng Y, de Jong RJ. Fibrinogen-bearing protein genes in the snail *Biomphalaria glabrata*: characterization of two novel genes and expression studies during ontogenesis and trematode infection. *Dev Comp Immunol* 2008;**32**:1119–30.

50. Zhang H, Wang L, Song L, Wang B, Mu C, Zhang Y. A fibrinogen-related protein from bay scallop *Argopecten irradians* involved in innate immunity as pattern recognition receptor. *Fish Shellfish Immunol* 2013;**35**:1988–92.

51. Knibbs RN, Osborne SE, Glick GD, Goldstein IJ. Binding determinants of the sialic acid-specific lectin from the slug *Limax flavus*. *J Biol Chem* 1993;**268**:18524–31.

52. Kurachi S, Song Z, Takagaki M, Yang Q, Winter HC, Kurachi K, Goldstein IJ. Sialic acid-binding lectin from the slug *Limax flavus*. Cloning, expression of the polypeptide, and tissue localization. *Eur J Biochem* 1998;**254**:217–22.

53. Kawabata SI, Iwanaga S. Role of lectins in the innate immunity of horseshoe crabs. *Dev Comp Immunol* 1999;**23**:391–400.

54. Gokudan S, Muta T, Tsuda R, Koori K, Kawahara T, Seki N, Mizunoe Y, Wai S, Iwanaga S, Kawabata S-I. Horseshoe crab acetyl group-recognizing lectins involved in innate immunity are structurally related to fibrinogen. *Proc Natl Acad Sci USA* 1999;**96** 10086:10091.

55. Sun JJ, Lan JF, Shi XZ, Yang MC, Yang HT, Zhao XF, Wang JX. A fibrinogen-related protein (FREP) is involved in the antibacterial immunity of *Marsupenaeus japonicus*. *Fish Shellfish Immunol* 2014;**39**(2):296–304.

56. Dong Y, Dimopoulos G. Anopheles fibrinogen-related proteins provide expanded pattern recognition capacity against bacteria and malaria parasites. *J Biol Chem* 2009;**284**:9835–44.

57. Cirimotich CM, Dong Y, Garver LS, Sim S, Dimopoulos G. Mosquito immune defenses against Plasmodium infection. *Dev Comp Immunol* 2010;**34**:387–95.

58. Wang X, Zhao Q, Christensen BM. Identification and characterization of the fibrinogen-like domain of fibrinogen-related proteins in the mosquito, *Anopheles gambiae*, and the fruitfly, *Drosophila melanogaster*, genomes. *BMC Genomics* 2005;**6**:114.

59. Middha S, Wang X. Evolution and potential function of fibrinogen-like domains across twelve Drosophila species. *BMC Genomics* 2008;**9**:260.

60. Baker NE, Mlodzik N, Rubin GM. Spacing differentiation in the developing Drosophila eye: a fibrinogen-related lateral inhibitor encoded by scabrous. *Science* 1990;**250**:1370–7.

Chapter 12

Genomic Instability and Shared Mechanisms for Gene Diversification in Two Distant Immune Gene Families: The Plant *NBS-LRR* Genes and the Echinoid *185/333* Genes

Matan Oren, Megan A. Barela Hudgell, Preethi Golconda, Cheng Man Lun, L. Courtney Smith
Department of Biological Sciences, The George Washington University, WA, United States

1   INTRODUCTION

One of the major challenges faced by immune systems is to generate a protein repertoire that is broad and competent enough to recognize the ever-diversifying array of pathogenic nonself. Eukaryotes have numerous strategies to achieve this. Innate immune systems consist of large families of pattern recognition receptors (PRRs) that identify different pathogen associated molecular patterns (PAMPs) with high specificity. Examples include (1) Toll-like receptors (TLRs)[1] found in most animals from Porifera to humans, with PAMP recognition function demonstrated in some species, including human, mouse, and fruit fly[2]; (2) fibrinogen-related proteins (FREPs) with antiparasite activities in mollusks[3]; (3) Down syndrome cell adhesion molecule (Dscam) in insects[4,5] and crustaceans[6,7] with opsonin function; and (4) variable domain-containing chitin binding proteins (VCBPs) in protochordates[8,9] that respond to gut microbes. The adaptive immune system in jawed vertebrates uses somatic recombination of gene segments to create enormous diversity of T cell and B cell receptors.[10] Alternatively, the adaptive immune system in the jawless vertebrates relies on a copy-choice mechanism to assemble sections of leucine-rich repeat (LRR) cassettes into a germline gene to create similar diversity of variable lymphocyte receptors.[11–13] On the other hand, innate immune systems have been suggested

The Evolution of the Immune System. http://dx.doi.org/10.1016/B978-0-12-801975-7.00012-8

to lack the flexibility of adaptive immunity to identify and respond to novel PAMPs that have either newly appeared, or have been newly introduced into a population, due to either environmental changes or as a result of the arms race with host immunity. Therefore, it is necessary for innate immune systems in eukaryotes to employ other types of swift genomic diversification mechanisms either within the lifespan of the host or between generations, to stay even in the arms race with the pathogens. Here, we discuss different aspects of genome diversification in two very distinct innate immune gene-families: the nucleotide binding site leucine rich repeat (*NBS-LRR*) genes in plants, and the *185/333* genes in echinoids. The first is abundant in many species of plants, is a subset of the resistance (*R*) genes, and appeared early in the plant lineage more than 500 million years ago[14] whereas the second is restricted to the echinoid lineage of echinoderms, and the extant genes are estimated to be only 2.7–10 million years old.[15,16] Although there are many differences between these two gene families, there are some striking similarities in the genomic structure and the gene diversity among and within species, which will be the focus of this review.

2 THE *NBS-LRR* GENE FAMILY IN HIGHER PLANTS

The immune response in plants consists of two arms: PAMP-triggered immunity (PTI) and effector-triggered immunity (ETI).[17,18] PTI relies on cell-surface-membrane mounted PRRs that extend into the apoplast and recognize and respond to microbial molecules. ETI functions most often in the plant cell cytoplasm, either acting directly by detecting pathogen virulence-factors called effectors, or acting indirectly by monitoring host proteins that have been altered by effector activity.[17,19] The guard hypothesis suggests that the indirect detection of effector activity is facilitated through a cytoplasmic complex of an R protein that functions as a guard for a host guardee protein. In normal conditions the guard/guardee complex is stable, but upon injection of effectors into the plant cell by a pathogen, the effectors alter the guardee, which is detected by the R protein guard, and induces a signaling pathway to activate the ETI response.[17,20] The indirect ETI response to changes in the guardee proteins maximizes the capacity of the plant host to detect the activity of a large variety of pathogens with a much smaller number of R proteins.[18,21] The key players in the ETI response are a diverse group of mostly intracellular R proteins[17,22] that are encoded by a few to hundreds of *R* genes that are present typically in clusters in every plant genome (Fig. 12.1A), with an expanded repertoire in flowering plants.[14,22] Most R proteins, although not all, are characterized by the presence of a nucleotide binding site (NBS) domain, a linker region, and a variable number of LRRs (Fig.12.1B, C).[23] There are 151 NBS-LRR proteins in the mouse-ear or thale cress, *Arabidopsis thaliana*, 458 in rice, 459 in wine grape, but only two in the much more primitive plant, the spike moss (reviewed in Ref. [14]). The NBS-LRR type of R proteins are divided into two major structurally distinct sub-groups, defined by the N-terminal domain, which is either a

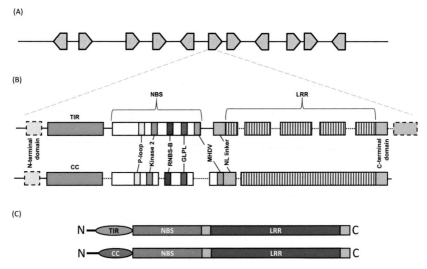

FIGURE 12.1 **An *R* gene cluster and the structures of the TNL and CNL genes and proteins.** (A) A representative homologous *R* gene cluster (not to scale). *R* genes are most often clustered within plant genomes, commonly in homologous clusters, with genes of similar structure and sequence. Each *gray polygon* represents an individual gene (introns and exons are not shown), and gene orientation is indicated by the pointed end of each polygon. Intergenic regions are represented by the *black line* and are not to scale. Gene clusters can vary in size and have different numbers of genes. The majority of genes range in size from 2 to 15 kb, with a maximum size of 44 kb.[25] (B) Representative structures of a Toll/interleukin-1 receptor domain (TIR)-NBS-LRR (TNL) gene and a coiled-coil domain (CC)-NBS-LRR (CNL) gene (not to scale). The structures of *R* genes are highly diverse, with an N-terminal domain (*light gray, dashed outline*) in some genes, a TIR domain in TNLs, or a CC domain in CNLs. The NBS domain has five key semi-conserved regions, including a P-loop, a Kinase 2 motif, and a Resistance Nucleotide Binding Site B (RNBS-B) motif,[26] plus two semi-conserved amino-acid motifs, GLPL and MHDV. Between the NBS domain and the LRRs is an NL linker (named for its location between the NBS and LRR regions). The LRRs can be encoded by either a single or by multiple exons, depending on the gene. The C-terminal domain is of variable lengths among genes, the first portion being encoded within the last LRR exon, and additional C-terminal regions can be encoded on multiple following exons (*blue, dashed outline*). Dotted horizontal lines represent introns that are present in some genes and absent in others. (C) Representative structure of TNL and CNL proteins. The domains that are present in both types of R proteins include the NBS, the NL linker, and the LRRs. The N-terminus is either a TIR or a CC, which defines the TNL or CNL type of R protein, respectively. *(Source: Part B modified from Refs. [27,28].)*

Toll/interleukin-1 receptor (TIR) domain in the TIR-NBS-LRR (TNL) type, or a coiled-coil (CC) domain in the CC-NBS-LRR (CNL) type (Fig. 12.1B, C) (reviewed in[21]). Binding of the LRRs of the TNL and CNL proteins to effector molecules, or to altered guardee proteins, triggers different downstream signaling cascades that lead to the hypersensitivity response (HR) in plants. HR is a rapid apoptotic reaction in infected cells, and those nearby, which functions to remove the availability of cytoplasmic nutrients to pathogens, and thereby restricts their growth and spread.[24]

3 THE *185/333* GENE FAMILY IN ECHINOIDS

The *185/333* gene family encodes a diversified repertoire of immune-response proteins in sea urchins. To date, the *185/333* gene families have only been identified in two species of sea urchins, *Strongylocentrotus purpuratus* (the California purple sea urchin)[15,16] and *Heliocidaris erythrogramma* (the Australian purple sea urchin).[29] However, these genes are likely present in most echinoids, as they have been identified in the genome sequences of *Strongylocentrotus franciscanus* and *Allocentrotus fragilis*[16] and *Lytechinus pictus* (K. Buckley, University of Toronto, personal communication). Among those, the most studied is the *Sp185/333* gene family in the California purple sea urchin, *S. purpuratus*, which was first identified because it showed significant up-regulation in response to immune challenge with heat-killed bacteria and PAMPs, including lipopolysaccharides (LPS), peptidoglycans (PGN), and β-1,3-glucan.[30–33] The family consists of up to 60 members; however, the gene number may vary among individuals[16] and among different species (K. Buckley, personal communication). The *Sp185/333* genes range in size from 1.2 to 2 kb and have only two exons separated by a small intron (380–413 nucleotides).[32,34] The first exon (51–54 nucleotides) encodes the hydrophobic leader, whereas the second encodes the mature protein that shows significant sequence diversity. Optimal alignments of genes and transcripts require the insertion of artificial gaps, which define the presence and absence of short blocks of sequence, known as *elements* (Fig. 12.2A). The combinations of different elements result in recognizable mosaics of elements, called *element patterns.*[31,32,34] This gene structure is persistent among sea urchin species studied to date, although the elements in *185/333* genes from different sea urchin species are not the same.[15,29] The predicted structure of the Sp185/333 proteins is a signal peptide at the N-terminus, a glycine-rich region with an arginine–glycine–aspartic acid (RGD) motif (suggestive of integrin binding), a histidine-rich region, and a C-terminal region (Fig. 12.2B). No secondary structure can be predicted based on the amino-acid sequence for any of the proteins deduced from the cDNA or gene sequences.[31–33,35] The *185/333* genes are expressed in specific subpopulations of sea urchin coelomocytes, and the encoded proteins appear to be localized internally in perinuclear vesicles in some phagocytes, and on the cell surface of small phagocytes.[29,36–38] In *S. purpuratus*, single phagocytes from immune-challenged sea urchins express a single *Sp185/333* message, inferring complex regulation of gene expression from the family and the production of a single Sp185/333 protein per cell.[38] It should be noted that although a genome sequence exists for an individual California purple sea urchin, the *Sp185/333* gene family is artificially underrepresented within this genome, likely due to computational assembly-contraction problems resulting from the variety of repeat sequences that are present between and within the genes (Fig. 12.2A). The size and organization of the *Sp185/333* gene family is currently known, based on gene and message

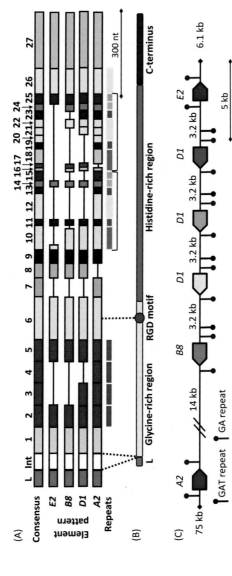

FIGURE 12.2 *Sp185/333 gene cluster, repeat-based alignment, element patterns and protein structure.* (A) Repeat-based alignment of the *Sp185/333* genes shown in (C). The alignment optimizes correspondence between repeats and elements whenever possible.[34] Optimal alignments require artificial gaps (*horizontal black lines*) that delineate individual *elements* shown as *different-colored rectangles*. The consensus of all possible elements are numbered across the top of the alignment. Each gene is composed of two exons; the first encodes the leader (L) and the second encodes the mature protein. Almost all genes have a single intron (int) of ~400 nt (not to scale). The mosaic combinations of presence or absence of different elements in the second exon defines the element pattern (*E2, B8, D1,* and *A2*). Elements that correlate with each of the six types of repeats are shown in *different-colored rectangles* at the bottom (type 1, *red;* type 2, *blue;* type 3, *yellow;* type 4, *green;* type 5, *pink;* type 6, *dark gray*); the brackets under the type 2 to type 6 repeats indicate the two duplicated regions. (B) The deduced Sp185/333 protein structure. The protein size and regions of the protein are correlated with the gene structure in (A); A2 (*red*), B8 (*orange*), three D1 (*yellow, green, blue*), and E2 (*purple*). The genes BK007096) are closely linked. Genes are indicated by element pattern and color; A2 (*red*), B8 (*orange*), three D1 (*yellow, green, blue*), and E2 (*purple*). The genes are located near the 3′ end of the BAC insert within 34 kB. Gene orientations are indicated and spacing is relative to the scale. GA microsatellites flank each gene and GAT microsatellites flank segmental duplications within which are positioned three D1 genes. (*Sources: Part A modified from [34]; part B modified from [39].*)

sequences, and on the assembled insert for one BAC clone (GenBank accession number BK007096), which contains six tightly clustered genes (Fig. 12.2C).[39]

4   GENE DIVERSIFICATION

There is ample evidence for rapid evolution in the *NBS-LRR* gene family in higher plants[14,40,41] and in the *185/333* gene family in sea urchins.[29,42] One has only to evaluate the variability of both the gene numbers among and within species, and the sequence diversity of the genes, to obtain a general understanding of the pace of diversification. The *NBS-LRR* gene family is one of the largest and most variable gene families in plants.[14] Although the common ancestor for the plant *NBS-LRR* genes is predicted to be much older than the common ancestor of the *Sp185/333* genes, the *NBS-LRR* family has continued to expand and diversify.[14] Many of its members exhibit allelic polymorphism,[18] and for some *NBS-LRR* loci, polymorphism within populations is as great as that characterized for the major histocompatibility complex in vertebrates.[40] The *NBS-LRR* genes show two general types of models for gene evolution: the majority are type I genes that show diversifying selection with a rapid rate of evolution and high sequence exchange among genes, and the rest are type II genes that show a slower rate of diversification correlating with less frequent exchanges.[20,22,27,40,43] These two models of gene evolution are not mutually exclusive, and *NBS-LRR* genes positioned within the same cluster can show signatures of both diversification rates.[27] It is noteworthy that the TNL class tends to show significantly higher evolution rates than the non-TNL genes, including the CNL class.[40] Within the TNL genes, sequences that encode the solvent-exposed regions of the LRRs (Fig. 12.1B) seem to be under the highest positive selection and show the highest levels of genetic diversification.[21] These regions show elevated ratios of the nonsynonymous versus synonymous substitutions (dN/dS). This is likely driven by the shared sequences among the LRRs, together with selection based on the function of the LRRs in pathogen-associated recognition.[43] In contrast, the region encoding the NBS domain undergoes purifying selection and is highly conserved, which is likely based on its functions in nucleotide binding, which is crucial for R protein function to initiate signaling in order to activate the protective HR.[21,23,44]

Similar to the *NBS-LRR* gene family, the *185/333* genes show exceptional diversity both among animals and among sea urchin species.[15,16,29,31,34,45] An unrooted phylogenetic tree of *185/333* sequences from *H. erythrogramma* and *S. purpuratus* shows a complete separation of sequences from the two species into different clades.[29] The recognizable element patterns in the second exon of the *Sp185/333* genes are composed of a mosaic of 25–27 different possible elements (depending on the alignment) that range in size from 12 to 258 nucleotides (Fig. 12.2A) and generate 51 different patterns that have been identified to date.[31,33,34] Similarly, the *He185/333* genes have 26 elements and 31 element patterns, based on the first report on this gene family.[29] The element patterns of the different *Sp185/333* genes impart high sequence diversity, but paradoxically, because they share element sequences, they are up to 88% identical.[16,34] Furthermore, although element sequences are shared among genes, identical sequences of full-length genes are not shared among individual sea urchins. This is because (1) only subsets of elements are shared among genes and among animals, (2) there is sequence diversity within different versions of the same element, and (3) there are sequence variations among intron from different genes. The *185/333* genes from both species show many nonsynonymous substitutions with respect to synonymous substitutions (dN/dS ratio) for some element sequences, indicating diversifying selection for these regions, whereas for other elements, a low dN/dS ratio, suggesting purifying selection, has been noted.[29,32,34] Furthermore, when *Sp185/333* gene sequences are compared, the level of diversity among the elements shows significant differences.[34] In general, the *185/333* and the *NBS-LRR* gene families portray sequence diversity patterns with exceptionally fast diversification rates and high dN/dS ratios for some regions within the genes, and slow diversification rates and low dN/dS ratios for other regions. For both families, a conserved basic structure of the genes that encode the functional regions of the proteins is maintained.

5   CLUSTERING AND TANDEM REPEATS

The *NBS-LRR* genes are unevenly distributed in the genome, and tend to be present in clusters that vary in size from 2 to 23 genes, with possibly more in single clusters (Fig. 12.1A).[14,28,43,46–51] For example, the rice Xa21 gene cluster has seven paralogs within 230 kb,[52] the tomato I2 cluster has seven paralogs within 90 kb,[53] and the RPW8 cluster in *Arabidopsis* has five paralogs within 13 kb.[54] *NBS-LRR* clusters can be homogeneous, with all members showing similar structure of either TNL or CNL genes (Fig. 12.1B, C), or can be heterogeneous with TNL and CNL genes mixed together.[55] Homogeneous *NBS-LRR* clusters that contain tandemly repeated genes are very common in many plant genomes. For example, ~40 homogeneous clusters are present in the *Arabidopsis* genome, compared to ~10 clusters that are heterogeneous.[49] There is evidence that the clustering of *NBS-LRR* genes is a major factor in the sequence diversification among the members of the family. The cluster size and gene copy number is positively correlated with sequence-exchange frequency among members of the cluster.[40,41,51] Furthermore, there are greater dN/dS ratios for paralogs in clusters compared to isolated paralogs.[51]

The published *Sp185/333* cluster consists of six closely linked *Sp185/333* genes within 34 kb. Five of the genes are tightly clustered within 20 kb and are 3.2 kb apart, whereas a peripheral sixth gene is located at a distance of 14 kb (Fig. 12.2C).[39] The peripheral genes are oriented in the same direction, whereas the four internal genes are oriented in the opposite direction. The cluster is composed of a mixture of homogeneous and heterogeneous genes based on the element patterns of the second exon (Fig. 12.2A). The three central genes all have a *D1* element pattern, and are positioned within three tandem segmental duplications of ~4.5 kb that show 99.7% sequence identity and are flanked by GAT microsatellites (Fig. 12.2C).[39] The near- identity among the *D1* genes and their flanking regions suggest very recent duplication events.[16,39]

Both the *R* and *185/333* gene families contain several types of repeats. The *NBS-LRR* genes contain exons that encode LRRs of 20–29 amino acids with a consensus sequence of LxxLxLxxNxL(T/S)GxIPxxLGxLxx, in which "L" is Leu, Ile, Val, or Phe, T/S is Thre or Ser, and "x" is any amino acid.[56–58] The number of LRRs can vary among *NBS-LRR* genes, ranging from 4 to 50 repeats.[27] For example, in *Arabidopsis,* the number of LRRs ranges from 8 to 25[28] and the *Resistance Gene Candidate 2 (RGC2)* genes in lettuce have 40 to 48 LRRs.[27] Although the LRRs have an established function for interaction with PAMPs or pathogen elicitors (reviewed in[17,59]), they also serve as an important component in creating genomic instability due to their repetitive nature, which leads to gene-family diversification. Evidence for the participation of LRRs in gene diversification processes lies within the differences in the LRRs among quickly diversifying type I *R* genes, compared to more slowly diversifying type II genes. The sequence identity of introns within type I genes vary between the 5' region and the 3' region of the gene (Fig. 12.1B). Introns within the LRR region have high sequence-identity when compared to each other, which may reflect higher rates of sequence exchanges within the LRR region. Introns within slowly evolving type II genes have low sequence identity, reflecting their lower rates of sequence-exchange events. TNLs have additional introns within the LRR coding regions that are absent from most known CNLs (Fig. 12.1B), which may be indicative of differences in the evolutionary history of the two gene types.[27,28] The greater number of introns within TNL genes versus CNL genes may indicate that TNL genes originated from a fusion of independent genes and are younger than CNL genes, which have few to no introns.[48] It is noteworthy that, although the CNL genes have lost their modular gene structure over time, the encoded proteins may maintain modular functions.

The repeats within the second exon of the *Sp185/333* genes allow two different alignments that are equally optimal.[34] The initial alignment is based on the cDNA sequences, and did not take into account the positions of the internal repeats.[32,33] The second alignment is repeat-based that optimized the correspondence of elements and repeats.[34] There are six types of imperfect repeats in the second exon that are both tandem and interspersed (Fig. 12.2A).[31,32,34,39] Depending on the gene, there are two to four type-1 repeats at the 5' end of the exon, plus multiple copies of type 2–6 repeats that are present in two duplications of the interspersed repeats, in addition to an extra type-3 repeat (Fig. 12.2A). In addition, there are GA microsatellites positioned on either side of each gene within the intergenic regions, and are located about 430 bp from the 5' end of each gene, and 300–700 bp from the 3' end (Fig. 12.2C).[39] The GAT microsatellites are positioned at the edges of three ~4.5 kb tandem segmental duplications that include three *D1* genes (Fig. 12.2C). Based on their positions at the edges of the duplicated regions, they may act as mediators of the duplication process.[39] Moreover, pairwise sequence comparisons among the clustered genes identified in the BAC insert show that the sequences between the ends of the coding regions and the nearby flanking GA microsatellite are much more conserved than the regions outside of the GA repeats.[39] This suggests that the microsatellites surrounding the *Sp185/333* genes and those surrounding the segmental duplications may promote diversification of the family through regional instability, including sequence duplication and limiting sequence homogenization from gene conversion.[16] Taken together, both the *185/333* and *R* gene families are characterized by clustering, repeats, and duplications. These features are found abundantly within the genomic structure for each of these innate immune gene-families, and are likely crucial for the processes that lead to gene diversification.

6   SPECULATIONS ON DIVERSIFICATION MECHANISMS OF THE *Sp185/333* GENES

The regions of the genome in which the *NBS-LRR* and the *Sp185/333* gene families are located, are very likely prone to genomic instability, which leads to gene sequence diversification. Gene diversification is initiated by mechanisms that regulate changes in the gene-copy number and organization of the whole family in which entire genes are duplicated, transferred to another location, deleted, or incur changes within the gene sequences (Fig. 12.3). The arms race between host and pathogen drives changes in host immune gene-sequence, which in turn drives functional adaptations in genes encoding effector proteins in pathogens, as demonstrated for the regions of the plant *R* genes that encode the LRRs. The variety of repetitive sequences in the *NBS-LRR* and *Sp185/333* gene families promote genomic instability and nucleotide mismatches that may take place when homologous chromosomes interact either during meiosis or DNA repair processes. Meiotic recombination and homologous DNA repair may be regarded as special events in which homologous chromosomes interact and promote sequence exchange. Several mechanisms that directly and indirectly lead to gene sequence rearrangements have been suggested for the *NBS-LRR* gene family. Based on the structural and diversification similarities of these two immune gene families, we speculate that these mechanisms apply to the *Sp185/333* genes as well. *NBS-LRR* genes are diversified by recombination between alleles and similar family members that result in new *R* genes with altered sequences. This spontaneous allele recombination is combined with selective pressures to detect PAMPs or elicitors, and results in gene variants with altered binding specificity. For example, individual L genes in flax that are derived from intragenic crossing-over show distinct phenotypes with regard to pathogen recognition.[60] Recombination in the *Sp185/333* genes has been detected computationally and is evident, not only between, but within elements and within the intron,[42] suggesting that recombination events can occur at

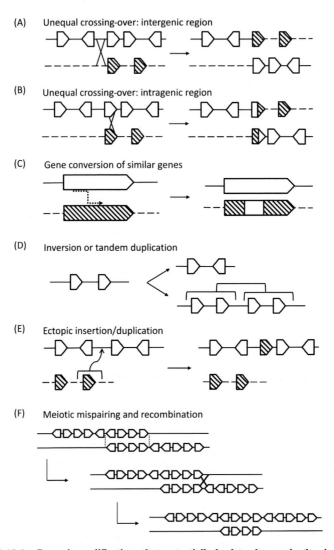

FIGURE 12.3 Genomic modifications that potentially lead to changes in the size of gene families, changes in the organization of clusters, and alterations to gene sequences. Genes are represented as *polygons* (*white* and *striped* genes are in nonallelic clusters), with the pointed end indicating gene orientation. The genomic DNA in which the genes are located is shown as a *solid* or *dashed horizontal line* representing nonallelic regions. The generation of diversity within clusters and sequence diversity within genes is illustrated. (A) An unequal crossing-over in an intergenic region between nonallelic clusters can alter the sizes of the clusters, and result in heterogeneous clusters. (B) Unequal crossing-over within genes in nonallelic clusters can generate recombinant genes, alter cluster sizes, and result in heterogeneous clusters. (C) Gene conversion results when the sequences of one gene are copied into a nonallelic gene of similar sequence. (D) Inversion changes the orientation of a gene within a cluster, whereas the tandem duplication of genes or sets of genes increases the size of a cluster. (E) A duplicated gene can be inserted into an ectopic location, generating a heterogeneous cluster. (F) Meiotic mispairing occurs when chromatids misalign in regions of allelic clusters of highly similar genes, with the outcome of more genes in one cluster and fewer in the allelic cluster. The recombination event is shown between genes, but can occur within genes, as in (B). The processes shown in (A), (B), (E), and (F) can increase and decrease gene-copy numbers in clusters and in gene families.

any point throughout the entire gene sequence and are not focused in hotspots. For example, there is no correlation between the patterns and numbers of the tandem type I repeats in the 5' end of the second exon and the patterns of the interspersed repeats located towards the 3' end of the exon (Fig. 12.1A). It has been suggested that highly similar sequences between duplicated genes within homologous clusters drive further diversification through processes such as unequal crossing-over (Fig. 12.3A, B),[61] resulting in unequal numbers and mispaired linked genes in the progeny, followed by processes that drive further diversification.[55] In both families, shared sequences among paralogs leads to a swift rate of recombination among the genes.

Gene conversion occurs either during meiosis or as a result of DNA repair processes when homologous sites show mismatches in base pairing. These mismatches are recognized and corrected by the DNA repair machinery to convert the sequence of one allele to the sequence of its homologous counterpart (Fig. 12.3C). Gene conversion is an important diversification mechanism in TNL genes that undergo rapid sequence diversification followed by pathogen-driven selection for function (reviewed in[22]). The *RGC2* type I genes in lettuce undergo rapid rates of gene conversion and recombination within the 3' end that encodes the LRRs, which have resulted in a large variety of *RGC2* genes.[27] Bioinformatic analysis of the *Arabadopsis* genome shows that gene-conversion events are driven by genes in clusters with sequence similarity.[61] The *Arabadopsis* gene-conversion events take place most commonly between genes that share 60–70% sequence identity, with most conversion events spanning 60–528 bp.[27,61,62] A greater tendency for gene conversion occurs when genes are proximal to each other, and is rarely found in genes dispersed farther away in the genome. It is not known whether gene conversion is a key mechanism for diversification in the *185/333* gene family. The structural components necessary for promoting gene conversion exist in the family, particularly given the significant sequence identity that is shared among the *Sp185/333* genes, which is based on shared element sequences.[34,39] Within a cluster, the presence of the microsatellites may initiate gene conversion, and then may limit the size of converted regions to block homogenization of the entire cluster.[39] Although it would be expected that higher sequence similarity would be present among tightly linked *Sp185/333* genes based on the likelihood of conversion occurring among proximal genes, comparisons among 121 genes of unknown linkage relationships from three *S. purpuratus* genomes show the same level of sequence similarity as genes of known linkage.[39] This lack of significant differences in the sequence diversity among clustered *Sp185/333* genes and 121 unique unlinked genes suggests that gene conversion may occur within the family among both local and more distant genes,[16] and that it occurs relatively swiftly within the family.

Both gene conversion and unequal crossing-over can drive gene duplication.[20] The most frequent duplication of whole *NBS-LRR* genes are tandem duplications, resulting in two similar genes in close proximity, which leads to the formation of a homogeneous gene cluster (Fig. 12.3D).[14,49,61] Gene duplication and ectopic insertion of either a small set of genes or single genes to a distant location on the same or on a different chromosome (Fig. 12.3E), may also contribute to the family sequence diversity, which includes the formation of heterogeneous clusters.[28] Chromosomal segmental duplication can affect large portions of plant genomes, and is involved in the expansion of *NBS-LRR* gene families.[28] Small segmental duplications in the *Sp185/333* gene cluster appears to be the source of the *D1* gene duplication.[39] Furthermore, duplications of the tandem type 1 repeats in the *Sp185/333* family (Fig. 12.2A) may have been derived from ancestral sequences through duplications of the repeats, in addition to recombination and deletions, based on a computational estimation of the evolutionary history of this region of the genes.[42] Finally, similar to the *NBS-LRR* gene families, meiotic mispairing (Fig. 12.3F), based on the close proximity of the *Sp185/333* genes within the cluster, in addition to the sequence similarities among the genes, has been speculated to drive changes in the size of the *Sp185/333* gene family.[16,39]

Transposable elements may also contribute to genomic instability, which may drive diversity in both single genes and gene clusters. It has been shown that some *NBS-LRR* genes are associated with transposable elements. For example, the rice Xa21 gene family contains a large number of transposable elements, including LTR-retrotransposons and miniature inverted repeat transposable elements (MITEs).[63] Fragments of transposable elements are also present within the *Sp185/333* gene cluster. A portion of a Gypsy 10 long terminal repeat (LTR) S element is positioned near the 3' end of the *A2* gene in association with the flanking GA microsatellite.[39] In addition, three tandem, incomplete Tc1-N1-SP DNA transposon fragments are positioned at the 5' end of the *E2* gene in association with the GA microsatellite. It is not known whether transposable elements contribute to the diversification of the *NBS-LRR* and the *Sp185/333* gene families. However, we speculate that the transposable elements may contribute to the instability of the genomic regions harboring the gene families, through unequal crossing-over promoted by the duplication of transposable elements in the vicinity of members of the families.

Gene fragments and pseudogenes are commonly found in tightly linked clusters of paralogous genes, including 25% of the sea urchin *SpTLR* genes.[64] It is thought that this is a result of duplication and recombination among similar genes that also promotes sequence diversification. The levels of *NBS-LRR* pseudogenes vary from one species of plant to another, but are generally abundant.[65] In *Arabadopisis*, 8.05% of the *NBS-LRR* genes are pseudogenes,[28] whereas 51.3% of the *NBS-LRR* gene family in two rice subspecies are pseudogenes.[65,66] Contrary to the *NBS-LRR* family and the sea urchin *SpTLR* family, only one pseudogene of 171 sequenced genes has been identified in the *Sp185/333* gene family.[34] The pseudogene had no intron, and had a deletion in part of the coding region in the second exon that introduces a frame shift. Curiously for a gene family with significant levels of shared sequence within and surrounding the genes, no gene fragments have been found in the genome. The unexpectedly low level of pseudogenes may be the result of rapid gene conversion (see previous sections) that may correct pseudogenes using sequences from nearby (and perhaps distant) genes, or alternatively by an unknown diversification regulation mechanism.

7 CONCLUSIONS

The *185/333* and the *NBS-LRR* gene families share several structural features, including inter- and intra-genic sequence repeats, duplicated genes, clustering, gene conversion, and diversifying selection in response to pathogens. These features are well established in the *NBS-LRR* gene family as components that are necessary for the initiation of a variety of diversification mechanisms. We find that the use of a comparative approach, even between echinoderms and higher plants, can be useful in understanding the biology of immune gene families, or for establishing hypotheses for how innate immune systems diversify and how potentially common mechanisms may function similarly in distantly related eukaryotes.

ACKNOWLEDGMENT

Funding to support the writing of this review was awarded by the United States National Science Foundation (IOS-1146124) to LCS.

REFERENCES

1. Janeway Jr CA, Medzhitov R. Innate immune recognition. *Ann Rev Immunol* 2002;**20**(1): 197–216.
2. Leulier F, Lemaitre B. Toll-like receptors—taking an evolutionary approach. *Nat Rev Genet* 2008;**9**(3):165–78.
3. Zhang S-M, Adema CM, Kepler TB, Loker ES. Diversification of Ig superfamily genes in an invertebrate. *Science* 2004;**305**(5681):251–4.
4. Schmucker D, Clemens JC, Shu H, Worby CA, Xiao J, Muda M, et al. *Drosophila* Dscam is an axon guidance receptor exhibiting extraordinary molecular diversity. *Cell* 2000;**101**(6): 671–84.
5. Watson FL, Püttmann-Holgado R, Thomas F, Lamar DL, Hughes M, Kondo M, et al. Extensive diversity of Ig-superfamily proteins in the immune system of insects. *Science* 2005;**309**(5742):1874–8.
6. Brites D, McTaggart S, Morris K, Anderson J, Thomas K, Colson I, et al. The Dscam homologue of the crustacean *Daphnia* is diversified by alternative splicing like in insects. *Mol Biol Evol* 2008;**25**(7):1429–39.
7. Ng TH, Chiang TA, Yeh TC, Wang HC. Review of DSCAM-mediated immunity in shrimp and other arthropods. *Dev Comp Immunol* 2014;**46**(2):129–38.
8. Dishaw LJ, Mueller MG, Gwatney N, Cannon JP, Haire RN, Litman RT, et al. Genomic complexity of the variable region-containing chitin-binding proteins in amphioxus. *BMC Genet* 2008;**9**(1):78.

9. Dishaw LJ, Giacomelli S, Melillo D, Zucchetti I, Haire RN, Natale L, et al. A role for variable region-containing chitin-binding proteins (VCBPs) in host gut–bacteria interactions. *Proc Natl Acad Sci* 2011;**108**(40):16747–52.

10. Litman GW, Rast JP, Fugmann SD. The origins of vertebrate adaptive immunity. *Nat Rev Immunol* 2010;**10**(8):543–53.

11. Alder MN, Rogozin IB, Iyer LM, Glazko GV, Cooper MD, Pancer Z. Diversity and function of adaptive immune receptors in a jawless vertebrate. *Science* 2005;**310**(5756):1970–3.

12. Herrin BR, Cooper MD. Alternative adaptive immunity in jawless vertebrates. *J Immunol* 2010;**185**(3):1367–74.

13. Boehm T, McCurley N, Sutoh Y, Schorpp M, Kasahara M, Cooper MD. VLR-based adaptive immunity. *Ann Rev Immunol* 2012;**30**:303–20.

14. Jacob F, Vernaldi S, Maekawa T. Evolution and conservation of plant NLR functions. *Front Immunol* 2013;**4**:297.

15. Ghosh J, Buckley KM, Nair SV, Raftos DA, Miller C, Majeske AJ, et al. Sp185/333: a novel family of genes and proteins involved in the purple sea urchin immune response. *Dev Comp Immunol* 2010;**34**(3):235–45.

16. Smith LC. Innate immune complexity in the purple sea urchin: diversity of the *Sp185/333* system. *Front Immunol* 2012;**3**:70.

17. Jones JD, Dangl JL. The plant immune system. *Nature* 2006;**444**(7117):323–9.

18. Maekawa T, Kufer TA, Schulze-Lefert P. NLR functions in plant and animal immune systems: so far and yet so close. *Nat Immunol* 2011;**12**(9):817–26.

19. Van Der Biezen EA, Jones JD. Plant disease-resistance proteins and the gene-for-gene concept. *Trend Biochem Sci* 1998;**23**(12):454–6.

20. Friedman AR, Baker BJ. The evolution of resistance genes in multi-protein plant resistance systems. *Curr Opin Genet Dev* 2007;**17**(6):493–9.

21. McHale L, Tan X, Koehl P, Michelmore RW. Plant NBS-LRR proteins: adaptable guards. *Genome Biol* 2006;**7**(4):212.

22. McDowell JM, Simon SA. Molecular diversity at the plant–pathogen interface. *Dev Comp Immunol* 2008;**32**(7):736–44.

23. Dangl JL, Jones JD. Plant pathogens and integrated defence responses to infection. *Nature* 2001;**411**(6839):826–33.

24. Lam E, Kato N, Lawton M. Programmed cell death, mitochondria and the plant hypersensitive response. *Nature* 2001;**411**(6839):848–53.

25. Nepal MP, Benson BV. CNL disease resistance genes in soybean and their evolutionary divergence. *Evol Bioinform Online* 2015;**11**:49.

26. Meyers BC, Dickerman AW, Michelmore RW, Sivaramakrishnan S, Sobral BW, Young ND. Plant disease resistance genes encode members of an ancient and diverse protein family within the nucleotide-binding superfamily. *Plant J* 1999;**20**(3):317–32.

27. Kuang H, Woo S-S, Meyers BC, Nevo E, Michelmore RW. Multiple genetic processes result in heterogeneous rates of evolution within the major cluster disease resistance genes in lettuce. *Plant Cell Online* 2004;**16**(11):2870–94.

28. Meyers BC, Kozik A, Griego A, Kuang H, Michelmore RW. Genome-wide analysis of NBS-LRR–encoding genes in *Arabidopsis*. *Plant Cell Online* 2003;**15**(4):809–34.

29. Roth MO, Wilkins AG, Cooke GM, Raftos DA, Nair SV. Characterization of the highly variable immune response gene family, *He185/333*, in the sea urchin, *Heliocidaris erythrogramma*. *PLoS ONE* 2014;**9**(10):e62079.

30. Rast JP, Pancer Z, Davidson EH. New approaches towards an understanding of deuterostome immunity. *Origin and evolution of the vertebrate immune system*. Springer; 2000. p. 3–16.

31. Nair SV, Del Valle H, Gross PS, Terwilliger DP, Smith LC. Macroarray analysis of coelomocyte gene expression in response to LPS in the sea urchin. Identification of unexpected immune diversity in an invertebrate. *Physiol Genomics* 2005;**22**(1):33–47.

32. Terwilliger DP, Buckley KM, Mehta D, Moorjani PG, Smith LC. Unexpected diversity displayed in cDNAs expressed by the immune cells of the purple sea urchin, *Strongylocentrotus purpuratus*. *Physiol Genomics* 2006;**26**(2):134–44.

33. Terwilliger DP, Buckley KM, Brockton V, Ritter NJ, Smith LC. Distinctive expression patterns of *185/333* genes in the purple sea urchin, *Strongylocentrotus purpuratus*: an unexpectedly diverse family of transcripts in response to LPS, β-1, 3-glucan, and dsRNA. *BMC Mol Biol* 2007;**8**(1):16.

34. Buckley KM, Smith LC. Extraordinary diversity among members of the large gene family, *185/333*, from the purple sea urchin, *Strongylocentrotus purpuratus*. *BMC Mol Biol* 2007;**8**(1):68.

35. Dheilly NM, Nair SV, Smith LC, Raftos DA. Highly variable immune-response proteins (185/333) from the sea urchin, *Strongylocentrotus purpuratus*: proteomic analysis identifies diversity within and between individuals. *J Immunol* 2009;**182**(4):2203–12.

36. Brockton V, Henson JH, Raftos DA, Majeske AJ, Kim Y-O, Smith LC. Localization and diversity of 185/333 proteins from the purple sea urchin–unexpected protein-size range and protein expression in a new coelomocyte type. *J Cell Sci* 2008;**121**(3):339–48.

37. Dheilly NM, Birch D, Nair SV, Raftos DA. Ultrastructural localization of highly variable 185/333 immune response proteins in the coelomocytes of the sea urchin, *Heliocidaris erythrogramma*. *Immunol Cell Biol* 2011;**89**(8):861–9.

38. Majeske AJ, Oren M, Sacchi S, Smith LC. Single sea urchin phagocytes express messages of a single sequence from the diverse *Sp185/333* gene family in response to bacterial challenge. *J Immunol* 2014;**193**(11):5678–88.

39. Miller CA, Buckley KM, Easley RL, Smith LC. An *Sp185/333* gene cluster from the purple sea urchin and putative microsatellite-mediated gene diversification. *BMC Genomics* 2010;**11**(1):575.

40. Chen Q, Han Z, Jiang H, Tian D, Yang S. Strong positive selection drives rapid diversification of *R*-genes in *Arabidopsis* relatives. *J Mol Evol* 2010;**70**(2):137–48.

41. Li J, Ding J, Zhang W, Zhang Y, Tang P, Chen J-Q, et al. Unique evolutionary pattern of numbers of gramineous NBS–LRR genes. *Mol Genet Genomics* 2010;**283**(5):427–38.

42. Buckley KM, Munshaw S, Kepler TB, Smith LC. The *185/333* gene family is a rapidly diversifying host-defense gene cluster in the purple sea urchin *Strongylocentrotus purpuratus*. *J Mol Biol* 2008;**379**(4):912–28.

43. Joshi RK, Nayak S. Perspectives of genomic diversification and molecular recombination towards *R*-gene evolution in plants. *Physiol Mol Biol Plants* 2013;**19**(1):1–9.

44. Krasileva KV, Dahlbeck D, Staskawicz BJ. Activation of an *Arabidopsis* resistance protein is specified by the *in planta* association of its leucine-rich repeat domain with the cognate oomycete effector. *Plant Cell Online* 2010;**22**(7):2444–58.

45. Smith LC. Diversification of innate immune genes: lessons from the purple sea urchin. *Dis Model Mech* 2010;**3**(5–6):274–9.

46. Kanazin V, Marek LF, Shoemaker RC. Resistance gene analogs are conserved and clustered in soybean. *Proc Natl Acad Sci* 1996;**93**(21):11746–50.

47. Michelmore RW, Meyers BC. Clusters of resistance genes in plants evolve by divergent selection and a birth-and-death process. *Genome Res* 1998;**8**(11):1113–30.

48. Shen KA, Meyers BC, Islam-Faridi MN, Chin DB, Stelly DM, Michelmore RW. Resistance gene candidates identified by PCR with degenerate oligonucleotide primers map to clusters of resistance genes in lettuce. *Mol Plant Microbe Interact* 1998;**11**(8):815–23.

49. Leister D. Tandem and segmental gene duplication and recombination in the evolution of plant disease resistance genes. *Trend Genet* 2004;**20**(3):116–22.

50. Zhou T, Wang Y, Chen J-Q, Araki H, Jing Z, Jiang K, et al. Genome-wide identification of NBS genes in japonica rice reveals significant expansion of divergent non-TIR NBS-LRR genes. *Mol Genet Genomics* 2004;**271**(4):402–15.

51. Guo Y-L, Fitz J, Schneeberger K, Ossowski S, Cao J, Weigel D. Genome-wide comparison of nucleotide-binding site-leucine-rich repeat-encoding genes in *Arabidopsis*. *Plant Physiol* 2011;**157**(2):757–69.

52. Song W-Y, Pi L-Y, Wang G-L, Gardner J, Holsten T, Ronald PC. Evolution of the rice Xa21 disease resistance gene family. *Plant Cell Online* 1997;**9**(8):1279–87.

53. Simons G, Groenendijk J, Wijbrandi J, Reijans M, Groenen J, Diergaarde P, et al. Dissection of the *Fusarium* I2 gene cluster in tomato reveals six homologs and one active gene copy. *Plant Cell Online* 1998;**10**(6):1055–68.

54. Xiao S, Ellwood S, Calis O, Patrick E, Li T, Coleman M, et al. Broad-spectrum mildew resistance in *Arabidopsis thaliana* mediated by RPW8. *Science* 2001;**291**(5501):118–20.

55. Baumgarten A, Cannon S, Spangler R, May G. Genome-level evolution of resistance genes in *Arabidopsis thaliana*. *Genetics* 2003;**165**(1):309–19.

56. Kajava A. Structural diversity of leucine-rich repeat proteins. *J Mol Biol* 1998;**277**(3):519–27.

57. Kobe B, Kajava AV. The leucine-rich repeat as a protein recognition motif. *Curr Opin Struct Biol* 2001;**11**(6):725–32.

58. Matsushima N, Miyashita H. Leucine-rich repeat (LRR) domains containing intervening motifs in plants. *Biomolecules* 2012;**2**(2):288–311.

59. Muthamilarasan M, Prasad M. Plant innate immunity: an updated insight into defense mechanism. *J Biosci* 2013;**38**(2):433–49.

60. Dodds PN, Lawrence GJ, Catanzariti A-M, Teh T, Wang C-I, Ayliffe MA, et al. Direct protein interaction underlies gene-for-gene specificity and coevolution of the flax resistance genes and flax rust avirulence genes. *Proc Natl Acad Sci* 2006;**103**(23):8888–93.

61. Mondragon-Palomino M, Gaut BS. Gene conversion and the evolution of three leucine-rich repeat gene families in *Arabidopsis thaliana*. *Mol Biol Evol* 2005;**22**(12):2444–56.

62. Xu S, Clark T, Zheng H, Vang S, Li R, Wong GK, et al. Gene conversion in the rice genome. *BMC Genomics* 2008;**9**(1):93.

63. Richter TE, Ronald PC. The evolution of disease resistance genes. *Plant Mol Evol* 2000;**42**(1):195–204.

64. Rast JP, Smith LC, Loza-Coll M, Hibino T, Litman GW. Genomic insights into the immune system of the sea urchin. *Science* 2006;**314**(5801):952–6.

65. Marone D, Russo MA, Laidò G, De Leonardis AM, Mastrangelo AM. Plant nucleotide binding site–leucine-rich repeat (NBS-LRR) genes: active guardians in host defense responses. *Int J Mol Sci* 2013;**14**(4):7302–26.

66. Luo S, Zhang Y, Hu Q, Chen J, Li K, Lu C, et al. Dynamic nucleotide-binding site and leucine-rich repeat-encoding genes in the grass family. *Plant physiol* 2012;**159**(1):197–210.

Chapter 13

The Evolution of the Toll-Like Receptor System

Carlos G.P. Voogdt, Jos P.M. van Putten

Department of Infectious Diseases and Immunology, Utrecht University, Utrecht, The Netherlands

1 INTRODUCTION

Ever since their emergence, multicellular hosts evolved strategies to survive in optimal symbiosis with parasitizing microorganisms. In turn, microbes continuously developed to evade the defensive barricades put up by their hosts. This ongoing evolutionary arms race has led to the development by the host of a sophisticated, germline-encoded immune system, commonly referred to as the innate immune system. The innate immune system distinguishes beneficial and harmful microbes and responds to environmental threats through an extensive arsenal of so-called pattern recognition receptors (PRR). Throughout host–microbe coevolution, these PRRs have evolved to recognize highly conserved microbe associated molecular patterns (MAMP). These cell-wall or nucleic-acid structures are essential for microbial survival, and hence difficult for the microbe to modify. Detection of these MAMPs enables the recognition of diverse microbes with a minimum set of receptors.

The best-studied family of PRRs are the Toll-like receptors (TLRs). TLRs are type I membrane-spanning glycoproteins that are typically composed of an extracellular domain (ECD), a transmembrane domain, and an intracellular signaling domain. Although the presence of TLR genes is conserved across the animal kingdom,[1] TLR structure and function have diversified in response to the changing habitat and environmental challenges. The discovery of TLRs started with the identification of a protein called Toll in the fruitfly *Drosophila melanogaster*. Toll was identified as a regulator during embryonic development.[2] Later, it was found that during an infection with fungi, the Toll protein was activated by its endogenous ligand, Spätzle. This activation initiated the production of antimicrobial peptides, thereby conferring immunity to fungi in *D. melanogaster*.[3] A search for proteins resembling Toll in other species resulted in the discovery of a murine Toll-like receptor (TLR4). TLR4 proved to be essential for the innate recognition of bacterial lipopolysaccharide (LPS).[4]

The Evolution of the Immune System. http://dx.doi.org/10.1016/B978-0-12-801975-7.00013-X

Since the discovery of TLR4 as the LPS receptor, many more TLRs with their respective microbial ligands have been identified and characterized in many different animals. The revolutionary advances in whole genome sequencing now allow studies on TLR evolution across diverse phyla. Here we will review current knowledge of the evolution of the TLR structure, diversity, and distribution across the animal kingdom, and the functions of TLRs in invertebrate and vertebrate animals, also in the context of ongoing host–microbe coevolution.

2 TLR STRUCTURE

2.1 Extracellular Domain

The extracellular domain of TLRs is composed of multiple consecutive leucine-rich repeats (LRR) that each consist of 22 to 29 amino acids with specifically placed hydrophobic residues. Upon folding, the LRRs form an arch-shaped structure in which closely packed β-sheets form the concave surface of the arch. The consecutive LRR motifs are typically flanked by an N- and C-terminal LRR (LRRNT and LRRCT, respectively) that often contain characteristically spaced cysteine residues. As also discussed in chapters: Lymphocyte Populations in Jawless Vertebrates: Insights Into the Origin and Evolution of Adaptive Immunity; Genomic Instability and Shared Mechanisms for Gene Diversification in Two Distant Immune Gene Families: The Plant NBS-LRR Genes and the Echinoid 185/333 Genes, the presence of LRR motifs in numerous proteins of animals, plants, fungi, bacteria, and viruses indicates that these motifs are of ancient origin and have remained important for protein–protein and receptor–ligand interactions throughout evolution.[5] In 2005, the crystal structure of the first TLR ECD (human TLR3) was resolved, and, since then, additional ECD structures of different vertebrate TLRs and of *D. melanogaster* Toll have been determined.[6–11] Results indicate that in all TLRs the extracellular LRR motifs form an arch-shaped structure that directly interacts with a particular microbial ligand, in contrast to *D. melanogaster* Toll that interacts with the endogenous cytokine Spätzle rather than directly with microbial ligands.

Throughout evolution, continuous diversification in the number and sequence of LRR motifs has resulted in an extensive family of structurally distinct TLRs.[12] Due to the structural diversity, the TLR family is able to recognize a large array of microbial ligands, ranging from lipids to proteins and nucleic-acid motifs. Upon interaction with a ligand, the LRRCT of two monomeric TLR molecules come into close proximity, with the LRRNTs spaced far apart. This results in the formation of a homo- or heterodimeric TLR complex that obtains a somewhat "M"-shaped configuration (Fig. 13.1).

One striking example of structure-based ligand specificity is the interaction of TLR2/1 and TLR2/6 heterodimers with bacterial lipoproteins. After binding triacylated lipoproteins, TLR2 forms a heterodimer with TLR1, whereas binding of diacylated lipoproteins leads to heterodimerization with TLR6. The

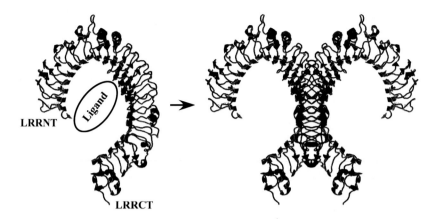

FIGURE 13.1 Upon binding of ligand to the arch-shaped ECD of a TLR, two TLRs will form a dimeric complex, bringing their LRRCT in close proximity, while the LRRNT are spaced far apart.

structural difference between TLR1 and TLR6 that allows for the discrimination of lipoproteins is the blocking of a lipid channel in TLR6 by only two phenylalanine residues. Substitution of these residues opens the lipid channel in TLR6 and makes the receptor receptive for binding triacylated lipoproteins, just like TLR1.[13] This shows that minute structural differences in the TLR ECD allows TLR family members to recognize ligands with great specificity.

2.2 Transmembrane Domain

TLRs are embedded in the membrane via a single-membrane spanning region of approximately 20 amino acids. The TLR family members that recognize lipid or protein ligands are generally positioned at the cell surface, whereas TLRs that bind nucleic acid motifs are located in endosomes. Some TLRs appear in a soluble form. The soluble TLRs originate from enzymatic cleavage of the full-length receptor (TLR2),[14] alternative splicing of the TLR gene (TLR4),[15] or from a separate gene (TLR5).[16] Both soluble TLR2 and TLR4 reduce the response of their membrane-bound form, and thus may act as decoy receptors that prevent an excessive response to their TLR ligands. Soluble TLR5, however, enhances the reactivity of membrane-bound TLR5 and might therefore aid in microbial detection. Soluble TLRs thus provide an additional form of structural TLR diversity.

2.3 Intracellular Domain

On the cytoplasmic side, TLRs contain a TIR domain, named after its structural and functional homology with *Drosophila* Toll and the Interleukin-1 receptor.

The evolutionary importance of the TIR domain is evidenced by its presence in multiple proteins of animals, plants, and even bacteria.[17] The TIR domain of TLRs is structurally composed of five alternating β-sheets and α-helices, connected by short loops that fold into a core of β-sheets surrounded by the α-helices.[18] Its function is to initiate downstream signaling upon ligand-induced receptor dimerization. Dimerization of TLRs brings their TIR domains in close proximity, creating a docking site for recruited adaptor proteins. The adaptor proteins also contain TIR domains and associate with TLRs through TIR–TIR domain interactions. In mammals, TLRs interact with five adaptor proteins: MyD88 (myeloid differentiation primary response protein 88), MAL or TIRAP (myeloid differentiation factor-88 adaptor-like protein), TRIF (TIR domain-containing adaptor protein inducing interferon β), TRAM (TIR domain-containing adaptor protein inducing interferon β-related adaptor molecule), and SARM (sterile α- and armadillo motif-containing protein). Based on the interaction with two major adaptor proteins, TLR signaling can be divided into two signaling routes. The MyD88-dependent route, used by all TLRs except for TLR3, results in early activation of the NF-κB (nuclear factor κB) transcription factor that drive the transcription of proinflammatory cytokines. The TRIF pathway used by TLR3 and (often) TLR4, activates IRF (interferon regulatory factor) transcription factors that stimulate transcription of type I interferon cytokines. The MAL and TRAM adaptors facilitate the interaction between MyD88 and TRIF and TLRs, whereas SARM functions as a negative regulator of the TRIF pathway.[19,20] Although considerably different in sequence and receptor makeup, both animals and plants use TIR domains and also LRR motifs in receptors involved in microbial recognition, implying that these structures may have originated before the divergence of the plant and animal kingdom.[1,21]

3 EVOLUTION AND DISTRIBUTION OF TLR GENES

3.1 Origin of TLRs

Bioinformatics analysis on whole genome data indicates that prokaryotes and fungi lack TLR orthologs. Within the kingdom of plants, receptors composed of LRR motifs attached to various signaling domains (so-called Receptor-like kinases or Nucleotide-binding site LRRs) are present, but show only low sequence similarity to TLRs. Functional studies indicate that these plant receptors respond to different microbial motifs and exploit fundamentally different signaling networks compared to animal TLRs. This indicates that the LRR-containing plant receptors are not ancient TLR orthologs, but rather form separate types of plant-specific receptors that have adapted a similar function as TLRs through the process of convergent evolution.[21,22] The origin of TLRs therefore lies in the animal kingdom (Metazoa).

At the root of the metazoan evolutionary tree is the phylum of sponges (Porifera) (Fig. 13.2).

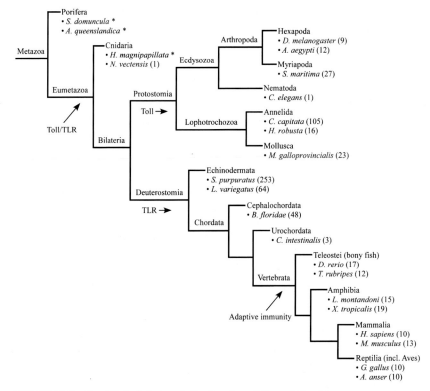

FIGURE 13.2   Simplified phylogeny indicating the relative relationship among some meta-zoans and the number of identified Toll and TLR genes in these species given in brackets. * Indicates TLR-related proteins in these species. The prototypical Toll/TLR has originated in the eumetazoan ancestor approximately 600 million years ago. Basal components of the adaptive immune system arose approximately 500 million years ago in early vertebrates. Echinoderms and nonvertebrate chordates show, in general, a large expansion of their TLR gene repertoire, a feature which may have evolved as an alternative to adaptive immunity. This phylogenic representation is not intended to include all species in which TLR genes have thus far been identified.

The sponge species *Suberites domuncula* and *Amphimedon queenslandica* do not contain typical TLRs, but do carry TLR-related genes. The predicted proteins contain a TIR and transmembrane domain, but have a very short ECD without canonical LRRs (*S. domuncula*[23]), or instead an extracellular immunoglobulin domain (*A. queenslandica*[24]). TLR-related proteins are also present in species of Cnidaria (jellyfish, sea anemones, corals, and Hydra), a sister phylum of Porifera. *Hydra magnipapillata* recognizes microbial ligands through interaction of two membrane proteins, one carrying a cytoplasmic TIR domain and the other carrying extracellular LRR motifs.[25] However, in the genome of a different cnidarian, *Nematostella vectensis* (sea anemone), a typical TLR gene (ie, with TIR and LRR domains), is present.[26] Typical TLR genes are also present in many species within the superphylum of Bilateria. The origin of TLRs therefore dates back to the eumetazoan (all animals except Porifera) ancestor, before the separation of Cnidaria and Bilateria, approximately 600 million years ago[1] (Fig. 13.2).

3.2 Structural Difference Between Protostomian and Deuterostomian TLRs

TLRs have been extensively conserved in bilaterian animals. The superphylum of Bilateria is divided in the protostomes (animals of which the embryonic blastophore forms the mouth) and in the deuterostomes (animals of which the embryonic blastophore forms the anus). Protostomes (including Ecdysozoa and Lophotrochozoa) carry genes encoding Toll proteins, which are structurally distinct from the deuterostomian TLRs. The protostomian Toll proteins generally contain two or more cysteine-rich clusters in the midst of their LRR motifs, whereas the deuterostome TLRs generally contain only one or two cysteine-rich clusters capping the LRR motifs (the LRRNT and LRRCT).[27] Exceptions are the *D. melanogaster* and *Anopheles gambiae* (Hexapoda) Toll-9, in which LRR motifs are more similar to deuterostomian TLRs than to other Toll proteins.[27] Conversely, some TLRs of the invertebrate deuterostome *Strongylocentrotus purpuratus* (sea urchin) are more similar to protostomian Tolls than to other TLRs.[28] Since the gene in the sea anemone *N. vectensis* (Cnidaria) shows a higher structural similarity to protostomian Toll than to deuterostomian TLR, it is likely that the structure of Toll represents the ancestral form, whereas in deuterostomes this ancestral form independently evolved to the TLR form.[1,27]

3.3 Toll and TLR Repertoire in Protostomes and Deuterostomes

Genomic data indicate that protostomes generally contain low to moderate numbers of Toll genes. Most arthropods (insects, crustaceans, myriapods, and chelicerates, belonging to the superphylum of Ecdysozoa) and some species of mollusks and annelids (superphylum Lophotrochozoa) have between 2 and 27 Toll genes.[1,29–33] No Toll genes have been detected yet in the lophotrochozoan Platyhelminthes, which may indicate that these animals have secondarily lost their ancestral Toll genes.[1] Among protostomes, extremes in the abundance of Toll genes exist. The nematode *Caenorhabditis elegans* has only one Toll gene, whereas the annelid worm *Capitella capitata* has 105 predicted Toll genes, an extensive repertoire likely created via many gene-duplication events.[33]

Interestingly, vertebrates (deuterostomes) contain roughly equal numbers of TLR genes, ranging from 10 TLRs in humans to 21 TLRs in amphibians. However, the invertebrate deuterostome *S. purpuratus* (Echinodermata) has massively expanded its repertoire to 253 TLR genes. Most of the sequence diversity in these genes exists in the LRR motifs, and the TLRs more resemble each other than TLR genes from other animals. This suggests that the vast TLR repertoire in the sea urchin results from gene duplication, conversion, and/or recombination events.[28,34] Independent expansion of the TLR repertoire seems to have occurred in the invertebrate deuterostome Amphioxus (*Branchiostoma floridae,* subphylum Cephalochordata), resulting in 48 TLR genes (mixed protostome- and deuterostome-like TLRs).[35] Perhaps these animals have compensated for their lack of an adaptive immune system by expanding their innate receptor diversity to cope with the diverse array of encountered microbial structures, a feature that may be of particular importance in the aquatic environment which these species inhabit.[36] In contrast, the aquatic living ascidian *Ciona intestinalis*, which is an urochordate closely related to vertebrates, has only three TLR genes.[37] Unlike vertebrate TLRs, two of the *Ciona intestinalis* TLRs recognize more than one type of ligand.[38] This multiligand recognition of these TLRs, together with an expansion of complement factors,[37] may have reduced the need for an expanded TLR repertoire in *C. intestinalis*.

3.4   Vertebrate TLR Phylogeny

Most knowledge on TLRs is based on studies of vertebrates (Fig. 13.3).

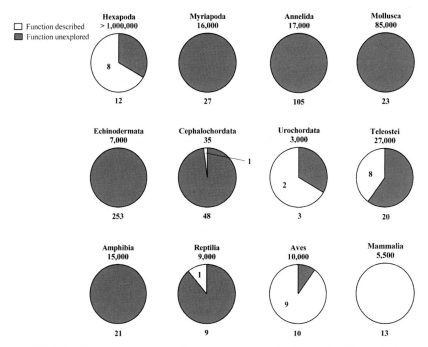

FIGURE 13.3   Knowledge on the function of the numerous TLR genes is still marginal and dominated by studies on vertebrate TLRs. The pie charts indicate the number of TLRs per animal group, with a known function (*white*) or without any functional data (*gray*). The highest number of TLR genes currently identified per animal group are given under each chart. The estimated number of species per group is given under the group name, to put our knowledge on TLR function in perspective with species diversity.

To date, 16 TLR genes have been identified in the lamprey (jawless verte-brate), 13 have been identified in mammals, 10 in birds, 21 in amphibians, and 20 in teleost fish.[31,39–41] Reptiles are predicted to have at least nine TLR genes. Based on sequence homology, most vertebrate TLRs can be grouped into six major families[42] that, in general, have retained the ability to recognize distinct ligands. The large TLR1 family, consisting of TLR1, 2, 6, 10, 14, 15, 16, 18, and 25 recognizes lipoproteins (eg, di- and tri-acylated lipopeptides). A typical members of this family are TLR15 that is activated by microbial proteolytic cleavage[43] and TLR10 that functions as a negative regulator of TLR2.[44] The TLR3, 4, and 5 families recognize double-stranded RNA, LPS, and bacterial flagellin, respectively. The family of TLR7, including TLR7, 8, and 9, recognize nucleic acid motifs. The sixth major family contains TLR11, 12, 13, 19, 20, 21, 22, 23, and 26.[42,45] The receptors in this family that are functionally character-ized, sense either protein (TLR11 and TLR12 respond to profilin of the proto-zoan *Toxoplasma gondii*[46,47]) or nucleic acid motifs, like the TLR7 family.[48] Especially from the large TLR1 and TLR11 families, some TLR genes appear to have been lost in various lineages, perhaps due to functional redundancy. Yet, almost all vertebrate species carry at least one gene from each of the major TLR families, underscoring the importance of innate recognition of a diverse array of microbial ligands.

An interesting exception to the conservation of the vertebrate TLR repertoire is the lack of TLR4 in some teleost fish, such as *Takifugu rubripes*. TLR4, com-bined with its coreceptors MD-2 and CD14, recognizes LPS, and this is of critical importance in the mammalian immune response to bacterial infections.[4] Some fish, including zebrafish (*Danio rerio*) and common carp (*Cyprinus carpio*), do have multiple TLR4 copies but lack the TLR4 coreceptor genes.[49] As a result, LPS sensing in fish is not mediated by TLR4. Instead, fish TLR4 appears to be a negative regulator of the proinflammatory NF-kB transcription factor.[50] The factors driving this divergent evolution are unknown and may await analy-sis of TLR4 in intermediate amphibian and reptile species.

Another example of dynamic TLR evolution in vertebrates is TLR15 in the clade of Diapsida (reptiles and birds). TLR15 is only present in avian and reptil-ian genomes, and its TIR domain is related to members of the TLR1 family.[51] However, unlike TLR1 family members that recognize lipopeptides, extensive sequence diversification of the TLR15 LRR motifs has led to the unique ability of this receptor to become activated by microbial proteases.[43] Why only diapsid animals have developed this trait, and whether it provides these animals with a significant immunological benefit is unknown.

4   TLR FUNCTION

Current knowledge on the evolution of Tolls and TLRs mainly results from pre-dictions based on genome analysis. As evolution is primarily function-driven, the challenge is to corroborate the predictions with functional evidence. At this time,

TLR-related proteins in Porifera have not been functionally characterized, and the only functional studies on cnidarian TLRs have been performed in Hydra. Hydra recognizes bacterial flagellin via an intermolecular interaction between the LRR motif and TIR domain containing proteins.[25] In addition, Hydra deficient in the primary TLR adaptor protein MyD88 are more susceptible to infection with *Pseudomonas aeruginosa*.[52] Although limited, these functional studies suggest that ever since its origin in the eumetazoan ancestor, the TLR system of Hydra functions in the host response to microorganisms. After the divergence of bilaterian animals, TLRs evolved independently in the protostomes and deuterostomes, which has led to functional diversification of the Toll and TLR systems.

4.1   Protostome Toll Function

Most knowledge of the function of protostomian Tolls comes from studies on the arthropod *D. melanogaster* (Hexapoda, Insecta), which has nine Toll genes. *D. melanogaster* Toll-1 (or simply, Toll) regulates the formation of the dorso-ventral axis in the fruit-fly embryo,[2] but is also involved in other developmental processes, including the regulation of organogenesis, alignment, and migration of cardioblasts in the embryonic heart and neural-network development.[1] In addition, Toll-1 initiates the synthesis of antimicrobial peptides from the fat body (equivalent of vertebrate liver) in adult flies after fungal infection.[3] Although less well-characterized, other *D. melanogaster* Tolls also play a role in either development or immunity; Toll-2, -6, and -8 are involved in regulating the anterior–posterior axis formation in the fly embryo,[53] whereas Toll-3, -8, and -9 are involved in the elimination of unfit cells from the developing embryo.[54] Toll-5 is phylogenetically most similar to Toll-1 and shares the ability to activate the promoter of an antimicrobial peptide gene.[55] Interestingly, Toll-9 is structurally more similar to deuterostomian TLRs, suggesting a function in fly immunity, but functional studies on this Toll produced inconsistent results.[56,57]

Functional studies on Tolls have also been performed in other insects. In the mosquito *Aedes aegypti*, Toll-5A, a gene duplicate homologous to *D. melanogaster* Toll-5, is also involved in immunity, as deduced from increased susceptibility of the Toll-5A knockdown mutant to the fungus *Beauveria bassiana*.[58] Other arthropods, including crustaceans, myriapods, and chelicerates, contain roughly equal numbers of Toll genes compared to insects, but their function has not been determined.[30]

Studies on Toll in the protostomian phylum Nematoda have been limited to the model nematode *C. elegans*. *C. elegans* contains only one Toll gene (TOL-1) and lacks the MyD88 adaptor protein and NF-κB transcription factor. Loss of function of the TOL-1 gene causes severe developmental defects, as well as increased susceptibility to bacterial infection,[59–61] suggesting a dual (MyD88 and NF-κB-independent) function of *C. elegans* Toll in development and in interaction with microbes, although the latter function appears less pronounced than in other protostomes like *D. melanogaster*.

For species of the protostomian superphylum Lophotrochozoa, functional studies on Tolls and TLRs have not been reported, although genes encoding Tolls, TLRs, and signaling molecules, including MyD88 and NF-κB transcription factor, have been identified[31,62] and are subject to regulation upon bacterial and fungal infection.[32,63] As functional studies on arthropod and nematode Tolls have revealed diverse and specialized functions for a structurally highly related family of proteins, the study on Toll function in lophotrochozoans may provide key insights in the original function of Toll proteins in the protostomian ancestor, and the events that have driven functional diversification of protostomian Tolls.

4.2 Invertebrate Deuterostome TLR Function

Investigation of the function of TLRs and TLR-signaling molecules in diverse deuterostomian animals is still in its infancy. TLR gene-expression profiling in various tissues during different life stadia or after infection indicate that the identified genes are expressed. The presence of TLR transcript in immune cells but not sea urchin (Echinodermata) embryos suggests that TLRs play a role in the sea urchin immune system.[64] Cephalochordates like amphioxus also have many putative TLR genes, most of which are not yet functionally explored (Fig. 13.3). The TLR1 receptor of Chinese amphioxus (*Branchiostoma belcheri tsingtauense*) functionally interacts with an amphioxus MyD88 adaptor and activates NF-κB in a human-cell background.[65] As the amphioxus genome is predicted to encode NF-κB orthologs,[35] this TLR may play a role in the amphioxus immune system. The amphioxus TLR is expressed in microbe-interacting tissues, including gills and the gut, and also during the gastrula stage of embryogenesis, which may indicate an additional role for this TLR in amphioxus development. The presence of MyD88 and NF-kB orthologs in both amphioxus and vertebrates suggests that the TLR signaling pathway as known in arthropods has likely been conserved in all deuterostomes.

Two of the three TLRs of the urochordate *C. intestinalis* recognize diverse microbial ligands (including flagellin and nucleic acids) and activate NF-κB in human cells. These ligands also induce expression of the proinflammatory cytokine Tumor Necrosis Factor alpha (an ancient and highly conserved inflammatory mediator) in the *C. intestinalis* gastrointestinal tract, suggesting that the TLRs have an immunomodulatory function.[38] The role of the TLRs in *C. intestinalis* development has not been investigated.

4.3 Vertebrate TLR Function

In vertebrates, the different TLRs are variably expressed in virtually all cell types. The TLRs are considered to scan the environment for microbial ligands and to orchestrate an adequate immune defense. These events are relatively rapid and of low specificity, and form the basis of the innate immune response.

Activation of TLRs ultimately results in enhanced production of antimicrobial peptides and proinflammatory cytokines and chemokines that attract and activate professional immune cells like neutrophils and macrophages.[66] T and B lymphocytes also express TLRs. TLR activation in diverse T-cell subsets promotes proliferation, migration, and proinflammatory cytokine production.[67] In B-cells, activation of TLRs also induces the production of cytokines as well as the expression of costimulatory molecules and differentiation of B-cells into immunoglobulin-producing plasma cells.[68] As indicated in several parts of this book, the immunoglobulin-based adaptive immune system is unique to vertebrates, and provides a much slower but more specific immune response than the innate response.

Besides microbial ligands, TLRs also respond to endogenous danger signals, the so-called damage associated molecular patterns (DAMPs). Endogenous activators include, among others, heat shock protein 60 (HSP60),[69] extracellular matrix components, antimicrobial peptides, and self-nucleic acid motifs. DAMP activation of TLRs can promote a potent inflammatory response that causes excessive and detrimental immune stimulation. Indeed, the presence of high levels of endogenous TLR ligands are associated with several autoimmune diseases.[70] The protostomian Toll receptors may also respond to endogenous danger signals. DAMPs released in *D. melanogaster* hemolymph result in the proteolytic cleavage of endogenous pro-Spätzle to form mature Spätzle, which binds to Toll-1 and initiates Toll signaling.[71]

Overall, the apparent role of invertebrate and vertebrate deuterostomian TLRs in immunity, together with the immune function of the studied Hydra TLR-like molecules and some protostomian Tolls, strongly suggests that a role in immunity is one of the ancestral functions of these receptors. Whereas Toll has expanded its function to regulate development, TLRs in vertebrates seem to have expanded their function to initiate and regulate the vertebrate-specific adaptive immune response. However, evidence is growing that vertebrate TLRs may also have additional functions. In cardiomyocytes, TLR9 activation reduces ATP synthesis via a MyD88- independent pathway, increasing stress tolerance in these cells. This could be beneficial during myocardial ischemia.[72] TLR9 may also be involved in correct neuron and muscle development, as mice lacking TLR9 show abnormalities in sensitivity, activity, and coordination.[73] Other TLRs, including TLR2, 3, and 8, negatively regulate the proliferation of neuronal progenitor cells as well as the outgrowth of axons from neurons in the developing mouse brain.[74] Stimulation of these TLRs in neurons does not activate the transcription factors that drive the immune responses, suggesting that TLRs in neurons function via an (unknown) different signaling network.[74] These vertebrate TLR functions may resemble, to some extent, the functions of Tolls in *D. melanogaster* neuronal development. Besides its role in embryonic axis formation, Toll-1 of *D. melanogaster* is also involved in proper development of motor neurons and musculature,[75] and Toll-6 and Toll-7 are receptors for neurotrophic factors.[76]

5 MICROBE-DRIVEN TLR EVOLUTION

5.1 Microbial Methods to Avoid Detection by TLRs

Throughout evolution, microbes and their hosts are in a Red Queen's race to prevent their own extinction. In order to survive and reproduce, microbes have to invent strategies to resist or evade host defenses, whereas hosts have to retaliate these strategies to prevent becoming overexploited. This also holds true for TLRs. One of the primary functions of TLRs is to detect microbes and to limit their numbers via activation of the immune system. Microbes, on the other hand, have evolved a great variety of tools to evade the TLR system.

One of the microbial evasion strategies is the degradation of TLR ligand. Some bacterial species, including the opportunistic pathogen *P. aeruginosa,* are motile by using a flagellum, which is composed of monomeric flagellin subunits. These flagellin subunits are potent activators of TLR5. However to avoid activation of TLR5, *P. aeruginosa* secretes an alkaline protease (AprA), which degrades released monomeric flagellins (but not intact flagella), thus preventing activation of TLR5 and the development of an innate immune response. *P. aeruginosa* AprA cleaves flagellin in a domain that is conserved across bacterial species, and therefore also degrades flagellins of other bacterial species.[77] Homologs of AprA have been identified in other flagellated bacteria, suggesting that flagellin degradation may be an evolutionary successful bacterial strategy for TLR5 evasion.

Microbes may also display virulence factors that physically block TLR recognition. Superantigen-like proteins (SSL3 and 4) of *Staphylococcus aureus* directly interact with the ECD of human and murine TLR2. This interaction presumably blocks the TLR2 ligand-binding pocket and hence prevents TLR2 from recognizing *S. aureus* cell-wall components. As a result, innate immune cells incubated with the SSLs and subsequentially stimulated with TLR2 ligands show greatly impaired production of proinflammatory cytokines.[78,79]

When microbes fail to escape recognition by TLRs, activation of the immune system may still be prevented by interfering with the TLR signaling cascade. Bacteria may engage host inhibitory receptors, which overrule activating receptors like TLRs.[80] Alternatively, *S. aureus* secretes a TIR domain-containing protein (TirS), which interferes with TLR signaling and impairs NF-κB activation and cytokine production.[81] Viruses also use molecular mimicry of signaling domains or degradation of molecules to interrupt TLR signaling.[82]

The most obvious microbial strategy to avoid detection by TLRs is to alter the structure of main TLR ligands such as flagellins or LPS. Flagellin subunits of β- and γ-proteobacteria (eg, the genus *Salmonella*) are recognized by TLR5 and evoke an immune response.[83] However, flagellin of α- and ε-proteobacteria (eg, the genus *Helicobacter*) is structurally different and lacks the TLR5 binding site, thus preventing detection by TLR5.[84] Similarly, bacteria may alter their lipid A, which is the part of LPS that is recognized by TLR4, and thus impair detection by the TLR4/MD-2/CD14 receptor complex.[85] At temperatures of its flea host (21 to 27°C), *Yersinia pestis* produces a lipid A structure that contains six acyl chains that potently activates TLR4. After transfer of *Y. pestis* to its 37°C mammalian host via a flea bite, *Y. pestis* produces tetra-acylated lipid A, which no longer activates TLR4 and enables *Y. pestis* to evade host immune activation.[86] The abilities of microbes to alter TLR ligand structures are however limited, as the ligands typically consist of conserved molecular patterns that are critical for microbial survival. This was nicely illustrated by substituting the TLR5 binding site in *Salmonella* flagellin with amino acids from *Helicobacter* flagellin. The *Salmonella* flagellin with *Helicobacter* amino acids could no longer be detected by TLR5, but at the cost of a loss of bacterial motility.[84]

5.2   Purifying Selection on TLRs

The diversification of microbes and their TLR evasion strategies exert a selective pressure on the evolution of the TLR system. The "direction" of this selective pressure can be determined using phylogeny-based analyses of site-specific codon substitutions. By comparing TLR sequences among species, a site is identified to undergo positive selection when the ratio of nonsynonymous over synonymous codon substitutions is > 1. This indicates that a site has remained polymorphic and may provide a fitness advantage through adaptive evolution. When the ratio of nonsynonymous over synonymous codon substitutions is < 1, the codon shows no or little variation across species and has undergone purifying selection. This indicates that polymorphisms in such a site would generally be detrimental, and hence the site evolves under functional constraint.[87] Evolution under functional constraint is seen in TLR adaptor proteins, especially MyD88 and TRIF, due to their nonredundant role in signal transduction.[88,89] The TLR adaptors interact with multiple proteins, and therefore polymorphisms would almost certainly impair their interaction with some of these proteins.[19] Maintaining function also dictates the evolution of the TIR domain[88,90] because it shows a high level of identity across diverse species, and substituting even a single important site in the TIR domain can render the TLR inactive.[4,91] In addition, the ECD of nucleic acid sensing TLRs (eg, TLR3, 7, 8, and 9) harbors polymorphisms, but these are rarely found in the ligand-binding region, indicating that ligand binding by these TLRs also evolves under functional constraint.[92–95] The reason for this constraint is likely the very similar structure of microbial and host nucleic acids, which poses the risk of inducing autoimmune responses. Through purifying selection, detrimental polymorphisms that may have increased the affinity to self-nucleic acids have likely been expelled from the population, thereby minimizing the risk of recognizing self-nucleic acids while maintaining adequate sensing of microbial nucleic acids.

5.3   Positive Selection on TLRs

In contrast to nucleic acid sensing intracellular TLRs, the ECD of surface-exposed TLRs (eg, TLR2, 4, and 5) displays a strong diversifying evolution driven by positive selection of advantageous mutations. Genomic data from diverse species has allowed the identification of positively selected sites in TLR genes among primates,[92] birds,[39,93] rodents,[94] cattle,[96] pigs,[97] and fish.[98] Most of these sites are located either near to or directly in the ligand-binding region. The highly polymorphic makeup of TLR ligand-binding regions in different hosts may have been driven by antagonistic coevolution with host-specific pathogens and/or the necessity to discriminate between host-specific commensals and pathogens.[99] Support for this diversifying evolution includes crystallography studies on both the human[100] and mouse[101] TLR4/MD2 complex that indicate that binding of LPS involves species-specific residues and functional studies that demonstrate that mouse TLR4 is activated by both hexa- and penta-acylated LPS,[102,103] whereas human TLR4 only responds to hexa-acylated LPS.

Diversifying evolution may also explain the differential TLR5 response to flagellin in different species. Most of the zebrafish TLR5 residues physically interacting with *Salmonella flagellin*[10] are poorly conserved across vertebrates. Furthermore, functional studies indicate that chicken and mouse TLR5 are more sensitive than human TLR5 to flagellin of *S. enterica* serovar Typhimurium.[91] The recently discovered TLR5 of the reptile *Anolis carolinensis* (Carolina anole) proved to be more sensitive than human TLR5 to flagellins of *P. aeruginosa* (unpublished results).[104] The species-specific recognition of TLR ligands, which has likely developed as a result of host-specific adaptations to coevolving microbial communities, may form a basis for the differential susceptibility or resistance to infection as seen among host species. Understanding the evolution of species-specific TLR functioning may thus aid in unveiling fundamental concepts behind zoonotic diseases.

6 CONCLUDING REMARKS

TLRs are among the most extensively studied innate immune receptors. Yet, there still remains much to be discovered about the evolution of this receptor family. One topic that merits more in-depth investigation is the greatly expanded number of TLR genes present in early invertebrate deuterostomes. Functional characterizations of (combinations of) TLR genes from these animals may provide evidence of independent evolution of a highly specific, sophisticated microbial recognition system based on innate immune receptors that is similar to the immunoglobulin-based adaptive immune system of vertebrates.

Another intriguing issue is the role and evolution of deuterostome TLRs beyond the immune system. Deciphering the roles for Tolls and TLRs in different organismal systems may question our view of the original function of the TLR system. Among the protostomes, the Lophotrochozoa seem to deserve more attention to elucidate the functions of the TLR genes in this superphylum.[1] Potential roles for TLRs outside the immune system may also be studied in more species of Cnidaria and early deuterostomes, so that the positional origin of TLR functions can be more accurately estimated.

Finally, understanding of the evolution of TLRs would be greatly aided by much broader functional studies involving ligands from a large variety of microbes. Phylogeny-based analyses of molecular TLR evolution are able to predict residues with potential relevance for TLR function. Functional studies may provide experimental evidence and unveil the selective pressures that are at the basis of the purifying or diversifying selection of TLRs. Combined, these analyses could be instrumental in deciphering the molecular basis for antagonistic host-specific coevolution with microbes, and the resistance to disease that naturally follows. Such knowledge may be of particular interest in animal breeding to select for disease-resistant genotypes,[93] as well as in predicting an individual's susceptibility to disease.

REFERENCES

1. Leulier F, Lemaitre B. Toll-like receptors—taking an evolutionary approach. *Nat Rev Genet* 2008;**9**:165–78.
2. Anderson KV, Jürgens G, Nüsslein-Volhard C. Establishment of dorsal-ventral polarity in the *Drosophila* embryo: genetic studies on the role of the Toll gene product. *Cell* 1985;**42**:779–89.
3. Lemaitre B, Nicolas E, Michaut L, Reichhart J-M, Hoffmann JA. The dorsoventral regulatory gene cassette spätzle/Toll/cactus controls the potent antifungal response in *Drosophila* adults. *Cell* 1996;**86**:973–83.
4. Poltorak A, He X, Smirnova I, Liu M-Y, Huffel CV, Du X, et al. Defective LPS signaling in C3H/HeJ and C57BL/10ScCr mice: mutations in Tlr4 gene. *Science* 1998;**282**:2085–8.
5. Buchanan SGSC, Gay NJ. Structural and functional diversity in the leucine-rich repeat family of proteins. *Prog Biophys Mol Biol* 1996;**65**:1–44.
6. Bell JK, Botos I, Hall PR, Askins J, Shiloach J, Segal DM, et al. The molecular structure of the Toll-like receptor 3 ligand-binding domain. *Proc Natl Acad Sci USA* 2005;**102**:10976–80.
7. Choe J, Kelker MS, Wilson IA. Crystal structure of human Toll-like receptor 3 (TLR3) ectodomain. *Science* 2005;**309**:581–5.
8. Ohto U, Tanji H, Shimizu T. Structure and function of toll-like receptor 8. *Microbes Infect* 2014;**16**:273–82.
9. Ohto U, Shibata T, Tanji H, Ishida H, Krayukhina E, Uchiyama S, et al. Structural basis of CpG and inhibitory DNA recognition by Toll-like receptor 9. *Nature* 2015;**520**:702–5.
10. Yoon SI, Kurnasov O, Natarajan V, Hong M, Gudkov AV, Osterman AL, et al. Structural basis of TLR5-flagellin recognition and signaling. *Science* 2012;**335**:859–64.
11. Parthier C, Stelter M, Ursel C, Fandrich U, Lilie H, Breithaupt C, et al. Structure of the Toll-Spätzle complex, a molecular hub in *Drosophila* development and innate immunity. *Proc Natl Acad Sci USA* 2014;**111**:6281–6.
12. Matsushima N, Tanaka T, Enkhbayar P, Mikami T, Taga M, Yamada K, et al. Comparative sequence analysis of leucine-rich repeats (LRRs) within vertebrate toll-like receptors. *BMC Genomics* 2007;**8**:124.
13. Kang JY, Nan X, Jin MS, Youn S-J, Ryu YH, Mah S, et al. Recognition of lipopeptide patterns by Toll-like receptor 2-Toll-like receptor 6 heterodimer. *Immunity* 2009;**31**:873–84.
14. LeBouder E, Rey-Nores JE, Rushmere NK, Grigorov M, Lawn SD, Affolter M, et al. Soluble forms of Toll-like receptor (TLR)2 capable of modulating TLR2 signaling are present in human plasma and breast milk. *J Immunol* 2003;**171**:6680–9.

15. Iwami K, Matsuguchi T, Masuda A, Kikuchi T, Musikacharoen T, Yoshikai Y. Cutting Edge: naturally occurring soluble form of mouse Toll-like receptor 4 inhibits lipopolysaccharide signaling. *J Immunol* 2000;**165**:6682–6.
16. Tsujita T, Tsukada H, Nakao M, Oshiumi H, Matsumoto M, Seya T. Sensing bacterial flagellin by membrane and soluble orthologs of Toll-like receptor 5 in Rainbow Trout (*Onchorhynchus mikiss*). *J Biol Chem* 2004;**279**:48588–97.
17. Ve T, Williams SJ, Kobe B. Structure and function of Toll/interleukin-1 receptor/resistance protein (TIR) domains. *Apoptosis* 2014;**20**:250–61.
18. Xu Y, Tao X, Shen B, Horng T, Medzhitov R, Manley JL, et al. Structural basis for signal transduction by the Toll/interleukin-1 receptor domains. *Nature* 2000;**408**:111–5.
19. O'Neill LAJ, Bowie AG. The family of five: TIR-domain-containing adaptors in Toll-like receptor signalling. *Nat Rev Immunol* 2007;**7**:353–64.
20. Gay NJ, Symmons MF, Gangloff M, Bryant CE. Assembly and localization of Toll-like receptor signalling complexes. *Nat Rev Immunol* 2014;**14**:546–58.
21. Ausubel FM. Are innate immune signaling pathways in plants and animals conserved? *Nat Immunol* 2005;**6**:973–9.
22. Boller T, Felix G. A renaissance of elicitors: perception of microbe-associated molecular patterns and danger signals by pattern-recognition receptors. *Annu Rev Plant Biol* 2009;**60**:379–406.
23. Wiens M, Korzhev M, Perović-Ottstadt S, Luthringer B, Brandt D, Klein S, et al. Toll-like receptors are part of the innate immune defense system of sponges (Demospongiae: Porifera). *Mol Biol Evol* 2007;**24**:792–804.
24. Gauthier MEA, Pasquier LDu, Degnan BM. The genome of the sponge *Amphimedon queenslandica* provides new perspectives into the origin of Toll-like and interleukin 1 receptor pathways. *Evol Dev* 2010;**12**:519–33.
25. Bosch TCG, Augustin R, Anton-Erxleben F, Fraune S, Hemmrich G, Zill H, et al. Uncovering the evolutionary history of innate immunity: the simple metazoan Hydra uses epithelial cells for host defence. *Dev Comp Immunol* 2009;**33**:559–69.
26. Miller DJ, Hemmrich G, Ball EE, Hayward DC, Khalturin K, Funayama N, et al. The innate immune repertoire in Cnidaria—ancestral complexity and stochastic gene loss. *Genome Biol* 2007;**8**:R59.
27. Imler J-L, Zheng L. Biology of Toll receptors: lessons from insects and mammals. *J Leukoc Biol* 2004;**75**:18–26.
28. Rast JP, Smith LC, Loza-Coll M, Hibino T, Litman GW. Genomic insights into the immune system of the sea urchin. *Science* 2006;**314**:952–6.
29. Waterhouse RM, Kriventseva EV, Meister S, Xi Z, Alvarez KS, Bartholomay LC, et al. Evolutionary dynamics of immune-related genes and pathways in disease-vector mosquitoes. *Science* 2007;**316**:1738–43.
30. Palmer WJ, Jiggins FM. Comparative genomics reveals the origins and diversity of arthropod immune systems. *Mol Biol Evol* 2015;**8**:2111–29.
31. Rauta PR, Samanta M, Dash HR, Nayak B, Das S. Toll-like receptors (TLRs) in aquatic animals: signaling pathways, expressions and immune responses. *Immunol Lett* 2014;**158**:14–24.
32. Toubiana M, Gerdol M, Rosani U, Pallavicini A, Venier P, Roch P. Toll-like receptors and MyD88 adaptors in Mytilus:complete cds and gene expression levels. *Dev Comp Immunol* 2013;**40**:158–66.
33. Davidson CR, Best NM, Francis JW, Cooper EL, Wood TC. Toll-like receptor genes (TLRs) from *Capitella capitata* and *Helobdella robusta* (Annelida). *Dev Comp Immunol* 2008;**32**:608–12.

34. Buckley KM, Rast JP. Dynamic evolution of toll-like receptor multigene families in echinoderms. *Front Immunol* 2012;**3**:136.
35. Huang S, Yuan S, Guo L, Yu Y, Li J, Wu T, et al. Genomic analysis of the immune gene repertoire of amphioxus reveals extraordinary innate complexity and diversity. *Genome Res* 2008;**18**:1112–26.
36. Ward AE, Rosenthal BM. Evolutionary responses of innate immunity to adaptive immunity. *Infect Genet Evol* 2014;**21**:492–6.
37. Azumi K, Santis RD, Tomaso AD, Rigoutsos I, Yoshizaki F, Pinto MR, et al. Genomic analysis of immunity in a Urochordate and the emergence of the vertebrate immune system: 'waiting for Godot'. *Immunogenetics* 2003;**55**:570–81.
38. Sasaki N, Ogasawara M, Sekiguchi T, Kusumoto S, Satake H. Toll-like receptors of the Ascidian *Ciona intestinalis* prototypes with hybrid functionalities of vertebrate Toll-like receptors. *J Biol Chem* 2009;**284**:27336–43.
39. Alcaide M, Edwards SV. Molecular evolution of the Toll-like receptor multigene family in birds. *Mol Biol Evol* 2011;**28**:1703–15.
40. Babik W, Dudek K, Fijarczyk A, Pabijan M, Stuglik M, Szkotak R, et al. Constraint and adaptation in newt Toll-like receptor genes. *Genome Biol Evol* 2015;**7**:81–95.
41. Kasamatsu J, Oshiumi H, Matsumoto M, Kasahara M, Seya T. Phylogenetic and expression analysis of lamprey toll-like receptors. *Dev Comp Immunol* 2010;**34**:855–65.
42. Roach JC, Glusman G, Rowen L, Kaur A, Purcell MK, Smith KD, et al. The evolution of vertebrate Toll-like receptors. *Proc Natl Acad Sci USA* 2005;**102**:9577–82.
43. Zoete MRde, Bouwman LI, Keestra AM, van Putten JPM. Cleavage and activation of a Toll-like receptor by microbial proteases. *Proc Natl Acad Sci USA* 2011;**108**:4968–73.
44. Oosting M, Cheng S-C, Bolscher JM, Vestering-Stenger R, Plantinga TS, Verschueren IC, et al. Human TLR10 is an anti-inflammatory pattern-recognition receptor. *Proc Natl Acad Sci USA* 2014;**111**:E4478–84.
45. Quiniou SMA, Boudinot P, Bengtén E. Comprehensive survey and genomic characterization of Toll-like receptors (TLRs) in channel catfish, *Ictalurus punctatus*: identification of novel fish TLRs. *Immunogenetics* 2013;**65**:511–30.
46. Kucera K, Koblansky AA, Saunders LP, Frederick KB, De La Cruz EM, Ghosh S, et al. Structure-based analysis of *Toxoplasma gondii* profilin: a parasite-specific motif is required for recognition by Toll-like receptor 11. *J Mol Biol* 2010;**403**:616–29.
47. Raetz M, Kibardin A, Sturge CR, Pifer R, Li H, Burstein E, et al. Cooperation of TLR12 and TLR11 in the IRF8-dependent IL-12 response to *Toxoplasma gondii* profilin. *J Immunol* 2013;**191**:4818–27.
48. Keestra AM, Zoete MRde, Bouwman LI, van Putten JPM. Chicken TLR21 is an innate CpG DNA receptor distinct from mammalian TLR9. *J Immunol* 2010;**185**:460–7.
49. Kanwal Z, Wiegertjes GF, Veneman WJ, Meijer AH, Spaink HP. Comparative studies of Toll-like receptor signalling using zebrafish. *Dev Comp Immunol* 2014;**46**:35–52.
50. Sepulcre MP, Alcaraz-Pérez F, López-Muñoz A, Roca FJ, Meseguer J, Cayuela ML, et al. Evolution of lipopolysaccharide (LPS) recognition and signaling: Fish TLR4 does not recognize LPS and negatively regulates NF-κB activation. *J Immunol* 2009;**182**:1836–45.
51. Boyd AC, Peroval MY, Hammond JA, Prickett MD, Young JR, Smith AL. TLR15 is unique to avian and reptilian lineages and recognizes a yeast-derived agonist. *J Immunol* 2012;**189**:4930–8.
52. Franzenburg S, Fraune S, Künzel S, Baines JF, Domazet-Lošo T, Bosch TCG. MyD88-deficient Hydra reveal an ancient function of TLR signaling in sensing bacterial colonizers. *Proc Natl Acad Sci USA* 2012;**109**:19374–9.

53. Paré AC, Vichas A, Fincher CT, Mirman Z, Farrell DL, Mainieri A, et al. A positional Toll receptor code directs convergent extension in *Drosophila*. *Nature* 2014;**515**:523–7.

54. Meyer SN, Amoyel M, Bergantiños C, de la Cova C, Schertel C, Basler K, et al. An ancient defense system eliminates unfit cells from developing tissues during cell competition. *Science* 2014;**346**:1258236.

55. Tauszig S, Jouanguy E, Hoffmann JA, Imler J-L. Toll-related receptors and the control of antimicrobial peptide expression in *Drosophila*. *Proc Natl Acad Sci USA* 2000;**97**:10520–5.

56. Ooi JY, Yagi Y, Hu X, Ip YT. The *Drosophila* Toll-9 activates a constitutive antimicrobial defense. *EMBO Rep* 2002;**3**:82–7.

57. Narbonne-Reveau K, Charroux B, Royet J. Lack of an antibacterial response defect in *Drosophila* Toll-9 mutant. *PLoS One* 2011;**6**:e17470.

58. Shin SW, Bian G, Raikhel AS. A Toll receptor and a cytokine, Toll5A and Spz1C, are involved in Toll antifungal immune signaling in the mosquito *Aedes aegypti*. *J Biol Chem* 2006;**281**:39388–95.

59. Pujol N, Link EM, Liu LX, Kurz CL, Alloing G, Tan M-W, et al. A reverse genetic analysis of components of the Toll signaling pathway in *Caenorhabditis elegans*. *Curr Biol* 2001;**11**:809–21.

60. Tenor JL, Aballay A. A conserved Toll-like receptor is required for *Caenorhabditis elegans* innate immunity. *EMBO Rep* 2008;**9**:103–9.

61. Pradel E, Zhang Y, Pujol N, Matsuyama T, Bargmann CI, Ewbank JJ. Detection and avoidance of a natural product from the pathogenic bacterium *Serratia marcescens* by *Caenorhabditis elegans*. *Proc Natl Acad Sci USA* 2007;**104**:2295–300.

62. Halanych KM, Kocot KM. Repurposed transcriptomic data facilitate discovery of innate immunity Toll-like receptor (TLR) genes across Lophotrochozoa. *Biol Bull* 2014;**227**:201–9.

63. Zhang S-M, Coultas KA. Identification and characterization of five transcription factors that are associated with evolutionarily conserved immune signaling pathways in the schistosome-transmitting snail *Biomphalaria glabrata*. *Mol Immunol* 2011;**48**:1868–81.

64. Buckley KM, Rast JP. Diversity of animal immune receptors and the origins of recognition complexity in the deuterostomes. *Dev Comp Immunol* 2015;**49**:179–89.

65. Yuan S, Huang S, Zhang W, Wu T, Dong M, Yu Y, et al. An amphioxus TLR with dynamic embryonic expression pattern responses to pathogens and activates NF-κB pathway via MyD88. *Mol Immunol* 2009;**46**:2348–56.

66. Takeuchi O, Akira S. Pattern recognition receptors and inflammation. *Cell* 2010;**140**:805–20.

67. Reynolds JM, Dong C. Toll-like receptor regulation of effector T lymphocyte function. *Trends Immunol* 2013;**34**:511–9.

68. Buchta CM, Bishop GA. Toll-like receptors and B cells: functions and mechanisms. *Immunol Res* 2014;**59**:12–22.

69. Ohashi K, Burkart V, Flohé S, Kolb H. Cutting edge: heat shock protein 60 is a putative endogenous ligand of the Toll-like receptor-4 complex. *J Immunol* 2000;**164**:558–61.

70. Piccinini AM, Midwood KS. DAMPening inflammation by modulating TLR signalling. *Mediat Inflamm* 2010;**2010**:e672395.

71. Ming M, Obata F, Kuranaga E, Miura M. Persephone/Spätzle pathogen sensors mediate the activation of Toll receptor signaling in response to endogenous danger signals in apoptosis-deficient *Drosophila*. *J Biol Chem* 2014;**289**:7558–68.

72. Shintani Y, Drexler HC, Kioka H, Terracciano CM, Coppen SR, Imamura H, et al. Toll-like receptor 9 protects non-immune cells from stress by modulating mitochondrial ATP synthesis through the inhibition of SERCA2. *EMBO Rep* 2014;**15**:438–45.

73. Khariv V, Pang K, Servatius RJ, David BT, Goodus MT, Beck KD, et al. Toll-like receptor 9 deficiency impacts sensory and motor behaviors. *Brain Behav Immun* 2013;**32**:164–72.

74. Okun E, Griffioen KJ, Mattson MP. Toll-like receptor signaling in neural plasticity and disease. *Trends Neurosci* 2011;**34**:269–81.

75. Halfon MS, Hashimoto C, Keshishian H. The *Drosophila* Toll gene functions zygotically and is necessary for proper motoneuron and muscle development. *Dev Biol* 1995;**169**:151–67.

76. McIlroy G, Foldi I, Aurikko J, Wentzell JS, Lim MA, Fenton JC, et al. Toll-6 and Toll-7 function as neurotrophin receptors in the *Drosophila melanogaster* CNS. *Nat Neurosci* 2013;**16**:1248–56.

77. Bardoel BW, van der Ent S, Pel MJC, Tommassen J, Pieterse CMJ, van Kessel KPM, et al. Pseudomonas evades immune recognition of flagellin in both mammals and plants. *PLoS Pathog* 2011;**7**:e1002206.

78. Bardoel BW, Vos R, Bouman T, Aerts PC, Bestebroer J, Huizinga EG, et al. Evasion of Toll-like receptor 2 activation by staphylococcal superantigen-like protein 3. *J Mol Med* 2012;**90**:1109–20.

79. Yokoyama R, Itoh S, Kamoshida G, Takii T, Fujii S, Tsuji T, et al. Staphylococcal Superantigen-like protein 3 binds to the Toll-like receptor 2 extracellular domain and inhibits cytokine production induced by *Staphylococcus aureus*, cell wall component, or lipopeptides in murine macrophages. *Infect Immun* 2012;**80**:2816–25.

80. Van Avondt K, van Sorge NM, Meyaard L. Bacterial immune evasion through manipulation of host inhibitory immune signaling. *PLoS Pathog* 2015;**11**:e1004644.

81. Askarian F, van Sorge NM, Sangvik M, Beasley FC, Henriksen JR, Sollid JUE, et al. A *Staphylococcus aureus* TIR domain protein virulence factor blocks TLR2-mediated NF-κB signaling. *J Innate Immun* 2014;**6**:485–98.

82. Bowie AG, Unterholzner L. Viral evasion and subversion of pattern-recognition receptor signalling. *Nat Rev Immunol* 2008;**8**:911–22.

83. Hayashi F, Smith KD, Ozinsky A, Hawn TR, Yi EC, Goodlett DR, et al. The innate immune response to bacterial flagellin is mediated by Toll-like receptor 5. *Nature* 2001;**410**:1099–103.

84. Andersen-Nissen E, Smith KD, Strobe KL, Barrett SLR, Cookson BT, Logan SM, et al. Evasion of Toll-like receptor 5 by flagellated bacteria. *Proc Natl Acad Sci USA* 2005;**102**:9247–52.

85. Maeshima N, Fernandez RC. Recognition of lipid A variants by the TLR4-MD-2 receptor complex. *Front Cell Infect Microbiol* 2013;**3**:3.

86. Montminy SW, Khan N, McGrath S, Walkowicz MJ, Sharp F, Conlon JE, et al. Virulence factors of *Yersinia pestis* are overcome by a strong lipopolysaccharide response. *Nat Immunol* 2006;**7**:1066–73.

87. Yang Z, Nielsen R. Codon-substitution models for detecting molecular adaptation at individual sites along specific lineages. *Mol Biol Evol* 2002;**19**:908–17.

88. Nakajima T, Ohtani H, Satta Y, Uno Y, Akari H, Ishida T, et al. Natural selection in the TLR-related genes in the course of primate evolution. *Immunogenetics* 2008;**60**:727–35.

89. Fornarino S, Laval G, Barreiro LB, Manry J, Vasseur E, Quintana-Murci L. Evolution of the TIR domain-containing adaptors in humans: swinging between constraint and adaptation. *Mol Biol Evol* 2011;**28**:3087–97.

90. Mikami T, Miyashita H, Takatsuka S, Kuroki Y, Matsushima N. Molecular evolution of vertebrate Toll-like receptors: evolutionary rate difference between their leucine-rich repeats and their TIR domains. *Gene* 2012;**503**:235–43.

91. Keestra AM, de Zoete MR, van Aubel RAMH, van Putten JPM. Functional characterization of chicken TLR5 reveals species-specific recognition of flagellin. *Mol Immunol* 2008;**45**:1298–307.

92. Wlasiuk G, Nachman MW. Adaptation and constraint at Toll-like receptors in primates. *Mol Biol Evol* 2010;**27**:2172–86.

93. Vinkler M, Bainová H, Bryja J. Protein evolution of Toll-like receptors 4, 5 and 7 within Galloanserae birds. *Genet Sel Evol* 2014;**46**:72.

94. Forn sková A, Vinkler M, Pagès M, Galan M, Jousselin E, Cerqueira F, et al. Contrasted evolutionary histories of two Toll-like receptors (Tlr4 and Tlr7) in wild rodents (MURINAE). *BMC Evol Biol* 2013;**13**:194.

95. Webb AE, Gerek ZN, Morgan CC, Walsh TA, Loscher CE, Edwards SV, et al. Adaptive evolution as a predictor of species-specific innate immune response. *Mol Biol Evol* 2015;**32**:1717–29.

96. Jann OC, Werling D, Chang J-S, Haig D, Glass EJ. Molecular evolution of bovine Toll-like receptor 2 suggests substitutions of functional relevance. *BMC Evol Biol* 2008;**8**:288.

97. Darfour-Oduro KA, Megens H-J, Roca AL, Groenen MAM, Schook LB. Adaptive evolution of Toll-like receptors (TLRs) in the family Suidae. *PLoS One* 2015;**10**:e0124069.

98. Sundaram AYM, Consuegra S, Kiron V, Fernandes JMO. Positive selection pressure within teleost toll-like receptors tlr21 and tlr22 subfamilies and their response to temperature stress and microbial components in zebrafish. *Mol Biol Rep* 2012;**39**:8965–75.

99. Werling D, Jann OC, Offord V, Glass EJ, Coffey TJ. Variation matters: TLR structure and species-specific pathogen recognition. *Trends Immunol* 2009;**30**:124–30.

100. Park BS, Song DH, Kim HM, Choi B-S, Lee H, Lee J-O. The structural basis of lipopolysaccharide recognition by the TLR4–MD-2 complex. *Nature* 2009;**458**:1191–5.

101. Ohto U, Fukase K, Miyake K, Shimizu T. Structural basis of species-specific endotoxin sensing by innate immune receptor TLR4/MD-2. *Proc Natl Acad Sci USA* 2012;**109**:7421–6.

102. Hajjar AM, Ernst RK, Tsai JH, Wilson CB, Miller SI. Human Toll-like receptor 4 recognizes host-specific LPS modifications. *Nature Immunol* 2002;**3**:354–9.

103. Steeghs L, Keestra AM, van Mourik A, Uronen-Hansson H, van der Ley P, Callard R, et al. Differential activation of human and mouse Toll-like receptor 4 by the adjuvant candidate LpxL1 of *Neisseria meningitidis*. *Infect Immun* 2008;**76**:3801–7.

104. Voogdt CGP, Bouwman LI, Kik MJL, Wagenaar JA, van Putten JPM. Reptile Toll-like receptor 5 unveils adaptive evolution of bacterial flagellin recognition. *Sci Rep* 2016;**6**:19046.

Chapter 14

The Evolution of Major Histocompatibility Complex in Teleosts

Masaru Nonaka, Mayumi I. Nonaka
Department of Biological Sciences, Graduate School of Science,
The University of Tokyo, Tokyo, Japan

1   GENOME ORGANIZATION

The human major histocompatibility complex (MHC) extends over four mega-base pairs, and contains more than 100 genes.[1] The MHC's proper function is believed to present peptides to T lymphocytes, which is performed by the alpha chains of MHC class I molecules encoded in the class I region, and the alpha and beta chains of MHC class II molecules encoded in the class II region. In addition, there are several genes with immunological functions (eg, complement Bf, C2, and C4) in the class III region of the mammalian MHC, although the physiological or evolutionary significance of this clustering of immunologically important genes has yet to be clarified. Phylogenetic studies of MHC gene organization, using the representative species of each vertebrate class, revealed that the avian chicken,[2] amphibian *Xenopus*,[3] and cartilaginous-fish shark[4] have a centrally organized MHC, in which the class I, II, and III genes are linked similarly to the mammalian MHC (Fig. 14.1A). As cartilaginous fishes are considered to be the most ancient extant group to possess the MHC, such a central organization appears to be the original configuration of the MHC, which is conserved by most vertebrate groups. However, in all the teleost species analyzed thus far, class I alpha chain and class II alpha or beta chain genes are not linked[5–8] (Fig. 14.1B). These results suggest that vigorous genomic rearrangements occurred in the MHC region of a common ancestor of teleost. Recent genomic analyses indicate that the linkage between class I and II genes is conserved in the basal ray-finned fish, such as the spotted gar, *Lepisosteus oculatus*,[9] and the bichir, *Polypterus senegals* (N.T. Fujito and M. Nonaka, unpublished), suggesting that the linkage between the MHC class I and II genes was conserved in the common ancestor of ray-finned fish, and was broken in the teleost lineage after the divergence of these basal ray-finned fish. It is tempting

The Evolution of the Immune System. http://dx.doi.org/10.1016/B978-0-12-801975-7.00014-1

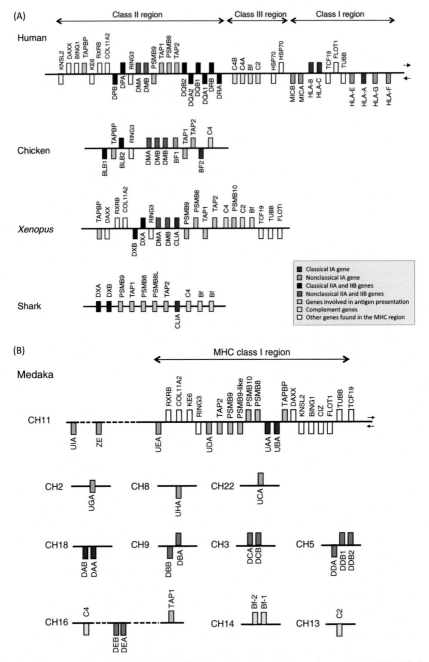

FIGURE 14.1 Organization of the MHC class I region of the various animals. The brief genomic organization of the MHC region of human, chicken, *Xenopus,* and shark (A), and teleost medaka (B) are schematically shown. The genomic organization of human MHC region is generally conserved in other vertebrates, except for medaka. In the medaka, the MHC class II genes and the genes in the human class III region, such as complement C4, C2, and factor B genes, are not located in the MHC region but spread over several chromosomes. The general feature of the medaka MHC region is well-conserved among various teleost species.

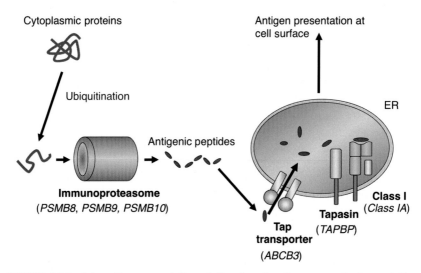

FIGURE 14.2 **Schematic representation of the class I antigen processing/presentation pathway.** Molecules involved in the class I antigen processing/presentation pathway are shown in bold, and the encoding genes present in the medaka MHC class I region are shown in italic in parentheses. As schematically shown here, there is no close structural similarity among immunoproteasome subunits, TAP subunits, tapasin, and class IA molecules.

to speculate that the dispersal of the MHC genes to several teleost chromosomes was triggered by the postulated teleost-specific tetraploidization[10] and the following large-scale genome rearrangement, although the direct evidence to show their direct causal relationship is still missing.

Despite the absence of the linkage between the MHC class I and II genes, the teleost classical class I genes show a curious linkage with the genes directly involved in class I antigen processing/presentation, defining the teleost MHC class I region[11–13] (Fig. 14.1B). These genes are *proteasome subunit beta type-8* (*PSMB8*), *PSMB9,* and *PSMB10* encoding subunits of the immunoproteasome responsible for production of the antigenic peptides, ATP-binding cassette, subfamily B (MDR/TAP), member 3 (*ABCB3*), and TAP binding protein (TAPBP). *ABCB3* encodes a subunit of TAP (transporter associated with antigen presentation) responsible for peptide transportation into the endoplasmic reticulum lumen, and *TAPBP* encodes tapasin, believed to help peptide loading to the class I molecule by mediating interaction between class I and TAP molecules (Fig. 14.2). There is no structural similarity among the TAP, immunoproteasome, and tapasin molecules. Therefore, the linked genes in the teleost MHC class I region are structurally unrelated, but functionally they are intimately linked genes. Most of these genes are also present in the mammalian MHC region. However, some of them are not closely linked in the placental mammalian MHC, where the class I genes and the TAP/immunoproteasome subunit genes are separated by the class III region, which spans approximately 1 M bases (Fig. 14.1A). The close linkage between the class I and *PSMB8* genes is conserved by the shark, ray-finned fish, amphibian *Xenopus*, reptilian anole, and basal mammals such as the platypus and wallaby. These results suggest that the close linkage between the class I gene and the genes directly involved in the class I antigen processing/presentation pathway is the original configuration of the MHC, and that the MHC of placental mammals who have lost this close linkage represents a derived situation.

Another example of the linkage between the structurally unrelated but functionally intimately linked genes found in the MHC is the linkage of the complement *factor B* (*Bf*), *C2*, and *C4* genes, whose role has been described in detail in "The Evolution of Complement System Functions and Pathways in Vertebrates." The *Bf* and *C2* genes are gene-duplication products, and these two genes show a close structural similarity. On the other hand, the *C4* gene has a similar structure to the *C3* and *C5* genes, which are totally different from the *Bf* and *C2* structure. However, *C2* and *C4* are closely linked functionally because they assemble to form the classical pathway *C3* convertase. The linkage between the *C4* and *Bf/C2* genes is conserved in shark, amphibian *Xenopus*, reptilian anoles, and mammals, whereas it is broken in all teleost fish analyzed thus far (Fig. 14.1B). Again, this linkage is conserved in bichir (N.T. Fujito and M. Nonaka, unpublished), suggesting that the linkages between the class I and II genes and between the *C4* and *Bf/C2* genes had broken simultaneously by the gross genome rearrangement that is believed to have occurred in the teleost common ancestor.

These results suggest that the original MHC configuration was the linkage among the class I genes, the class II genes, and the class III complement genes, as well as the close linkage among the class I antigen processing/presentation genes. The former linkage seems to be broken at the early stage of teleost evolution, whereas the latter linkage was retained by most teleost. On the other hand, the close linkage among the class I antigen processing/presentation genes was disrupted in the placental mammalian lineage.

2 CLASS I

The MHC class I molecules have been identified in all vertebrates except for the jawless fishes such as lampreys, suggesting that they had been established in the common ancestor of Gnathostomata after the divergence of Agnatha in concert with other molecules involved in the adaptive immune system. Agnathan immunity and its functioning in absence of MHC is presented in "Lymphocyte Populations in Jawless Vertebrates: Insights Into the Origin and Evolution of Adaptive Immunity." The MHC class I molecule is composed of two polypeptide chains: (1) an α chain encoded by the *IA* gene, and (2) a β-2 microgrobulin encoded by the *B2M* gene (Fig. 14.3A). The α chain has three extracellular domains, termed α1, α2, and α3, and a transmembrane and a cytoplasmic tail

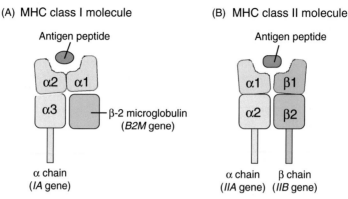

FIGURE 14.3 **Domain structure of the MHC class I and II molecules.** Both MHC class I and II molecules are heterodimer composed of the α and β chains. They have four extracellular domains, and peptide-binding groove is formed by the two membrane-distal domains, α1 and α2 in the case of class I, and α1 and β1 in the case of class II.

region. The β-2 microgrobulin polypeptide chain is instead composed of one IgC domain and binds to the α chain noncovalently. Most animals possess multiple copies of the *IA* gene within and outside the MHC region, whereas the *B2M* gene is located outside the MHC region in all species investigated so far, except for shark.[14]

The *IA* genes are classified into two categories: classical (Ia) and nonclassical (Ib). The products of the Ia genes, such as human leukocyte antigen (*HLA*)-*A*, *HLA-B,* and *HLA-C* are expressed on most cell surfaces and functions in the presentation of intracellular peptide antigens, including the peptides derived from foreign pathogens to cytotoxic CD8[+] T cells, which kill the infected cells directly. The α1 and α2 domains form a peptide-binding site and are highly polymorphic with many allelic products, which could bind various peptide antigens, whereas the α3 domain is not variable. The α3 domain interacts with the CD8 molecule, expressed on the cytotoxic T lymphocytes during recognition of the MHC class I molecules by those cells. The Ia genes are located within the MHC region in all animals, and are linked to the genes encoding the molecules directly involved in class I antigen presentation, such as immunoproteasome subunits, TAP transporter, and TAPBP. In contrast, the Ib genes are not polymorphic and are expressed in more restricted tissues. In addition, most of the amino-acid residues assigned as important for binding of the antigen peptides in the Ia molecule[15] are often substituted by other amino acids in the Ib molecules, suggesting that Ib molecules are not involved in antigen presentation. The Ib genes contain two types of genes; one is represented by the evolutionarily ancient gene-duplication products such as the human *MHC class I chain-related* (*MIC*) genes and *MHC class I-related* (*MR1*) genes, which have evolved independently from the Ia genes. The other type of Ib gene is represented by relatively recent gene-duplication products such as the human *HLA-E, HLA-F,* and *HLA-G.* Although the precise functions of the Ib molecules are not understood fully, the Ib genes are important for evolutionary study of the *IA* genes.[16]

In the teleost, the *IA* genes have been analyzed in various species and many *IA* genes are detected in each species. They are classified into several lineages by phylogenetic analysis. The most popular lineage is the U lineage, identified in all teleost species analyzed, and includes both Ia and Ib genes. The U lineage is also identified in the basal ray-finned fishes such as sturgeon[17] and spotted gar.[18] The other lineages, such as the Z lineage, include only Ib genes and have expanded mainly in the basal teleost, such as cyprinids and salmonids,[19–21] suggesting that these lineages had been established in the early days of the teleost evolution but diminished during diversification of later species, although the ZE gene in the Z lineage has been identified in a few higher teleosts, such as fugu, flounder, and medaka. Interestingly, the $\alpha 1$ and $\alpha 2$ domains of the ZE gene cluster with those of an *IA* gene of lungfish in the phylogenetic analysis.[22,23] However, no genes in the other lineages, including the U lineage, cluster with any *IA* genes of other vertebrates.

The most characteristic feature in the evolution of the teleost *IA* genes is the differential evolution of the three extracellular domains found in the U lineage.[22] In other vertebrates, the Ia and recently duplicated Ib genes evolved generally in a species-specific manner in all three domains, and orthologous relationships of the genes are found only among the closely related species. However, phylogenetic analysis of the teleost *IA* genes showed that the $\alpha 1$, $\alpha 2$, and $\alpha 3$ domains evolved in a quite different manner, and that the orthologous relationships among the distantly related species have been maintained in the $\alpha 1$ domain, whereas the $\alpha 3$ domain experienced sequence homogenization among the loci. Fig. 14.4 shows the phylogenetic trees constructed separately for the $\alpha 1$ and $\alpha 3$ domains, using the nucleotide sequences of various teleost Ia genes and some Ib genes. The $\alpha 1$ domains of the teleost *IA* genes, except for the zebrafish, formed four deeply diverged lineages, termed L1, L2, L3, and L4, supported with high bootstrap values (Fig. 14.4A). L1 included the genes from all acanthopterygians analyzed thus far and salmonids, suggesting that this group is the major lineage of the euteleost *IA* genes. L2 included the genes from the medaka and its close relatives such as Amazon molly and platyfish. L3 included the genes from all acanthopterygians, such as molly, platyfish, tilapia, cichlids, and pufferfish. L4 included the genes from the medaka, molly, tilapia, and salmonids. Three lineages except for L3 included the Ia genes. These results clearly showed the orthologous relationships among the various euteleost *IA* genes. Lineages L1 and L4 contain acanthopterygians and salmonids, indicating that the establishment of these lineages predated the divergence of the acanthopterygians and salmonids, which occurred approximately 260 million years ago.[24] Similarly, the establishment of L2 and L3 predated at least the divergence of medaka and molly or platyfish at 135 million years ago, and of medaka and pufferfish at 180 million years ago, respectively. The *IA* genes of zebrafish were

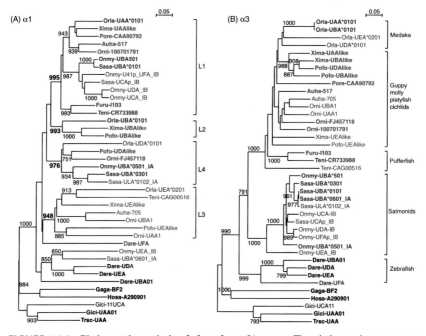

FIGURE 14.4   Phylogenetic analysis of the teleost *IA* genes. The phylogenetic trees were constructed by the NJ method, using the nucleotide sequences of various teleost *IA* genes in the U lineage separately for the α1 (A) and α3 (B) domains. The numbers on each branch represent the >750 bootstrap values calculated from 1000 replications. The genes used were the Ia and Ib genes, detected in the MHC class I region of medaka (22), fugu (11), platyfish (NCBI, genome database), guppy (NCBI, genome database), Amazon molly (NCBI, genome database), tilapia (NCBI, genome database), salmonids[25,26] and zebrafish,[13,27] and some unmapped *IA* genes from tilapia and cichlid. In the genes whose locus number is apparent, one allele from one locus was used in the phylogenetic trees, except for the salmonid Ia genes. Salmonids possess only one Ia gene, termed *UBA*, but it is exceptionally highly polymorphic in both Atlantic salmon and rainbow trout.[28-31] Therefore, several alleles were added for the salmonid *UBA*. In addition, because Atlantic salmon and rainbow trout contain two MHC class I regions generated by tetraploidization, these regions are distinguished as _IA and _IB. The putative classical genes are shown in bold. The *IA* genes of sharks and some other vertebrates were added as outgroups. The accession numbers are as follows: medaka, Orla-UAA*0101, Orla-UBA*0101, and Orla-UDA*0101 (AB183488), Orla-UEA*0201 (BA000027); guppy, Pore-CAA90792 (Z54086); Amazon molly, Pofo-UBAlike (XM_007564296), Pofo-UDAlike (XM_007564294), Pofo-UEAlike (XM_007564324); platyfish, Xima-UAAlike (XM_005808181), Xima-UBAlike (XM_005802885), Xima-UEAlike (XM_005808195); cichlid, Auha-517 (AF038550), Auha-705 (AF038551); Nile tilapia, Orni-UAA1 and Orni-UBA1 (AB270897), Orni-100701791 (XM_003459617); pufferfish, Furu-I103 (AJ271723), Teni-CR733988 (CR733988), Teni-CAG00516 (CAAE01014601); Atlantic salmon, Sasa-UBA*0601_IA (AF504013), Sasa-UBA*0101 (AF504019), Sasa-UBA*0301 (AF504022), Sasa-ULA_IA (EF441211), Sasa-UCAp_IB (EF427379); rainbow trout, Onmy-UBA*0501_IA (AB162342), Onmy-UBA*501 (AF287488), Onmy-UCA_IB, Onmy-UDA_IB, Onmy-UEA_IB, and Onmy-UFAp_IB (AB162343); zebrafish, Dare-UBA01 (Z46777), Dare-UDA and Dare-UFA(AL672151), Dare-UEA (BC097061); nurse shark, Gici-UAA01 (AF220063), Gici-11_UCA (AF028557); banded houndshark, Trsc-UAA (AF034327); chicken, Gaga-BF2 (AB426152); and human, Hosa-A*290901 (AM944568).

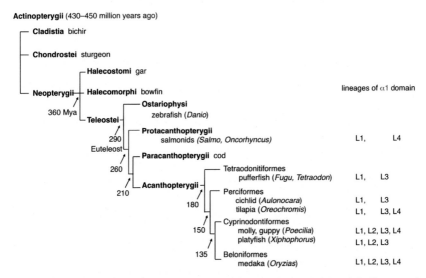

FIGURE 14.5   **Evolutionary relationships of the teleost species analyzed and the lineages of the α1 domain detected.** The divergence times estimated by whole mitogenome sequences (24) are shown at each branch in million years ago.

not included in any of the four lineages, and some of them clustered with some salmonid genes with a rather lower bootstrap value, suggesting that the mode of the diversification of teleost *IA* genes was different in the early days of fish evolution. The results are summarized in Fig. 14.5.

In contrast, the α3 domain clustered by species or related fish groups with no exceptions, regardless of Ia or Ib types, suggesting that homogenization occurred among multiple loci within each species after speciation (Fig. 14.4B). The topology of the phylogenetic tree is the same as that believed to be true for the species evolution (also see Fig. 14.5). Because the α3 domain is known as a constant domain interacting with CD8 on cytotoxic T cells, homogenization might be necessary for retaining the potential for CD8 binding, as well as binding of the β2M. On the other hand, the α2 domains showed no lineages with high bootstrap values, in contrast to the α1 domains, suggesting that partial gene conversion or unequal crossing-over occurred among multiple loci during the divergence of teleosts (data not shown).[22]

The conservation of orthologous relationships of the teleost Ia genes for over 260 million years ago is exceptionally long. The orthologs of the human Ia genes, *HLA-A* and *HLA-B,* are found in macaques, and the orthologs of the human Ib genes, *HLA-E* and *HLA-F,* are found in new world monkeys. The *HLA-F* locus was estimated to have occurred at about 46–66 million years ago.[32] However, it is hard to detect orthology between more distantly related species of the mammals. In marsupials, some Ib genes show orthology between the opossum and wallaby that diverged about 80 million years ago,[33] but it is difficult to detect one-to-one orthology between the Ia genes of these species.

It is probable that differential evolution of three α domains contributed to the long-term conservation of the α1 domain, the diversification of the α2 domain, and the homogenization of the α3 domain. It is speculated that genetic events such as recombination and/or gene conversion have occurred frequently in the teleost *IA* genes, in addition to gene duplication and deletion. Such genetic events also contributed to the allelic diversification, as seen in the salmonid Ia gene. Salmonids possess only one Ia gene termed *UBA*. However, the α1 domains of the *UBA* alleles were detected in at least two of four ancient lineages, and one was out of the lineages (Fig. 14.4A), suggesting that a sequence of an α1 domain of other loci was introduced into salmonid *UBA* as an allele. Interallelic recombination between the exons encoding the α1 and α2 domains has been observed in the medaka[34] and salmonids.[28,35]

The teleost MHC class I region differs from other vertebrates in that it contains no class II genes and no class III region, and that the *IA* genes are linked more closely with the antigen-processing genes essential for antigen presentation by the class I molecules. The tight linkage of the Ia genes and the antigen-processing genes within approximately 150 kb might facilitate coevolution of these genes, possibly providing the genetic basis for the dynamic evolution of the teleost Ia genes.

3   CLASS II

The MHC class II molecules are cell-surface glycoproteins, which bind peptides of extracellular origin, and display them to CD4+ T cells.[36] The MHC class II molecules consist of two noncovalently-associated polypeptide chains, the α and β chains, which comprise two extracellular domains, α1 and α2, or β1 and β2, respectively, a connecting peptide, a transmembrane region, and a cytoplasmic tail (Fig. 14.3B). The mammalian MHC class II genes are classified into two categories, classical and nonclassical. The classical MHC class II genes are polymorphic, polygenic, and are constitutively expressed in professional antigen-presenting cells, such as B cells, macrophages, and dendritic cells. Interferon-γ, secreted upon infection by Th1 T cells and NK cells, induces the expression of the classical MHC class II molecules in various other cell types. The α1 and β1 domains of the classical MHC class II molecules are highly variable, and are encoded by class IIA (*DXA*) and class IIB (*DXB*) genes, respectively, where *D* stands for class II, *X* for an unspecified class-II family, and *A* or *B* for the α or β subclass.[37] The classical MHC class II genes are present in all jawed vertebrates analyzed to date, with the exception of Atlantic cod.[38] In addition to the classical MHC class II genes, most jawed vertebrates possess the nonclassical MHC class II genes. Although the basic structure of the nonclassical molecules are similar to their classical counterparts, they are not polymorphic, and some of them play roles other than presenting peptides to T cells. The functions of most of them remain poorly understood.

A newly synthesized classical MHC class II molecule, HLA-DP, -DQ, or -DR in humans, is transported from the endoplasmic reticulum to the MHC class II compartment (MIIC) of endosomal compartments by binding to a protein called the invariant chain (Ii), which blocks the peptide-binding groove of a classical MHC class II molecule so that other endogenous peptides cannot bind to the groove. In the MIIC, the Ii is cleaved by a cysteine protease, cathepsin, leaving a short fragment, called the class II-associated invariant-chain peptide (CLIP). Subsequently, the nonclassical class II molecule, HLA-DM, binds to the class II–CLIP complex and helps the class II molecule to load antigen peptides. After appropriate binding of a peptide to a class II molecule, the class II–peptide complex is transported to the cell surface, where it displays the peptide to CD4[+] T cells.[39,40] The DM genes have been identified not only in mammals but also in chickens and frogs, indicating phylogenetic conservation of its role to help peptide loading throughout tetrapods.

Compared to the class I genes, information on the class II genes of ray-finned fish is limited, although class II genes have been cloned from spotted gar, Ostariophysi (catfish, zebrafish, and carp), Protacanthopterygii (salmon and trout), and Acanthopterygii (fugu, stickleback, cichlid, sea bass, etc.). These class II genes of ray-finned fish, both class IIA and class IIB genes, are classified into several lineages; one lineage called the A lineage[41] or the DA group[9] contains all the classical class II genes identified from ray-finned fish thus far. From the primitive ray-finned-fish spotted gar, several class IIA and IIB genes have been identified.[9] However, none of them belonged to the A lineage, and it is still an open question as to whether spotted gar has the classical MHC class II genes or not. Interestingly, these identified class II genes of spotted gar are linked to each other, and linked with the classical MHC class I gene, suggesting that the non-linkage between the MHC class I and class II genes was established only within the teleost lineage. Zebrafish belonging to Ostariophysi has both A lineage and non-A lineage MHC class II genes. However, the exact number of these genes is still not clear since the genome assembly (Zebrafish Genome Project (http://www.sanger.ac.uk/resources/zebrafish/genomeproject.html/; Wellcome Trust Sanger Institute, UK) is still imperfect, and it is difficult to discriminate between alleles and loci. In Atlantic salmon, there are one pair of A lineage class II genes, IIA and IIB, and several non-A lineage class II genes. Some of them, located on chromosomes 2 and 5, are believed to have been generated by the salmonid-specific whole genome duplication. In *Xiphophorus* fishes, two divergent, unlinked class IIB genes, *DAB* and *DXB*, were identified.[42] In Nile tilapia, expression of several classical class IIA and IIB genes, and at least one nonclassical class IIA gene, are reported, and the number of expressed classical genes is different, depending on the haplotype.[43] Sato et al.[44] reported that Nile tilapia have two divergent families of class II genes, the IIa and IIb families, which differ in their chromosomal locations, and might have split before the separation of the teleost orders and experienced a different mode of evolution. Recently, Atlantic cod was shown to have no CD4, class II, or Ii genes.[38] The most comprehensive analysis of MHC class II genes was performed in medaka, using the in-depth and draft genome information for the highly diverged inbred strains Hd-rR and HNI, respectively (http://www.shigen.nig.ac.jp/medaka/genome/top.jsp; Hyodo-Taniguchi and Sakaizumi, 1993). Medaka has five pairs of expressed class II genes, comprising one IIA and one IIB gene, located on chromosomes 3, 5, 9, 16, and 18 (Fig. 14.1B). None of them are linked with the class I genes. Three pairs of the class II genes on chromosomes 3, 9, and 18 belong to the A lineage, and one of them on chromosome 18 shows a high degree of polymorphism, indicating that only this pair are classical class II genes.

The most characteristic feature of the teleost MHC class II genes is the absence of the *DM* gene. The DM molecules encoded by the *DM* genes, which reside in the MHC region of all tetrapod species analyzed thus far plays a pivotal role in the class II antigen presentation pathway in peptide editing and stabilization of the classical class II molecules. Thus the absence of the *DM* gene in the ray-finned fish suggests that the ray-finned fish possess quite different MHC class II antigen presentation system. Molecular mechanism of this system is still mostly unknown, and it is interesting to clarify whether some nonclassical class II genes of ray-finned fish are involved in class II antigen presentation or not.

4 PSMB8

PSMB8 is a catalytic subunit of immunoproteasome, which processes intracellular proteins into potentially antigenic peptides that bind with MHC class I molecules in the endoplasmic reticulum lumen. The MHC class I bound with peptides in the endoplasmic reticulum is transported to the cell surface to present antigens to the cytotoxic T lymphocytes.[45] The 20S proteasome, a catalytic core of the larger 26S proteasome, is a large complex composed of four stacks of two outer α-rings and two inner β-rings containing seven α and seven β subunits, respectively.[46,47] Among them, only three beta subunits have catalytic activity. In the constitutive proteasome, PSMB5, PSMB6, and PSMB7 are responsible for chymotrypsin-like, caspase-like, and trypsin-like activities, respectively. Upon immunological reaction, secreted IFN-γ induces PSMB8, PSMB9, and PSMB10 that replace with PSMB5, PSMB6, and PSMB7, respectively.[48,49] Immunoproteasomes formed by replacement of these three subunits show a higher activity to cleave the C-terminal side of hydrophobic amino acids or basic amino acids.[50] PSMB8-deficient mice show reduced cell-surface expression of MHC class I molecules and increased susceptibility to pathogens.[51] In contrast, two missense mutations of the human *PSMB8* gene, one affecting only the chymotrypsin-like activity and the other affecting all three peptidase activities, are reported to cause autoinflammation and lipodystrophy in homozygotic carriers, without increasing their susceptibility to pathogens.[52–54] These reports suggest that PSMB8 plays some roles outside of the class I antigen processing-pathway, and that the full physiological function of PSMB8 is still to be understood.

Dichotomous types of PSMB8 have been reported from sharks, ray-finned fish, and tetrapods. These two types possess either bulky aromatic amino-acid residues such as Phe and Tyr (termed F type), or smaller amino-acid residues such as Ala and Val (termed A type) at the 31st position of the mature protein.[55–61] The 31st residue of PSMB8 is located at the entrance of the S1 pocket and is believed to affect cleaving specificity.[47,60] Only the A-type allele of the PSMB8 gene has been reported from placental mammals, and human PSMB8 possessing Val at the 31st position has been reported to show chymotrypsin-like specificity, which cleaves the C-terminal side of large hydrophobic amino-acid residues.[52] Although the cleaving specificity of F-type PSMB8 has not been directly analyzed, 3D modeling predicted elastase-like specificity cleaving the C-terminal side of smaller neutral amino-acid residues.[60]

These two types of the PSMB8 gene show curious evolution in the ray-finned fish lineage. As shown in Fig. 14.6, the A- and F-type PSMB8 of basal ray-finned fish such as bichir (Polypteriformes), butterfly fish (Osteoglossiformes), zebrafish (Cypriniformes), salmon and trout (Salmoniformes), and pond smelt (Osmeriformes) formed type-specific clusters, termed A- and F-lineage, respectively.[55,59] The allelic status of the A- and F-type PSMB8 was demonstrated in bichir and zebrafish by segregation analysis[59] and genome analysis, demonstrating that *PSMB8* is a single-copy gene in these species (N.T. Fujito and M. Nonaka, unpublished). These results indicate that the A- and F-type PSMB8 represent an extremely long-term trans-species polymorphism (TSP) that has been maintained for more than 400 million years since the divergence of Polypteriformes from the teleost lineage.[55,59,60] TSP originally described with the mammalian class I and II genes is believed to be maintained by balancing selection, such as overdominance selection, where heterozygous individuals show a higher fitness than homozygous individuals of either alleles.[62] All TSPs reported thus far continued for less than 100 million years, indicating that the dimorphism of the *PSMB8* gene of basal ray-finned fish maintained more than 400 million years should be under unprecedentedly strong balancing selection. In contrast, all *PSMB8* sequences of higher ray-finned fish such as mirror dory (Zeiformes), soldierfish (Beryciformes), medaka (Beloniformes), and puffer fish (Tetraodontiformes) are included in the A lineage. Although the possibility that the presence of the F lineage alleles in these groups were overlooked due to an insufficient number of analyzed samples cannot be totally excluded, these results suggest that the F lineage was lost in the higher teleost lineage after the divergence of Osmeriformes, but before the divergence of Zeiformes.[59] Interestingly, however, both the A- and F-type PSMB8 are present in some Beloniformes and Tetraodontiformes fish, and both the A- and F-type alleles of these species belong to the A lineage. Phylogenetic analysis indicates that the A- and F-type alleles of each species form a species-specific cluster, suggesting that the F-type alleles were revived multiple times independently within the A lineage, although the loss of the F lineage occurred only once

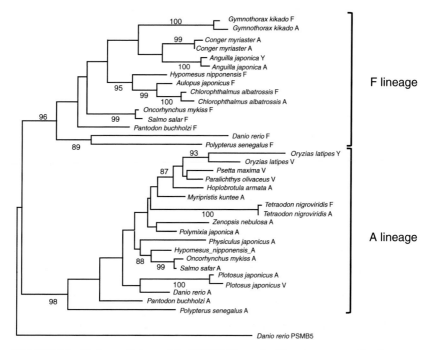

FIGURE 14.6   Phylogenetic trees of the PSMB8. The nucleotide sequences encoding the mature protein were aligned with Clustal X and evolutionary analysis was conducted in MEGA6.0. The phylogenetic trees were constructed by the maximum likelihood (ML) method, based on the general time-reversible model. Bootstrap percentages were determined with 100 bootstrap replications, and only bootstrap values more than 80% are shown. The letter after the name of species shows the 31st residue of mature peptide. The *PSMB5* sequences of zebrafish (*D. rerio*, NM_131151) was used as an outgroup. Accession numbers of the used *PSMB8* sequences are: *Pantodon buchholzi* (F, AB890134, A, AB890135), *Gymnothorax kidako* (F, AB890125, A, AB890124), *Conger myriaster* (V, AB890131, A, AB890130), *Anguilla japonica* (Y, AB890133, A, AB890132), *Hypomesus nipponensis* (F, AB890137, A, AB890136), *Polypterus senegalus* (F, AB686529; A, AB686530), *Danio rerio* (F, NM_001017791; A, NM_131392), *Salmo salar* (F, BT060153; A, NM_001123535), *Oncorhynchus mykiss* (F, BT073071; A, AB162343), *Oryzias latipes* (Y, D89725; V, NM_001184952), and *Tetraodon nigroviridis* (F, CR691449, A, CR697191). Other sequences are unpublished data of M. Noro and M. Nonaka.

in the common ancestor. The opposite situation is observed in Anguilliformes and Aulopiformes. Out of three Anguilliformes species analyzed, *Gymnothorax kikado* and *Anguilla japonica* possess both the A- and F-type alleles, and the *Conger myriaster* possesses only the A-type allele. All these alleles belong to the F lineage irrespective of their types, suggesting that the A lineage had been lost in the common ancestor of Anguilliformes, and A-type allele revived at least three times independently within the F lineage.[59] Two Aulopiformes species, *Aulopus japonicus* and *Chlorophthalmus albatrossis,* show a similar evolutionary pattern of the PSMB8 gene (Fig.14.6). Both the long-term trans-species dimorphism and recurrent recovery of dimorphism indicate that the PSMB8 dimorphism is under

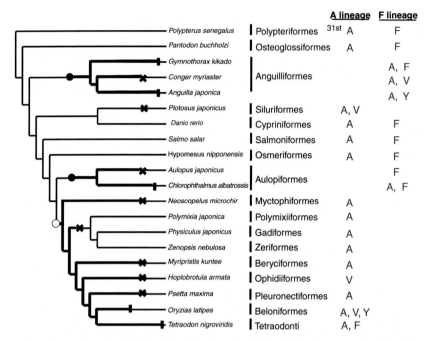

FIGURE 14.7   The evolutionary history of PSMB8, based on interallelic sequence homogenization scenario. The phylogenetic tree of ray-finned fish discussed here[63,64] is schematically shown at left, and A-type (^{31}A or ^{31}V) and F-type (^{31}F or ^{31}Y) alleles identified in each species are shown in red and blue, respectively, separately for the A- and F- lineages at right. Symbols on the phylogenetic tree represent the evolutionary events of PSMB8 dimorphism as follows: closed circle, interallelic sequence homogenization replacing most parts of the A lineage sequences with the F lineage sequences; open circle, interallelic sequence homogenization replacing most parts of the F lineage sequences with the A lineage sequences; vertical bar, intermission of continuous interallelic sequence homogenization; cross, loss of A- or F-type; black heavy line, continuous interallelic sequence homogenization. The timing of intermission of interallelic sequence homogenization was inferred from the nucleotide sequence diversity between the A- and F-type alleles.

exceptionally strong balancing selection.[57,59,60] However, if the balancing selection is so strong, it is strange that the original dimorphism based on the ancient A and F lineages has been lost at least four times during vertebrate evolution: the loss of the F lineage in higher teleosts and tetrapods, and the loss of the A lineage in Anguilliformes and Aulopiformes. An alternative explanation of the phylogenetic tree compatible with the continuous maintenance of the PSMB8 dimorphism is interallelic sequence homogenization excluding the 31st amino acid-encoding region,[56,59] as schematically shown in Fig. 14.7. Evidence for recent interallelic sequence homogenizations have been reported from Anguilliformes[59] and tetrapods.[56] Thus, interallelic sequence homogenization does not seem to be an exceptionally rare event. It is tempting to speculate that the evolutionary event underlying the apparent loss of the A lineage in the common ancestor of Anguilliformes and Aulopiformes, and apparent loss of the F lineage in the common ancestor of higher teleost and in the common ancestor of tetrapods, were also interallelic sequence homogenization except for the close vicinity of the 31st residue. Once such interallelic sequence homogenization occurred between the A and F lineage sequences, the A and F alleles should show a high degree of sequence identity that could facilitate further interallelic sequence homogenization. However, if sequence homogenization has not occurred for a while just by chance, the nucleotide sequences of the A and F alleles could diverge so much that sequence homogenization cannot occur easily anymore. Sequence homogenization in each species after speciation could generate the phylogenetic pattern, apparently suggesting recurrent recoveries of dimorphism, as shown in Fig. 14.7. Whether the evolution of the *PSMB8* dimorphism actually followed this sequence homogenization scenario, or the recurrent recoveries scenario, has yet to be clarified. However, the totally unprecedented pattern of evolution of the *PSMB8* dimorphism suggests the presence of an exceptionally strong balancing selection that has maintained the PSMB8 dimorphism of basal ray-finned fish for more than 400 million years. Although the molecular basis for this balancing selection has yet to be clarified, there is a curious correlation between the PSMB8 dimorphism and the close linkage between the *PSMB8* and *MHC* class *I* genes. The close linkage between these two genes is conserved by most jawed vertebrate groups except for birds, who lost the *PSMB8* gene itself, and placental mammals. Since all *PSMB8* genes of placental mammals analyzed thus far do not show dimorphism, the close linkage between the *MHC* class *I* and *PSMB8* genes seems to have meaning only in the presence of the PSMB8 dimorphism. One possible explanation is that the close linkage between the *MHC* class *I* and *PSMB8* genes facilitates coevolution of these two genes.

5 CONCLUSIONS

The teleost MHC is characterized by the tight linkage of the classical class I gene with the genes directly involved in class I antigen processing/presentation. The linkage between the class *I* and *PSMB8* genes is of special interest, since this linkage seems to have enabled exceptionally dynamic evolution of these genes in teleosts. The most important evolutionary meaning of the vertebrate MHC could be to provide a genome region for the class I antigen processing/presentation genes to perform coevolution.

REFERENCES

1. Consortium TMs. Complete sequence and gene map of a human major histocompatibility complex. The MHC sequencing consortium. *Nature* 1999;**401**(6756):921–3.
2. Kaufman J, Milne S, Gobel TW, Walker BA, Jacob JP, Auffray C, et al. The chicken B locus is a minimal essential major histocompatibility complex. *Nature* 1999;**401**(6756):923–5.
3. Nonaka M, Namikawa C, Kato Y, Sasaki M, Salter-Cid L, Flajnik MF. Major histocompatibility complex gene mapping in the amphibian Xenopus implies a primordial organization. *Proc Natl Acad Sci USA* 1997;**94**(11):5789–91.

4. Flajnik MF, Ohta Y, Namikawa-Yamada C, Nonaka M. Insight into the primordial MHC from studies in ectothermic vertebrates. *Immunol Rev* 1999;**167**:59–67.

5. Bingulac-Popovic J, Figueroa F, Sato A, Talbot WS, Johnson SL, Gates M, et al. Mapping of mhc class I and class II regions to different linkage groups in the zebrafish. *Danio Rerio, Immunogenet* 1997;**46**(2):129–34.

6. Hansen JD, Strassburger P, Thorgaard GH, Young WP, Du Pasquier L. Expression, linkage, and polymorphism of MHC-related genes in rainbow trout, oncorhynchus mykiss. *J Immunol* 1999;**163**(2):774–86.

7. Naruse K, Fukamachi S, Mitani H, Kondo M, Matsuoka T, Kondo S, et al. A detailed linkage map of medaka, oryzias latipes: comparative genomics and genome evolution. *Genetics* 2000;**154**(4):1773–84.

8. Sato A, Figueroa F, Murray BW, Malaga-Trillo E, Zaleska-Rutczynska Z, Sultmann H, et al. Nonlinkage of major histocompatibility complex class I and class II loci in bony fishes. *Immunogenetics* 2000;**51**(2):108–16.

9. Dijkstra JM, Grimholt U, Leong J, Koop BF, Hashimoto K. Comprehensive analysis of MHC class II genes in teleost fish genomes reveals dispensability of the peptide-loading DM system in a large part of vertebrates. *BMC Evol Biol* 2013;**13**:260.

10. Postlethwait JH, Woods IG, Ngo-Hazelett P, Yan YL, Kelly PD, Chu F, et al. Zebrafish comparative genomics and the origins of vertebrate chromosomes. *Genome Res* 2000;**10**(12):1890–902.

11. Clark MS, Shaw L, Kelly A, Snell P, Elgar G. Characterization of the MHC class I region of the Japanese pufferfish (*Fugu rubripes*). *Immunogenetics* 2001;**52**(3–4):174–85.

12. Matsuo MY, Asakawa S, Shimizu N, Kimura H, Nonaka M. Nucleotide sequence of the MHC class I genomic region of a teleost, the medaka (*Oryzias latipes*). *Immunogenetics* 2002;**53**(10–11): 930–40.

13. Michalova V, Murray BW, Sultmann H, Klein J. A contig map of the Mhc class I genomic region in the zebrafish reveals ancient synteny. *J Immunol* 2000;**164**(10):5296–305.

14. Ohta Y, Shiina T, Lohr RL, Hosomichi K, Pollin TI, Heist EJ, et al. Primordial linkage of beta2-microglobulin to the MHC. *J Immunol* 2011;**186**(6):3563–71.

15. Madden DR, Gorga JC, Strominger JL, Wiley DC. The three-dimensional structure of HLA-B27 at 2.1 A resolution suggests a general mechanism for tight peptide binding to MHC. *Cell* 1992;**70**(6):1035–48.

16. Rodgers JR, Cook RG. MHC class Ib molecules bridge innate and acquired immunity. *Nat Rev Immunol* 2005;**5**(6):459–71.

17. Wang D, Zhong L, Wei Q, Gan X, He S. Evolution of MHC class I genes in two ancient fish, paddlefish (*Polyodon spathula*) and Chinese sturgeon (*Acipenser sinensis*). *FEBS Lett* 2010;**584**(15):3331–9.

18. Grimholt U, Tsukamoto K, Azuma T, Leong J, Koop BF, Dijkstra JM. A comprehensive analysis of teleost MHC class I sequences. *BMC Evol Biol* 2015;**15**:32.

19. Lukacs MF, Harstad H, Bakke HG, Beetz-Sargent M, McKinnel L, Lubieniecki KP, et al. Comprehensive analysis of MHC class I genes from the U-, S-, and Z-lineages in Atlantic salmon. *BMC Genomics* 2010;**11**:154.

20. Kruiswijk CP, Hermsen TT, Westphal AH, Savelkoul HFJ, Stet RJM. A novel functional class I lineage in zebrafish (*Danio rerio*), carp (*Cyprinus carpio*), and large barbus (*Barbus intermedius*) showing an unusual conservation of the peptide-binding domains. *J Immunol* 2002;**169**:1936–47.

21. McConnell SC, Restaino AC, de Jong JL. Multiple divergent haplotypes express completely distinct sets of class I MHC genes in zebrafish. *Immunogenetics* 2014;**66**(3):199–213.

22. Nonaka MI, Aizawa K, Mitani H, Bannai HP, Nonaka M. Retained orthologous relationships of the MHC class I genes during euteleost evolution. *Mol Biol Evol* 2011;**28**(11):3099–112.
23. Sato A, Sultmann H, Mayer WE, Klein J. Mhc class I gene of African lungfish. *Immunogenetics* 2000;**51**(6):491–5.
24. Setiamarga DH, Miya M, Yamanoue Y, Azuma Y, Inoue JG, Ishiguro NB, et al. Divergence time of the two regional medaka populations in Japan as a new time scale for comparative genomics of vertebrates. *Biol Lett* 2009;**5**(6):812–6.
25. Shiina T, Dijkstra JM, Shimizu S, Watanabe A, Yanagiya K, Kiryu I, et al. Interchromosomal duplication of major histocompatibility complex class I regions in rainbow trout (*Oncorhynchus mykiss*), a species with a presumably recent tetraploid ancestry. *Immunogenetics* 2005;**56**(12):878–93.
26. Lukacs MF, Harstad H, Grimholt U, Beetz-Sargent M, Cooper GA, Reid L, et al. Genomic organization of duplicated major histocompatibility complex class I regions in Atlantic salmon (*Salmo salar*). *BMC Genomics* 2007;**8**:251.
27. Sambrook JG, Figueroa F, Beck S. A genome-wide survey of major histocompatibility complex (MHC) genes and their paralogues in zebrafish. *BMC Genomics* 2005;**6**:152.
28. Aoyagi K, Dijkstra JM, Xia C, Denda I, Ototake M, Hashimoto K, et al. Classical MHC class I genes composed of highly divergent sequence lineages share a single locus in rainbow trout (*Oncorhynchus mykiss*). *J Immunol* 2002;**168**(1):260–73.
29. Grimholt U, Drablos F, Jorgensen SM, Hoyheim B, Stet RJ. The major histocompatibility class I locus in atlantic salmon (*Salmo salar* L.): polymorphism, linkage analysis and protein modelling. *Immunogenetics* 2002;**54**(8):570–81.
30. Miller KM, Li S, Ming TJ, Kaukinen KH, Schulze AD. The salmonid MHC class I: more ancient loci uncovered. *Immunogenetics* 2006;**58**(7):571–89.
31. Kiryu I, Dijkstra JM, Sarder RI, Fujiwara A, Yoshiura Y, Ototake M. New MHC class Ia domain lineages in rainbow trout (*Oncorhynchus mykiss*) which are shared with other fish species. *Fish Shellfish Immunol* 2005;**18**(3):243–54.
32. Adams EJ, Parham P. Species-specific evolution of MHC class I genes in the higher primates. *Immunol Rev* 2001;**183**:41–64.
33. Siddle HV, Deakin JE, Coggill P, Hart E, Cheng Y, Wong ES, et al. MHC-linked and un-linked class I genes in the wallaby. *BMC Genomics* 2009;**10**:310.
34. Nonaka MI, Nonaka M. Evolutionary analysis of two classical MHC class I loci of the medaka fish, oryzias latipes: haplotype-specific genomic diversity, locus-specific polymorphisms, and interlocus homogenization. *Immunogenetics* 2010;**62**(5):319–32.
35. Shum BP, Guethlein L, Flodin LR, Adkison MA, Hedrick RP, Nehring RB, et al. Modes of salmonid MHC class I and II evolution differ from the primate paradigm. *J Immunol* 2001;**166**(5):3297–308.
36. Neefjes J, Jongsma ML, Paul P, Bakke O. Towards a systems understanding of MHC class I and MHC class II antigen presentation. *Nat Rev Immunol* 2011;**11**(12):823–36.
37. Klein J, Bontrop RE, Dawkins RL, Erlich HA, Gyllensten UB, Heise ER, et al. Nomenclature for the major histocompatibility complexes of different species: a proposal. *Immunogenetics* 1990;**31**(4):217–9.
38. Star B, Nederbragt AJ, Jentoft S, Grimholt U, Malmstrom M, Gregers TF, et al. The genome sequence of Atlantic cod reveals a unique immune system. *Nature* 2011;**477**(7363):207–10.
39. Denzin LK, Cresswell P. HLA-DM induces CLIP dissociation from MHC class II alpha beta dimers and facilitates peptide loading. *Cell* 1995;**82**(1):155–65.
40. Hiltbold EM, Roche PA. Trafficking of MHC class II molecules in the late secretory pathway. *Curr Opin Immunol* 2002;**14**(1):30–5.

41. Bannai HP, Nonaka M. Comprehensive analysis of medaka major histocompatibility complex (MHC) class II g{Bannai, 2013 #396}enes: implications for evolution in teleosts. *Immunogenetics* 2013;**65**(12):883–95.

42. McConnell T, Godwin UB, Norton SF, Nairn RS, Kazianis S, Morizot DC. Identification and mapping of two divergent, unlinked major histocompatibility complex class II B genes in xiphophorus fishes. *Genetics* 1998;**149**(4):1921–34.

43. Murray BW, Shintani S, Sultmann H, Klein J. Major histocompatibility complex class II A genes in cichlid fishes: identification, expression, linkage relationships, and haplotype variation. *Immunogenetics* 2000;**51**(7):576–86.

44. Sato A, Dongak R, Hao L, Shintani S, Sato T. Organization of Mhc class II A and B genes in the tilapiine fish oreochromis. *Immunogenetics* 2012;**64**(9):679–90.

45. Rock KL, Goldberg AL. Degradation of cell proteins and the generation of MHC class I-presented peptides. *Ann Rev Immunol* 1999;**17**:739–79.

46. Groll M, Ditzel L, Lowe J, Stock D, Bochtler M, Bartunik HD, et al. Structure of 20S proteasome from yeast at 2.4 A resolution. *Nature* 1997;**386**(6624):463–71.

47. Unno M, Mizushima T, Morimoto Y, Tomisugi Y, Tanaka K, Yasuoka N, et al. The structure of the mammalian 20S proteasome at 2.75 A resolution. *Structure* 2002;**10**(5):609–18.

48. Akiyama K, Yokota K, Kagawa S, Shimbara N, Tamura T, Akioka H, et al. cDNA cloning and interferon gamma down-regulation of proteasomal subunits X and Y. *Science* 1994;**265**(5176):1231–4.

49. Fruh K, Gossen M, Wang K, Bujard H, Peterson PA, Yang Y. Displacement of housekeeping proteasome subunits by MHC-encoded LMPs: a newly discovered mechanism for modulating the multicatalytic proteinase complex. *Embo J* 1994;**13**(14):3236–44.

50. Tanaka K, Kasahara M. The MHC class I ligand-generating system: roles of immunoproteasomes and the interferon-gamma-inducible proteasome activator PA28. *Immunol Rev* 1998;**163**:161–76.

51. Fehling HJ, Swat W, Laplace C, Kuhn R, Rajewsky K, Muller U, et al. MHC class I expression in mice lacking the proteasome subunit LMP-7. *Science* 1994;**265**(5176):1234–7.

52. Agarwal AK, Xing C, DeMartino GN, Mizrachi D, Hernandez MD, Sousa AB, et al. PSMB8 encoding the beta5i proteasome subunit is mutated in joint contractures, muscle atrophy, microcytic anemia, and panniculitis-induced lipodystrophy syndrome. *Am J Hum Genet* 2010;**87**(6):866–72.

53. Arima K, Kinoshita A, Mishima H, Kanazawa N, Kaneko T, Mizushima T, et al. Proteasome assembly defect due to a proteasome subunit beta type 8 (PSMB8) mutation causes the autoinflammatory disorder, Nakajo–Nishimura syndrome. *Proc Natl Acad Sci USA* 2011;**108**(36):14914–9.

54. Kitamura A, Maekawa Y, Uehara H, Izumi K, Kawachi I, Nishizawa M, et al. A mutation in the immunoproteasome subunit PSMB8 causes autoinflammation and lipodystrophy in humans. *J Clin Investig* 2011;**121**(10):4150–60.

55. Fujito NT, Nonaka M. Highly divergent dimorphic alleles of the proteasome subunit beta type-8 (PSMB8) gene of the bichir polypterus senegalus: implication for evolution of the PSMB8 gene of jawed vertebrates. *Immunogenetics* 2012;**64**(6):447–53.

56. Huang CH, Tanaka Y, Fujito NT, Nonaka M. Dimorphisms of the proteasome subunit beta type 8 gene (PSMB8) of ectothermic tetrapods originated in multiple independent evolutionary events. *Immunogenetics* 2013;**65**(11):811–21.

57. Miura F, Tsukamoto K, Mehta RB, Naruse K, Magtoon W, Nonaka M. Transspecies dimorphic allelic lineages of the proteasome subunit {beta}-type 8 gene (PSMB8) in the teleost genus oryzias. *Proc Natl Acad Sci USA* 2010;.

58. Nonaka M, Yamada-Namikawa C, Flajnik MF, Du Pasquier L. Trans-species polymorphism of the major histocompatibility complex-encoded proteasome subunit LMP7 in an amphibian genus, xenopus. *Immunogenetics* 2000;**51**(3):186–92.
59. Noro M, Nonaka M. Evolution of dimorphisms of the proteasome subunit beta type 8 gene (PSMB8) in basal ray-finned fish. *Immunogenetics* 2014;**66**(5):325–34.
60. Tsukamoto K, Miura F, Fujito NT, Yoshizaki G, Nonaka M. Long-lived dichotomous lineages of the proteasome subunit beta type 8 (PSMB8) gene surviving more than 500 million years as alleles or paralogs. *Mol Biol Evol* 2012;**29**(10):3071–9.
61. Tsukamoto K, Sakaizumi M, Hata M, Sawara Y, Eah J, Kim CB, et al. Dichotomous haplotypic lineages of the immunoproteasome subunit genes, PSMB8 and PSMB10, in the MHC class I region of a teleost medaka, oryzias latipes. *Mol Biol Evol* 2009;**26**(4):769–81.
62. Klein J, Sato A, Nikolaidis N. MHC, TSP, and the origin of species: from immunogenetics to evolutionary genetics. *Ann Rev Genet* 2007;**41**:281–304.
63. Inoue JG, Miya M, Tsukamoto K, Nishida M. A mitogenomic perspective on the basal teleostean phylogeny: resolving higher-level relationships with longer DNA sequences. *Mol Phylogenet Evol* 2001;**20**(2):275–85.
64. Miya M, Takeshima H, Endo H, Ishiguro NB, Inoue JG, Mukai T, et al. Major patterns of higher teleostean phylogenies: a new perspective based on 100 complete mitochondrial DNA sequences. *Mol Phylogenet Evol* 2003;**26**(1):121–38.

Subject Index

A

Activation pathways, 152
Adaptive immune responses, 1
Adaptive immune system (AIS), 51, 151
Adenosine 5′-triphosphate (ATP), 88
Adhesion molecules, 56
Adrenaline, 231
Aedes aegypti, 319
Aeromonas hydrophilia, 89
Aeromonas salmonicida, 91
Agglutinins, 51, 52
Agnathan lymphocytes, 56
    presumed role of populations, eliminating
        pathogens, 58
Agnathan T-like cells, antigen recognition
        by, 57
AIS. *See* Adaptive immune system (AIS)
Allantoicase, 218
Allocentrotus fragilis, 298
Amphibians, 74, 78, 282
    antibody activity, 74
    B cell populations, 74
    IFNs, 184
    Ig heavy-chain isotypes, 74
    production of IL-2 by T cells, 78
    T lymphocytes, 78
    in vitro culturing of CD4/CD8
        thymocytes, 78
Amphimedon queenslandica, 260, 315
Amphioxus, 316
AMPs. *See* Antimicrobial peptides (AMPs)
Anaphylatoxin receptors, 162
Angiopoietin, 279
Anguilla anguilla, 112
Anolis carolinensis, 75, 127, 324
Anopheles gambiae, 256, 257
Anopheles gambiae, 241
Antibacterial activity, 39
Antigen receptors, 51
Antimicrobial peptides (AMPs), 2
Apoptosis, 51, 111
Apoptosis-inducing ligand (APRIL), 122
Appendicularians, 29
Appendicularias, 29

B

APRIL. *See* Apoptosis-inducing ligand (APRIL)
Arabidopsis thaliana, 296
Argopecten irradians, 17
Arthropoda, 6, 288
Aryl hydrocarbon receptor (AHR), 56
Ascaridia galli, 111
Ascidiacea, 29
Ascidian circulation, 30
Ascidian hemocytes, 31
    and oxidative stress response, 40
Ascidian pigmentation, 33
Ascidians, 29
Astakines, 5
ATP-synthase, 5
Australian purple sea urchin, 298
AUUUA destabilization sequence, 92
Avian type I IFNs, 184

Bacterial mimicry, 290
Bacteriovorax marinus, 277
BAPs. *See* Bioactive peptides (BAPs)
BCAP. *See* B-cell adaptor protein (BCAP)
B-cell adaptor protein (BCAP), 57
B-cell CLL/lymphoma 6 (BCL6), 57
B-cell receptor-associated protein (BCAP), 52
B-cell receptors (BCRs), 52, 71, 295
B cells, 59, 70, 72
    amphibians, 74
    bony fish, 73
    cartilaginous fish, 72
    reptiles, 75
BCR gene, 54
BCRs. *See* B-cell receptors (BCRs)
Beauveria bassiana, 319
Bf/C2 genes, 334
Bf/C2-like molecules, 161
β-1,3-glucan, 4, 298
Bichir, 342
Bilaterians, 288, 315
    insects, 289
    pancrustacea-crustaceans, 289
    phylum arthropoda, 288
    phylum mollusca, 288

T follicular helper (Tfh) cells, 99
TGF. *See* Transforming growth factor (TGF)
Thaliaceans, 29
Thalia democratica, 40
Th cell markers CD4, T-bet, and GATA3, 100
Th1-like response, 92
Thymoids, 61
β-Thymosins, 5
Thyrotropin (TSH), 227
Tipartite motif-containing (TRIM) protein, 191
TIR. *See* Toll/interleukin-1 receptor (TIR)
TIR domain-containing protein (TirS), 322
TIR-NBS-LRR (TNL), 296
TirS. *See* TIR domain-containing protein
(TirS)
TIR–TIR domain interactions, 313
TLRs. *See* Toll-like receptors (TLRs)
T lymphocytes. *See* T cells
TNF family, 116
    amphibians, 126
    basal vertebrates, 118
    birds, 126
    cephalochordates, 118
    cyclostomata, 118
    fish, 119
        remaining TNFSF members, 124–126
        TNFSF1-3, 119–122
        TNFSF13 and 13B, 122–124
    primitive chordates, 118
    protostomian invertebrates, 116
    reptiles, 126
    urochordates, 118
TNF-like weak inducer of apoptosis
(TWEAK), 125
TNF receptors, 38
TNFSF2 genes, 120, 127
TNFSF members within vertebrates, 117
TNL. *See* TIR-NBS-LRR (TNL)
Toll/interleukin-1 receptor (TIR), 296
Toll-like receptor 3 (TLR3), 56
Toll-like receptors (TLRs), 57, 69, 173, 311
    distribution, 314
    evolution, 314
    family, 175–177
    function, 318
        invertebrate deuterostome TLR, 320
        protostome toll, 319
        vertebrate TLR, 320
    microbe-driven evolution, 322
        detection avoidance methods, 322
        positive selection, 323
        purifying selection, 323
    origin, 314

protostomian and deuterostomian,
structural difference, 316
structure, 312
    extracellular domain, 312
    intracellular domain, 313
    transmembrane domain, 313
TLR-related proteins, 315
vertebrate phylogeny, 317
Toll proteins, 316
Toll signaling, 321
Toxoplasma gondii, 318
Trachemys scripta, 76
Trachidermus fasciatus, 283
Transcription factors, 6, 57
Transcriptome analysis, 39, 52
Transforming growth factor (TGF), 229
Transglutaminases (TGases), 5
Transmembrane (TM) domain, 207, 263, 313
Transmission electron microscopy, 2
Trans-species polymorphism (TSP), 342
Tridacna crocea, 18
Trophocytes, 33
Trout, 342
Trout rIL-15, 99
Trypanoplasma borreli, 90, 110
Trypanosoma carassi, 115
TSH. *See* Thyrotropin (TSH)
TSP. *See* Trans-species polymorphism (TSP)
Tumor necrosis factor alpha, 320
Tumor necrosis factor-alpha converting
enzyme (TACE), 119
Tumor necrosis factor superfamily (TNFSF),
116
Tunicates, 29
    hemocytes, immune role of, 33
    phylogenetic tree of, 30

U
Urochordates, 29

V
Vanadocytes, 33
Variable domain-containing chitin binding
proteins (VCBPs), 295
Variable lymphocyte receptor B (VLRB), 160
Variable lymphocyte receptors (VLR), 52
V-binding proteins, 33
VCBPs. *See* Variable domain-containing chitin
binding proteins (VCBPs)
Vertebrates
    antigen-receptors, 244
    IFNs and IFN receptors, 182

Printed in the United States
By Bookmasters